VEGAN BETRAYAL

Love, lies, and hunger in a

plants-only world

MARA J. KAHN

Little Boat Books

This book is not intended as a substitute for the health recommendations of registered dieticians, nutritionists, naturopaths or other professional providers. Some individuals who expressed their beliefs and opinions remain anonymous to protect their privacy.

Published by Little Boat Press
Boulder, Colorado, USA
Current Edition: June 2017

LIBRARY OF CONGRESS CATALOGING-IN-PUBLICATION DATA

Kahn, Mara J.
  Vegan betrayal: love, lies and hunger in a plants-only world / Mara Kahn
    p. cm.

Includes biographical references.
  ISBN: 978-0-9903413-2-1
  1. Food 2. Agriculture 3. Evolution 4. Memoir I. Title

Printed with recycled paper.

10 9 8 7 6 5 4 3 2 1

Designed by Susan France

Printed in the United States of America

for Laura

Wisdom arises in an atmosphere of open inquiry.
It's essential not to close down inquiry.

—Sangha Dassa

CONTENTS

VEGAN BETRAYAL

FAILURE TO THRIVE

W E HAVE BEEN SEDUCED by a beautiful idea, a utopian fable. Eat plants only, they keep telling us, and you'll not only enjoy excellent health but have no blood on your hands.

Our young people have been listening; veganism has grabbed millions by the heart and the throat. Those who aren't loudly preaching are quietly caring about the plight of animals and the planet. These are admirable intentions, grounded in a noble *philosophy*, but what advocates need to start talking about is *physiology*— and the startling lack of evidence for healthy vegan outcomes. Short-term studies? Not many and not always positive. Life-long? Nada.

Vegans-for-life are flying on blind faith. Not a single human population has endured on an all-plants diet. Not one traditional culture has ever elected to eat this way—and for sound nutritional reasons. Veganism is, in a word, *untested*. Except it is now being tested on the bodies of our daughters, sons, friends and lovers, maybe even you. Credible health and longevity statistics for this nouveau diet won't be available for several generations, but with a 70% dropout rate, the evidence is mounting that all is not well in Vegan World (Asher et al).

At the outset, you may indeed lose weight or recover from bad eating habits on this restrictive diet. Over time, however, plants-only doesn't work in our bodies any better than it does in nature or agriculture. Yet the faithful keep insisting: "One world, one diet! Nobody needs to eat animals!" Before the ascent of veganism, vegetarians put out a similar message, but they're older and wiser now and many have a far different story to tell. And it's not the one being told by the best-selling but misleading *The China Study*.

Praise or blame our distant ancestors but we *need* the distinct nutrients offered by animals—"carninutrients" they're called, some of them recently discovered— and isolated supplements or synthetics can never replace the complex synergy of nutrient-dense whole foods. Innate genetic and biochemical factors also influence your body's response to diet: which foods to eat and which to avoid for optimal health and disease prevention. Some individuals are doing well on a vegan diet, thus far anyway, while others are suffering, despite supplementation. Some are suffering greatly, their health compromised and their quality of life diminished. This is the fatal flaw in the vegan argument: their wild, unfounded assumption that all of us will stay healthy on a well-planned, all-plants diet. This is far from the truth, and millions of ex-vegans will attest to their sense of betrayal. Many of their disillusioned voices echo throughout this book.

The "Failure to Thrive" syndrome among dedicated, doing-it-right vegans is real. It is now recognized by an increasing number of medical doctors, including pro-vegan Michael Klaper, MD. Carb-sensitive types, people with cold-climate ancestry or high-protein needs, slender women over 35, and long-term vegans are especially vulnerable. Two of America's oldest vegans, the movement's original leaders, suffered and died from Parkinson's disease. The suspect? Lack of the brain-nourishing, essential fatty acid DHA, conspicuously scarce in plant food.

IT'S SEDUCTIVE TO BELIEVE, as well, that animals are not killed to put plant food on our tables. The truth, as always, is more complex. Depending on the crop and production methods, a vegan diet can bring death to more animals than an omnivore's—and more destruction to the soil and diversity of life. Does this mean we have to abandon our ethics every time we dine? Absolutely not. Contrary to the strident moralizing of animal rightists, be you veggie or omnie, there are principled ways to be an animal-honoring, earth-smart consumer.

This book is a cautionary tale, not an outright rejection of vegetarianism and its strict sister, veganism. It is a rejection of a too-often smug and self-righteous attitude: that an omnivore's diet is inherently unhealthy and unethical; that everyone on the planet can and should be a vegetarian—preferably a life-long vegan. These are misleading and potentially harmful beliefs.

There are many voices in this world that are not your own, urgently telling you what to do and how to think, especially concerning diet. By listening to your own inner voice and intelligent body, you will discover what is right for you. So if a well-meaning friend, veg'n preacher, or some skinny dude tries to convince you that theirs is the best diet for everyone and you too should jump on board, just smile and walk into the forest like wise people do—and figure it out for yourself. Their absolute conviction and pious insistence is flawed. I know because I used to be one of the most passionate among them.

1.

AT FIRST BITE

I AM ABOUT TO EAT a warm-blooded animal for the first time in over 25 years. My meal of choice is Colorado-raised bison on a whole-grain bun. Having mentally prepared myself for months, I carefully remove the dark, just-braised flesh and place it on a clean white plate, naked and alone. I want to face it directly: this steaming and tender, palm-size piece of prairie muscle. I want to reflect on the brawny, magnificent animal whose life abruptly ended so that I might eat and eat abundantly. And I want to remember the Arapaho who hunted bison on the Great Plains mere miles from where I sit alone at this kitchen table, who worshipped it, prayed to it, gave thanks to it and utilized every bone, muscle, organ, tendon and sinew of its dynamic, vigorous body.

Yet when the moment finally arrives, despite all this pre-dinner mindfulness, all I can bear to slice off and put inside my mouth is a bite of bison the size of my little fingernail. I'm sure to throw up if eat any more than this—even this minuscule piece of meat probably won't go down.

Our bodies never lie. The awareness of *Bison bison,* of warm succulent animal flesh inside my long-awaiting maw is overpowering, excruciating. Rarely, my mouth and gullet affirm in this bewildering moment, have I experienced anything so intense, so enlivening. More wary bites follow and surges of energy and alertness start to flood my bodily awareness as the potent neurotransmitters dopamine and norepinephrine kick in. I am astounded—expected nothing like this. Yet with each cautious swallow, this same forceful message is zinged to my brain by the complex network of neurons and transmitters embedded in my throat and gut.

How long has it been, my wise body is already chiding me, since you offered me food so nourishing? For how many years of crushing fatigue have you turned a deaf ear to my cries? Still wired to a beautiful ideology, my mind is desperately trying to deny what's happening. *You can't eat this and feel good. It's decaying flesh; it's rotten for your health; it's bad karma! You're a traitor, a turncoat, a brute. Listen to me! You can't love animals and then eat them!*

My decades-old rant continues as my impartial tongue, mouth, and esophagus examine the evidence. So far so good, yes, very good indeed. After being slowly and thoroughly masticated, the bison flesh is going down just fine. Time passes and it's irrefutable. My body is starting to sing, rejoicing in this long-denied fat and protein-rich nourishment. *Finally* my brain shuts up, jolted awake by the stunning reality of this never to be forgotten moment: my body feeling vibrant, energized, and alive in a way it hasn't felt in a pitifully long time.

Swiftly and unexpectedly, I am overcome by long suppressed memories of Sunday beef stew dinners and convivial family barbeques, my whole gregarious tribe in attendance: loving grandparents, aunts and uncles, cousins and siblings, proud parents and babbling babies, all gathered happily around the open-air fire. Not simply visual, these are powerful corporal remembrances of energy exchange and kinship, joy and community, pungent tastes and savory smells—ancestral ways of eating that are locked into the multi-faceted DNA of our lineage.

Buoyant, I observe my hypercritical mind making one final frantic attempt to negate the now unmistakable signs of a completely objective body. My body which knows *exactly* what it needs to thrive; my intelligent body which I ignored again and again these past long years of declining health and vanishing energy. Suddenly I feel an overwhelming urge to storm outside and go running. Leap over rocks and jump barricades! When was the last time I felt so exuberant, so alive?

Later that evening, sitting quietly in a state of gratitude, easily digesting my first red meat in decades, I realize this doesn't feel like food alone. *This feels like medicine.* Slowly the inevitable words are articulated by my well-satisfied tongue. How long have I been in denial?

2.

THE BEAUTIFUL VEGETARIAN

A VERY LONG TIME, I must confess. It was September in Paris, over thirty years ago. The azure skies were tranquil, the university students restless, and my placid 19-year-old life was about to be hurled into new realms, like a virgin flung to the lions. Hearing a commotion outside a friend's apartment one bright Sunday afternoon, I unbolted the door to find a resolute young woman climbing the building's twisting stairs. A French touring bike with Italian parts balanced lightly on her sturdy shoulders. "Linda Upland," she declared with a solid handshake, reaching the landing and nimbly setting down her purple and white-streaked Motobecane. "You didn't know I was arriving?"

She was 23 and California gorgeous, golden-haired and rosy-cheeked, with an earthiness in her strong athletic body and a confidence in her deep spontaneous laugh that left me thunderstruck, in awe. "What universe does she inhabit," I was already asking myself, "that I do not?" Having spent the summer cycling up the Pacific coast from San Francisco to Vancouver, turning east to peddle through Canada's amber fields all the way to Toronto, Linda had flown to London, ferried across the Channel, and just this day blown into Paris on two skinny wheels, still smelling like a fresh, sun-scoured beach. She was wholesome, free-loving, free-wheeling, astonishingly self-assured, and glowing with good health. She was a vegetarian.

She was, in sum, everything that this scrawny, reserved, hot dog-chomping Midwesterner most definitely was not. Hailing from corn and pork-laden central Illinois, I barely knew what the concept meant, let alone ever met a live veggie specimen. (There had been hushed rumors of one *right in our midst* at a Madison, Wisconsin journalism conference for high school seniors.) But Linda's radiant face and long lustrous hair sang out to me in wondrous, not weird, ways and her soaring, jovial energy seemed to bounce around the apartment walls like rainbow prisms of light. Yet she was grounded and affectionate, the quintessential Bay Area flower child who had frolicked and fornicated during the Summer of Love, garnishing cops with tangerine-tinted poppies at the world's first rock festival.

A homegrown hippie-veggie child, that was Linda, but with an enviable flare for adventure. She was the Renaissance Fair maiden, hawking sandalwood and rosehips; she was serene Saint Christina entrancing the local snakes to lick away her sweat; and she was Artemis running barefoot and braless through the redwood forest, a stag at her flank, excited male hounds at her feet.

Gazing down at my own skinny limbs, outfitted in tailored pants and button-up cardigan, I slowly pushed thick glasses up my long quivering nose—still full of Linda's windy, woodsy scent—and thought to myself, *hmmm*, something's up with this spirited, plant-eating young woman of which I know absolutely nothing, something I need to seriously ponder. Is it any wonder I had intuitively braced myself at the top of those Parisian stairs, mouth flapping open and brain on high alert, as this female force of nature ascended into my life?

3.

VEGAN HEALTH

EVERY DAY IN AMERICA, throngs of spanking new vegans—armed with *The China Study*—arise and go forth to the produce section of their local supermarket. Each has made a solemn vow to eliminate all animal products from his or her life. Ardent and youthful, most will feel fine during the first months of their vegan commitment. After that, however, they are venturing into unchartered territory.

Throughout history, deliberate plants-only eaters have been limited to sheep, goats, and the like, plus a smattering of monkish humans living in isolated religious communities. Of course, there have been *vegetarians* like my pal Linda since recorded time, but these people gladly incorporate dairy and/or eggs into their nutritional arsenal. Moreover, worldwide, most arrive at vegetarianism by way of their lineage and climate, not the persuasive devices of agenda-driven activists and a for-profit media.

The constant print/online bombardment is paying off. The most recent Gallup poll reveals that nearly 12 million American adults call themselves vegetarians, abandoning all meat, while an additional 5 million claim to consume zero animal products. Globally, the numbers are also escalating. Google hits for "vegan" keep zooming higher and you can now book a Holistic All-Vegan Caribbean Cruise, complete with "certified no-critters toiletries." We are, in fact, witnessing the largest, swiftest mass conversion to plants-only eating in human history, yet we have no idea of the ultimate health results of this experimental diet.*

These millions of new converts do not, by and large, live in the traditional home ground of vegetarianism: the warm Indus Valley and Mediterranean climes,

*In "How the Health Argument Fails Veganism," vegan promoter Virginia Messina, RD, states: "There isn't any health argument for veganism," noting that high-plant omnivorous diets can be healthy, so "we have to stretch the truth.....to overstate the benefits of vegan diets and sometimes minimize or dismiss the risks." Many vegan advocates do exactly that: exaggerate any benefits and stay quiet about the risks.

where the diet first flourished and is embedded in the cultural heritage and genetic stock. They hail from Los Angeles and Seattle, Austin and Atlanta, London and Berlin. For the most part, they are young, single, and female. Teens are foregoing chicken in favor of chickpeas; the Herbivorous Butcher is open for business in Minneapolis; and legume lovers in New York City can grab a Skyscraper Burger at the vegan fast-food chain, Blossom du Jour.

For all these young converts, veganism represents a smart dietary choice in an era of increasing obesity, diabetes, and heart disease. Eating more plants is associated with lower cholesterol levels, lower blood pressure and decreased risk of hypertension, along with higher levels of dietary fiber and the vitamins C, E, and folate. Perhaps even more persuasive are the beautiful faces and buff bodies of all those pro-veg celebrities splashed across our laptops and magazines. What can I say? The dazzling appearance of my blond, fast-pedaling California friend ignited my own youthful conversion.

Vegetarianism, and especially veganism, received a huge public boost in 2009 when the ADA, American Dietetic Association (now the Academy of Nutrition and Dietetics) published its revised official position on these restrictive diets: *Appropriately planned vegetarian diets, including total vegetarian or vegan diets, are healthful, nutritionally adequate, and may provide health benefits in the prevention and treatment of certain diseases.*

Veg diets even got a plug from the conservative Department of Agriculture, whose Dietary Guidelines now state that "vegetarian-style eating patterns have been associated with improved health outcomes." Well-publicized studies from Dean Ornish, for example, confirm a regression of coronary heart disease when individuals were placed on a vegetarian diet of less than 10% fat. And a small study by Caldwell Esselstyn of *Forks Over Knives* film-fame showed a reversal of advanced heart disease for patients on a low-fat vegan diet.

So why wouldn't *everyone* choose to be a vegetarian or, better yet, a loyal vegan for the rest of his or her life? Turns out there are many reasons, largely familial and cultural, but the very best reason for many of us *not* to become long-term vegans is the same one being hyped by all of the above: for our health.

RARELY IN ALL THE PRO-VEGAN literature will you find a discussion of the high dropout rate due to diminished strength and vitality as the years unfold: 70% of vegans ditch their diet; 86% of vegetarians, according to a large, respected study by the Humane Research Council (Asher). Nearly 1/3 of these vegans/vegetarians

6

(veg'ns) cite poor health as a prime factor, with 82% from this group confirming that their health improved within 2 days to 3 months once meat was reintroduced.

Nor is there recognition by advocates that a predictably high-carb/low-protein vegan diet is a disaster-in-waiting for the fast-oxidizing metabolic types among us with high-protein needs. And rarely will you find mention of the dearth of valid vegan health data. What few studies we do have, including Esselstyn's, are of low quality, with a small sample size and lack of controls. Even the ADA position paper offers disturbingly few studies specific to vegans. Sorry, but vegetarian research cannot be applied to vegans—whole different animal. The truth is this: not one respected study has shown a vegan diet to be healthy over the long-term, and most research uncovers troubling deficiencies.

What about all those recommendations to eat plentiful vegetables, fruits, and greens? They're about adding *more* plants to the American diet, not eating *only* plants, and it's deceitful for any vegan crusader to pretend they're the same thing. Perhaps even more disquieting is the lack of public awareness that the ADA's pro-veg'n position paper was authored by just two people: a long-time vegetarian evangelist and a tenacious vegan promoter.

Moreover, when research links lower disease rates with a high-plant diet, the right question is seldom asked. Lower disease rates *compared to what?* The answer, invariably, is a diet heavy in processed food, trans fats, refined grains and sugar; i.e., our sad, sick, deviant American diet. The Ornish studies, for instance, were of diseased adults up to age 75 with very poor eating and lifestyle habits—a fair description of former President Bill Clinton who took up the vegan diet a few years back (and has since abandoned it). Participants in the Esselstyn study were aging, ailing individuals on statin drugs. *What any of this has to do with healthy young people who embrace veganism is decidedly unclear.* Furthermore, positive results from the Ornish diet depended on the critical addition of daily exercise, stress management, and group therapy to arrive at its pro-veg'n conclusion.

Control for lifestyle habits and drug therapy, as every reliable nutrition study must, and *then* compare a vegetarian or vegan diet to one of whole plants and judicious amounts of wild-caught fish or pastured meat—like the seafood-loving Mediterranean diet or the animal-adoring French diet—and the health advantages either disappear or are greatly surpassed.

4.

LA BOUCHERIE

"WANT TO TAKE IT for a spin?" the lovely vegetarian Linda asked me, sensing my bug-eyed fascination with her ultra-sleek, panniers-equipped French bike. *Moi?* This clumsy bibliophile who rode a fat-tubed Huffy through the corn fields, straw basket duct-taped to the handlebars? Sure, I'd give it a go, but what on earth had she done with the kickstand?

Mostly, however, we walked—all over the City of Lights and Ivry-sur-Seine, the tough working-class neighborhood of Lasserre, our leftist, intellectual, meat-revering French friend. As for myself, I was taking a much-needed break from the blinkered world of academics. And since Lasserre was currently away traveling, Linda and I gratefully took over her cozy, low-rent flat, perched above a tatty 18th century red-brick warehouse. True to its bohemian spirit, the place offered no bathroom whatsoever, so we washed up in the kitchen sink and took turns sharing the ground floor *toilette*—basically a flushable hole in the floor—with a dozen scruffy, badass male laborers who gleefully grinned and grunted whenever one of us emerged from behind its baby blue door.

It was here, in Lasserre's snug apartment, under the enthusiastic tutelage of the wise and experienced Linda, that this uptight teen innocent from central Illinois—granddaughter of a Methodist minister, daughter of a no-nonsense church elder—received her initiation into the marvels of Zen Buddhism, vegetarianism, macro-biotics, in-house body piercings and mellow Afghani hashish, alternating with hearty swigs of bargain French wine. And let us not forget the always seductive Pink Floyd throbbing in the background.

Cautious and tentative at first, it didn't take long for my conservative Midwest roots to start spreading wildly, sucking up powerfully fresh and nourishing water, sprouting new and ever more exotic flowers. Within a few weeks I had devoured

Linda's entire portable library: paperbacks on Taoism and Hinduism, Gandhi and non-suffering, veggie philosophy and animal rights. It all made perfect sense, appealing to my ideals of justice and morality. Everything about vegetarianism felt right. I loved animals; why would I want to eat them? Why would I want them killed in the way these books described, in such a brutal, inhumane manner? Why would I want them killed at all, when I could eat plant food and emerge healthy and fit? Maybe, just maybe, if I stuck with it long enough, even radiantly healthy like Linda.

Then one lazy Saturday morning, lounging on floor pillows, inhaling orange slices and fresh chocolate croissants, Linda suddenly stood up and announced that my education was incomplete. "It's time for a tour of the local butcher shop," she insisted, gazing at me with those soothing Pacific-blue eyes. "Every meat eater needs to do this and the sooner the better." Say what? As in, like....*butchering animals??* My mind rebelled and my stomach lurched. *Could you grant me an exemption? Please!!* I begged her shamelessly, got down on my knees. After all, I'd grown up in a genteel urban setting. My mom shopped at superstores and my sis worked after school at the local Kroger deli. Post-church we'd drive there as a family to pick up silken-smooth, plastic-draped chicken breasts for our Sunday afternoon supper. No way was I ready for this lesson in carnivore reality.

THE NEIGHBORHOOD *boucherie* that Linda selected for my initiation adjoined a lively outdoor bazaar, just one of 80 roaming markets offered in Paris every day. Strolling happily among the crowded and colorful stalls—forgetting altogether the purpose of our journey—we admired row after row of white-fleshed peaches and polished yellow apples, artfully arranged alongside golden quince from the Rhône valley and shining figs from Provence. Fingering fresh baby leeks and the last of the summer truffles, we leaned close to sniff the fragrant lemon balm and lingered dreamily over baskets brimming with sunflowers.

Spotting fresh greens just around the bend, I nonchalantly meandered ahead, turned a tiny corner, a mere tuck in time, and found myself face to faceless with hanging corpses of eviscerated cows. A high-pitched gasp escaped my throat: part revulsion, part dissent. I visibly struggled for breath. *No! Not here! Not next to the baby spinach and Swiss chard!* Yes, yes, my little friend, right here, right now, squarely in front of your blameless, childlike eyes. Razor-edged, two-foot cleavers going at it, hacking and severing and slicing lean muscle off dense bone, right here on this people-packed street. On this table are tossed the thick flank, the middle haunch, and the fat rump. Now over here, on glistening display for all to inspect are the crimson cheeks, the shiny kidneys, the twelve-inch tongues. And here, decorated with curly kale, we have the shimmering calf brains and the wee lamb hearts, so recently torn from the living animals they appear to be throbbing. Blanched and beheaded chickens hang by their scrawny, just-plucked legs. And now come dancing before your virtuous, torn-open eyes: severed pigs' feet, or "trotters" as the French fondly call them, fat pink toes all lined up in a row.

This little piggy went to market....my analytical brain began to mock my insular innocence. Very quickly it pointed out all the browsing locals moving casually amid the swinging corpses, haggling for lower prices on boar heads and broccoli. Panic-stricken, my blinders ripped off, I could feel the blood slowly draining out of my head into my now stumbling feet, my carnivore vigor vanquished.

Linda caught up and glanced at me with those knowing, compassionate eyes. Astonishing, isn't it? For all my 19 years of existence, I had never correlated the abundance of meat continuously flowing across our family table—not directly, not REALLY—with these sinewy, blood-purged muscles of real animals swaying headless and heartless in the morning breeze. *You do comprehend that a turkey sandwich is a proud bird dismembered?* Sure, sort of, but not in any meaningful way, not before this very moment when the veil of obscurity was so abruptly snatched away. Same as 98% of Americans, I hadn't been raised on a farm with urea-pooping hens and brown-eyed bovines wandering around. Hamburger had always made its appearance saran-wrapped and grill-ready, as pliant and lifeless as pretty pink playdough.

Mere hours before, I now realized with full-on visceral distress, these animal parts before me had assembled as one—to trot, dine, snort, sleep or copulate back at the local French farm. Perhaps this very morning, these same creatures had felt the vast life force flowing through them, content to ruminate, gaze at the cloudless blue sky, delight in their own existence, catch a snooze, shoo away flies.

Yet at this exact instant, before my adolescent eyes, they were being crudely, perfunctorily butchered into bloody pieces of meat for human consumption. And I had to turn away, suddenly feeling so deceived, so estranged from my previous life of not-knowing. And in that split second of finally realizing the truth, in that awful moment of enlightenment, I knew that I would end up just like Linda: a devout vegetarian for life.

5.

THE ETHICAL VEGETARIAN

EVEN MORE CONVINCING than the veg'n health argument is the ethics factor. In survey after survey, both American and British, ethical concerns are cited as the dominant reason for abstention from animal products. Similar to my own reality zap, many of these mostly-urban veggies opted for an alternative diet after finally confronting the once-living reality of their daily dead meat.

But any long-overdue illumination about meat as butchered animal parts is just the beginning of an ethical eater's angst and revulsion. The real horror story is how today's industrial animals are treated and raised, living out their short, sad, suffering lives in servitude to factory farms and the gods of efficiency and profit. And whenever humans serve these gods alone, omitting compassion and common sense, we are on civilization's downward spiral to collapse.

I will not spare you the hideous details, even if you have read them before. Every person on the planet should be fully conscious of the source of his or her meat and the treatment of the animals prior to and during slaughter. It's upon learning the truth about industrial livestock operations—how these creatures are moved quickly and cruelly from birth to butcher—that many make the choice to turn veg'n, often within mere minutes of their awakening from blissful ignorance.

Even your average consumer now understands that most modern meat comes not from the charming pastoral farms of our collective childhood, farmers in bib overalls leading well-tended poultry and cattle to grass-thick pastures, but from Concentrated Animal Feeding Operations (CAFOs), where tens of thousands of critters are slammed together in vile, often filthy conditions. Read about the so-called life of the industrial chicken you're planning to eat for dinner tonight and you may be hard-pressed to choke down even one meaty mouthful.

Now imagine *you* are one of those "broilers" as they're called. Crammed into a warehouse-size structure with a thousand other birds, you can barely turn around, left to stand in your own feces while fending off anxious attacks from your antibiotic-pumped fellow chickens gone mad. There is no natural light, no adequate ventilation, and the toxic stench permeates everything but there's no escape; you are cornered. Trapped. Aggressive bird behavior is breaking out all over, so the factory farmer has a hasty, albeit excruciating solution: amputate toes and claws. Now you can't even walk. Hey, no problem! Because soon enough, even standing will be impossible as your legs collapse, unable to support your enormous weight, the result of a perversely sped-up growth pattern from bioengineered breeding.

If you happen to be an industrial egg layer, so sorry, you've got it even worse. Shoved into a wire cage with up to nine other hens, your allotted moving space is 70 square inches—that's like six adult humans smashed together in a shower stall. This translates to a lifetime without nesting, perching, foraging, preening or anything else resembling natural behavior. You can't even flap your wings or sit down to rest. Driven crazy by these suffocating conditions, you and your fellows turn cannibalistic, violently attacking one another.

No big deal, says the ever-clever factory farmer. I'll simply mutilate the lot of you by searing off your beaks without painkillers. Now stop bitchin' and just be glad you're female! The egg industry has no use whatsoever for newborn male chicks. Thrown aside, they're either pulverized in high-speed grinders or piled on top of each other and left to die of asphyxiation. But don't count on a long life as a girl bird. Once your egg production falls off, you too will be killed and sent to rendering plants because your flesh is "too battered to even go into canned soup," according to Compassion Over Killing's *Veg Starter Guide*. Well, at least you no longer have to suffer—you're outta here!

And if you're born a cow instead? You get to begin your life on open pasture. Wahoo! Six to ten months later, however, you're traumatically weaned from your momma (who mourns and bellows for days) and shipped to crowded feedlots for artificial fattening on food that nature didn't design for you—a grass-eater—to consume. This means federally-subsidized corn and cheap "fillers" like poultry litter: i.e., feces, feathers, sawdust, and god knows what-all scraped off factory floors. Be happy they're not still feeding you dead cow parts, a common practice until its connection to mad cow disease became sickeningly clear. But wait! In the US, chicken feed can contain dead cow parts, and feed most certainly gets spilled into the chickens' litter and that litter is fed to cows. Get the cannibalistic drift?

Could this disconnect from nature's plan for herbivores be any more brazen and idiotic? Not to worry, because on your alien corn and chicken-litter diet, you'll be pumped with antibiotics and a slew of other drugs to avert acidosis and potentially fatal bloat—part and parcel of a high-starch, artificial diet that sets you soaring from 80 pounds to half a ton in a little over a year, thick with marbled meat and Burger King bound. Fast food just keeps getting faster. Yet in trying to speed up anything and everything, humans are only hastening their own demise.

HERE'S THE REASON for this perversion of nature: government-subsidized corn is super cheap and fattens very quickly, allowing for your expedient slaughter and swift movement to market. It's all a game of speed because time is money and fatter animals in shorter times means ever more *money, money, money!* You and your buddies are no longer living, feeling beings. You are crude merchandise for profit. You are, as the farm report contends, commodities.

Veal may have the cruelest origins of all. As a newborn, you're torn from your mother's side and chained to a 2-foot wide stall where you spend your brief and terribly lonely life in solitary confinement, unable to walk, socialize, play in the sunlight or breathe fresh air. The resulting muscle atrophy creates the tender meat coveted by veal eaters, and the force-fed, iron-deficient milk substitute keeps you anemic. Thus, your flesh will be "desirably pale." But fear not; you'll be allowed to live to the ripe old age of 18 weeks before being shipped off for slaughter.

Surely it's better to be born a pig. If ever there existed an intelligent, curious creature, you are it! In the wild you take pleasure in trotting for miles, sniffing out edibles and mucking around in cool, muddy sloughs. As a factory piglet, though, you're confined to a crowded concrete pen which generates such acute frustration that you and your bros end up aggressively biting each others' butts and tails. Easy solution. The factory tech simply saws down teeth and whacks off tails! And if you are unlucky enough to be male, he'll also rip out your testicles—no pain-killers, of course. When slaughter time rolls around, you might even be conscious as they start to slit your throat and rip off your skin. *Tired of reading all this? Sick to your stomach? Good—that's the point.*

AND LET'S NOT FORGET the workers in these houses of hell who are likewise treated indecently, many of them recent immigrants, young single moms, or other economically desperate people willing to work for low wages in risky conditions. When journalist Susan Bourette went undercover in a large Canadian slaughterhouse, she exposed the truth of Big Meat and its underclass of workers who slave away on the kill floor, performing wretched and dangerous work on behalf of all factory-meat eaters. Lasting only four queasy days, Bourette toiled haplessly "in the bowels of a building with walls that sweat gristle and blood," she pens in *Meat: A Love Story*. "A modern-day chop house that serves up pork bellies and picnic roasts, loins and shoulders, and the odd human finger."

You know what that smell is? a factory veteran growled, inhaling deeply of the vile odor of mass slaughter just as Bourette was about to toss her cookies. *That's the smell of money.* "The internal logic of modern meatpacking is based on ever faster line speeds and low wages to extract bigger profits," confirms Bourette. From packed feedlots to massive processing plants, this brand of cruelty on an industrial scale—with little to zero regard for the animals involved—represents a new moral low in human existence.

I won't continue with the endless, horrendous details. They're in every animal rights manifesto, every veg beginner's guide. Yet it's critical to remind ourselves again and again that the modern corporate animal farm is one of the greatest evils ever devised by humanity and must be wiped off the face of the earth.

ANIMAL LIBERATIONISTS, vegetarians, and vegans: you have sounded the clarion call and for that we are eternally grateful. Now, however, it's time to get real. At 97% of the world's consumers, it is omnivores who hold the power to shut down factory farms, demand humane alternatives, and drive the new food revolution.

6.

OUR VOW UNTIL DEATH

I DIDN'T TELL LINDA about my no-meat vow at the farmer's market. We were too busy fending off males. For everywhere we went in Paris—Montmartre, the Louvre, Tuileries Garden—the men were sure to follow. French, British, Italian or Moroccan, it didn't seem to matter. They were on Linda's fragrant trail like bloodhounds pursuing an estrogen-lathered fox.

That same evening she finally succumbed to two tall, platinum-blond Danes sporting pedigree smiles, her chosen escorts to a lively brasserie. Veg dinners of any style or substance were tough to find in those days, but luckily this bar served traditional Mediterranean ratatouille as a refreshing first course: sautéed eggplant, tomatoes, zucchini and baby onions simmered to perfection in a jumbo pot with finely chopped basil, garlic, and herbes de Provence. The Scandinavian boys let my bashful, nerdy self tag along—no doubt out of pity.

Well, I showed them, ignorant elitists! Smashed on sweet Spanish wine, I began to expound on the virtues of pre-Einstein physics, followed by a rant on my personal concept of infinity. It's not outside of us, I kept repeating, but *inside* us, inside the atom, which—if you keep on dividing and dividing—goes on forever. Brilliantly structured, ever more miniature universes, one inside the other without end! This was pre-quark knowledge, for me anyway, and yet I was remarkably confident of my thesis. Confidence, in fact, seemed to be growing by the swigful. The blond young men nodded politely at the pale, egghead American, indulging me with quick winks and sly smiles as I proceeded to get stinkin' drunk for the first time in my highly sober, exceedingly virginal life.

By the time Linda left with the purebreds at nearly 2 AM and I found my lost, swoony way back to our cheap hotel for the night, I was feeling decidedly woeful.

15

I was also famished, having managed to get down only a few bites of baguette all day, following my meat-as-animal illumination. Moreover, the hotel carpet was so funky, the stained bed sheets so unappetizing, I decided to pitch Linda's teensy bike tent (toted around for just such emergencies) smack in the middle of our rented room, tossing in some threadbare blankets for company. Totally exhausted, stripped down to my granny panties and about to crawl in, I instinctively turned to find a smarmy middle-age man smack in my face, his unshaven visage sprouting a disgusting smile, his greasy breath reeking of dinner and dead animals. Too wasted to shriek, I slowly apprehended that this was the same hotel manager who had guided us to this very room that afternoon.

By now his grubby smile had visibly broadened in the pale window light. "Mademoiselle, where is your lovely friend Leeenda?" he leered, contemplating my slim hips and girlish breasts in the shadowy, suddenly airless room. "Hmmm, why this arrangement? *Pourquoi*?" he smirked, stroking the tent door, his black scraggly beard starting to quiver. "And would you like some help getting to sleep *ce soir*?" Out of nowhere remotely familiar, out of some mysterious, indefinite particle or place—probably a quark—materialized the most commanding baritone I'd ever heard in my life. "*Out of here! You blood-sucking leech!*" I barked, long skinny arms waving vigorously. "*Vite! Vite!*" the big new person inside of me bellowed as the pitiful, rejected man scurried out of the room and down the hall. Utterly amazed by my newly found voice, I turned the lock for the second time that night, jammed a banged-up dresser against the door, and settled into a deep, intoxicated, hungering sleep.

LATE THE NEXT DAY, wandering through woodsy and serene Père Lachaise to visit the graves of Jim Morrison and Edith Piaf—hearty meat eaters, still I adored them—it occurred to me that it was "now or never" to officially declare myself a vegetarian. Having hopped off the bus at Rue de la Réunion, Linda and I had ambled into the obscure east entrance of this arguably most famous cemetery in the world. Established by Napoleon in 1804, Père Lachaise is a hilly city of the dead, strewn with antiquated tombs and celebrated names. Chopin, Bernhardt, Wilde, Molière, on and on they go, far as the eye can see.

Tracing a gently rising-falling cobblestone path, we found ourselves lingering beneath towering shade trees, mesmerized by the sight and sounds of a nearby stonecutter at work. On bended knees and with infinite patience, he was chiseling

16

someone's name into a block of smooth black granite. Peering closer, we realized there were not yet enough carved letters to comprise a whole person. So whether man, woman or child, famous or unknown, we knew not, this someone who had already died or was perhaps this very hour facing death.

That fleeting moment is likewise engraved in my memory. The swift certainty of the workman's chisel cutting cold stone. The haunting hush between each firm strike. And the golden autumnal light streaming between the centuries-old linden trees, between the stonecutter's warm human body and ours. Linda offered me one of her homemade herbal rice balls and we ate in silence and gratitude.

We were bonded, she and I, the youth among the ancients, the living among the dead, bonded in the knowledge that we were young, aware, and fully alive. Bonded in our shared resolution to always and forever honor life. Never again would we live or dine unconsciously. Never again would we eat sentient animals who had been treated brutally and destroyed unwillingly, who had suffered and died to end up on our plate.

7.

YOUNG BITCHIN' FEMALES:
GET SKINNY!

ALL ACROSS THE NATION, teen girls are gossiping around messy tables in high school cafeterias. Their eye makeup is sophisticated, their noses skillfully pierced, and they're eating fake pepperoni pizza brought from home because they'd rather gag than swallow meat from real animals. They talk about food, calories, and lean blue-eyed jocks. The ones who aren't super skinny badly want to be. *I mean why eat dead animals when you don't have to? The way they're killed is so gross and inhumane! Just stop eating meat and you'll look and feel great!*

Exactly like Linda and myself decades ago, it's young females who command the leading edge in today's surge in vegetarianism, including 10% of girls ages 13 to 15. Some take the sacred vow even younger. Starting in the second grade, Cara refused to eat beef or pork because she felt so terrible for the animals. Her parents insisted their daughter eat chicken and fish for health reasons, but when she spotted squawking birds stuffed into cages in the back of a pickup, Cara announced that she would never again eat chicken in her life. "Having seen what she saw," her mom disclosed to *The Baltimore Sun*, "we knew there was no way we were going to change her mind."

No parental persuasion possible? Why is that? Well, no different than my own youthful paroxysms at the Paris meat market, today's tender-hearted young girls can't endure the thought of animals—especially adorable and familiar domestic animals—being penned up, slaughtered, and cut into chunks on their behalf. It's an emotive, passionate decision. Females are hard-wired to nurture, not butcher. Once they realize the actual source of their food and the saw-edged methods by which it ends up on their table, meat is instantly off the menu.

Even more noteworthy, a growing number of these girls are going vegan, swearing off all animal products forever, including dairy, eggs, honey, gelatin, even yeast. But are they replacing protein-dense, calcium-rich animal food with equally potent plants-only fare? And are they closely monitoring their healthy-fat needs and omega-3s? These are valid questions because teens are still growing and obtaining all the macro and micronutrients in optimal amounts is critical. Yet lunches bought by vegans in my daughter's high school revolved around pasta, chips, and diet pop. It's also discouraging to read the first two questions regarding specific foods in the book *Vegan & Vegetarian FAQ*: "Where can I find vegan marshmallows?" and "Where can I find vegan donuts?"

"But these are junk food vegans!" advocates correctly note, and vegan health outcomes can't be judged this way. Unfortunately, teens in general aren't known for making the most nutritious choices when it comes to meals and snacks. Take away the abundant and easily acquired calcium, protein, iron, zinc and vitamin B12 in animal products, and exacting food selection among teens becomes even more crucial. None of this is deterring the promotion and proliferation of veganism, however, with females continuing to outpace males.

Partial credit for the rise in girl vegans this past decade goes to *Skinny Bitch*, the runaway bestseller by Rory Freedman and Kim Barnouin that resonated with wannabe-thin young females across the globe. Sneaking in nasty tales of animal slaughter between cheeky, foul-mouthed, girl-power incantations, these two striking and yes, skinny escapees from the modeling world appeal to the vanity of teen girls as much as their values. *Eat like us and you will look like us* is their powerful message, and Freedman and Barnouin keep churning out more look-alike books to feed the skinny frenzy, including *Skinny Bitchin'* and *Skinny Bitch in the Kitch*, selling millions worldwide.

Sounds great, eh? Eat all vegan = get thin = get men! (You're not loveable otherwise is the harsh insinuation.) And save animals while doing it! Enormous caveat: Did you notice that neither Freedman nor Barnouin actually stated they were vegans in *Skinny Bitch?* In a 2010 interview, Freedman revealed she'd been vegan for less than one year when the book was published. Are you kidding me? That translates to a few months of being vegan, if at all, when the book was being written. A rather flimsy basis for marketing a radical new food regime, wouldn't you say?

Definitely not enough time to know the personal health effects of this inadequately studied diet. Definitely a risky mandate for converting possibly hundreds of thousands of young girls to a restricted pattern of eating heretofore followed by head-shaved, celibate monks. Detractors have called *Skinny Bitch* brazen vegan propaganda, its message ripped straight out of a pro-anorexia site. A shameless homage to modelesque bony hips. A ruthless put-down of non-skinnies as big fat pigs.

There it is, right on the first page of the book: Healthy = Skinny. But the truth is that being too thin is seriously *unhealthy*, increasing risk of anemia, lowered immunity, and broken bones. Studies reveal that following a restrictive diet to lose weight also increases hostility and aggression. Bitch indeed. Furthermore, over time, too-low calorie intake can generate malnourishment, persistent fatigue, and life-altering depression. Skinny females are also more likely to suffer from infertility and miscarriages; skinny males from sexual dysfunction and suicide. And there's more: thin people can be carrying around the most dangerous kind of fat, visceral fat that hides in tissues and organs. Skinny-fat these people are called and they're at high risk for inflammation and metabolic syndrome. Up to 40% of thin people have this syndrome, the road to type 2 diabetes. Overall, being underweight is more harmful to your health than being fat (Paradis; Ray; Thomas).

A meta-analysis of 50 respected studies revealed that too-lean people of all ages—18.5 BMI (body mass index) or lower—have nearly twice the risk of death from all causes compared to normal weight people. *Even obese individuals come out ahead of skinnies in all-cause mortality risk.* Odd, I didn't see these vital facts in all those *Skinny* books, did you?

Joel Ray, MD, the study's leader, cautions health authorities not to lead people into believing that thin equates with good health. But that's exactly what authors on a skinny mission are doing, and they should be spanked on their skinny little asses for doing so. Having a beneficial amount of muscle mass and fat for one's gender is a much more desirable physique, Dr. Ray confirms. Weight itself is not a marker of good health; physical and metabolic fitness are far more important.

SADLY, SUPER THIN continues to sell as "healthy and sexy" in our irrational, celeb-obsessed world. What's more, the much-hyped connection between veganism and skinnyism is rampant. Yet another glossy food magazine arrived at my house today with this popular editorial lead: *Go Vegan, Get Slim!* And you can't walk into a Barnes & Noble without being bombarded by veg books and cookbooks asserting that you, your family, and your best friends—even your rodent-shredding carnivorous cat—should jump right in and start living a guilt-free, gaunt vegan life.

Rarely in all these glowing *you-go-girl, just-do-it* vegan articles or ads is there the slightest mention of all the bright red flags being waved behind the flashy commercial seduction. Red flags like girls with eating disorders who hide behind vegetarianism—anorexic and bulimic females are 400% more likely to be veg'ns than omnivores (Aloufy; Bardone-Cone). Red flags like increased risk of anxiety, depression, and other mental health problems among vegetarians and low-meat consumers (Michalak). Also: teenage girls losing their menstrual periods; females *and* males not getting sufficient protein, fat, and calories during critical growth years; female vegans with lower bone mineral densities and substantially higher risk for fractures and osteoporosis (Pedersen; Appleby; Ambroszkiewicz).

Reliable research data on exclusively vegans is tough to find. What little exists on bone health, especially of long-term vegans, "is not as encouraging as one might hope," warn pro-veg authors Brenda Davis and Vesanto Melina in a rare admittance of cracks in the vegan world. More than half the studies cited in their book, *Becoming Vegan,* found "significantly lower bone density" in plants-only eaters compared to both meat eaters and lacto-ovo vegetarians. Even worse, the EPIC-Oxford Study revealed that vegans had a *37% higher incidence rate of bone fractures* as compared to omnivores.

Both veg and non-veg teens bolt down way too much processed food and soda, whose high levels of sodium and phosphoric acid, respectively, also contribute to calcium loss. (Sliced fake meats are sodium bombs, serving up an astounding 600-950 mg per three ounces.) Vegans, however, have specific risk factors for osteoporosis that meat eaters do not, including a tendency toward: too-low body weight; inadequate dietary calcium; inadequate collagen production; and a high-fiber diet that decreases calcium absorption. Moreover, their lower estrogen levels are linked to decreased bone density.

Females don't stop maturing until age 19 on average, yet some female vegans are eight years old, or even younger. How many of these girls—or their parents for that matter—realize that nearly 50% of their bone mass growth occurs between ages 8 and 18? Only 10% is added after that, reaching peak density by age 30. So it is imperative that adequate bone mass is achieved in the adolescent and teen years.

Furthermore, as your bones fill in and become denser your weight *must* go up, so girls who try to stay skinny and not gain pounds as they mature will not build enough bone mass. Called osteopenia ("less bone"), this serious condition is increasing among young women who follow low-calorie, vegan-type diets without adequate protein and fat to build bone collagen, putting themselves at higher risk for osteoporosis down the line. Despite these alarming results from EPIC-Oxford and other studies, the Academy of Nutrition and Dietetics continues to irresponsibly endorse a vegan diet as appropriate for all infants, children, and teens.

As far as heart disease, research on vegan outcomes is inconclusive. Data from four combined studies (two Seventh-day Adventist plus the EPIC-Oxford and Heidelberg studies) reveal that both fish eaters and dairy/egg eaters showed lower levels of heart disease incidence than vegans. The low vitamin D status of plants-only eaters is one risk factor, and additional research corroborates a "higher than expected risk for heart disease among some vegans," admit Davis and Melina.

Seriously low serum levels of long-chain omega-3 fatty acids—22-55% that of omnivores—may be responsible for the higher platelet aggregation also found in vegans (the first step in blood clot formations that can lodge in arteries and block blood flow, leading to heart attacks). These ultra-low omega-3 levels, especially of brain-protective DHA, may also be responsible for the higher veg'n death ratio for "mental and neurological diseases" found by the Oxford Study (2.5 times that of omnivores), as well as the Parkinson's disease that took the lives of two of the vegan movement's earliest advocates (Appleby; Fuhrman; Fabelo; Dyall). The abundance of pro-inflammatory omega-6s in plants, especially grains and refined vegetable oils, has also emerged as a serious health issue for plant eaters.

And while vegan stats for blood pressure, hypertension, and low-density lipoprotein (LDL) are commendable, homocysteine levels, an independent risk factor for heart disease, are consistently higher in vegetarians compared to omnivores, *with vegans having the highest levels of all.* Low levels of vitamin B12, missing in all plants, are probably causing vegans' elevated homocysteine levels, conditions linked to brain atrophy, dementia, and birth defects (Elmadfa; Obersby).

These are discouraging findings. Meanwhile, research on cancer and veganism is too limited to draw conclusions, and there's no credible evidence that an all-plants diets can prevent or reverse cancer. Many protective factors against this disease, such as conjugated linoleic acid (CLA) and coenzyme Q10, are found in efficacious amounts in animals only. Vegans can and do die from cancer, like musician Robin Gibb who was a dedicated vegan for decades. And Apple founder Steve Jobs, who had a lifetime obsession with extreme diets, including veganism and fruitarianism (high-fructose), died at 56 from pancreatic cancer. Indeed, new research reveals that fructose is readily metabolized by pancreatic cancer cells to increase their proliferation (H. Liu).

As for diabetes risk in vegans, this too is understudied. Recall that vegetarian research data cannot be assigned to vegans. So if you read or hear any pundits claiming that long-term vegans have reduced rates of diabetes, heart disease and cancer, ask to see the valid research—because it's doesn't exist. The Heidelberg Study, in fact, concluded that being a vegan is associated with "a higher mortality risk" than being a lacto-ovo vegetarian. Moreover, a vegetarian vs. omnivorous diet had "no effect on overall mortality" for health conscious people.

Think I'm slanting the evidence or picking on vegans? Quite the opposite. I have vegan friends and family members I adore. I want them all to live long and healthy lives. That's why I spent the last five years of my life digging deep into the exceedingly dry and stultifying nutrition literature (*the reason I turned this book into a story instead of a fact sheet*). We simply don't know enough about this constricted diet to be recommending it to the general population, let alone shouting out to teens and adolescents from every fitness magazine and celebrity cookbook: *Go Vegan!* The scientific evidence for a healthy, long-term outcome just isn't there. "Modern pioneers" is what promoters are calling today's vegans. Oh, they are pioneers alright. "Test animals" is more like it. You can be certain that future generations will be closely scrutinizing the lifetime health results of today's young vegans who have no such data to rely upon.

This diet is too new in the human experience in any kind of substantial numbers to validate results. (Look up "history of veganism" and you'll find about ten lines). Although a few large studies are finally underway—and that's a very good thing—everything we currently know about vegan health derives from very limited research that does not always separate short-term therapeutic vegans from committed lifers and frequently leaves out crucial information about actual food choices. Unbelievable, but research participants often fill out *one* food frequency questionnaire, at the onset, even if a study lasts for a number of years. Yet young people—and females of all ages—are notorious for their fast-track hopping from one in-vogue diet to the next. This past year alone, half the vegans I know have morphed into paleos.

If they present any studies at all, veg books and cookbooks usually cite only a few conducted on actual vegans. And research to date reveals vegan inadequacies or outright deficits in many key nutrients: iodine, iron, zinc, vitamins A (retinol), D3 and B12, selenium, taurine (now recognized as a functional nutrient), protein,

23

calcium, and EPA/DHA fatty acids, among others. Zealots will plead nutritional ignorance for the individuals studied, while continuing to argue that veganism is a healthy lifelong diet for all comers of all ages. *It's time to demand the evidence.*

THOUGH THE MAJORITY of converts are female, plenty of young males are taking the all-plants pledge. Others are contemplating going vegan, especially if they're dating one. Peer pressure, especially of the girlfriend variety, can be a powerfully persuasive force at this largely unverified, exploratory stage of life. What's more, male or female, youthful brains are still under construction.

Now don't get your rankles up; we're all a work in progress. But a profusion of brain studies over the past decade clearly show that neural insulation isn't complete until our mid-20s. Before that, literally, we're not all here. Our cortex's frontal lobes—the "control panel" of the brain that governs reason, insight and judgment—are not fully connected. This is the part of our brain that inquires, "What might be the long-term consequences of this action? What are possible negative results?" Youthful brain chemistry is also different: very excitable and responsive to new ideas. All this makes for emotional, sometimes impulsive young adults, impatient to explore and take on new risks—diet included.

So meat moguls of the world, beware. You better keep watch on the growing number of chic, skinny-by-intention young females who slurp spirulina smoothies and practice ashtanga yoga in designer hemp pants—because they are fiercely attached to their veg viewpoint and working hard on converting their boyfriends.

8

LIBERATION ROAD

To find your fearless best self: dine with shepherds, sleep on the earth.

—Mara O'Connell

Do 19-YEAR-OLD vegan virgins still exist? Still virtuous after a month in France, I lay atop Lasserre's thin, lumpy floor mattress, closed soft green eyes, and began my magical afternoon conjuring: lavender-scented fields, succulent ripe vineyards and most delicious of all, grape-smashing orgies with long-legged Scandinavian males. Oh what our bodies might do together if one (or more) were to glide naked beneath these white sheets right now. And yes, what *might* our bodies do? For that, even more than animal rights, was the question that tormented my tender, untested body and mind.

To make matters worse, Bertolucci's *Last Tango in Paris* was still showing around the capital city. Cinema-passionate Parisians had been talking about little else all year. Sucked in by all the hubbub, I queued up for a ticket and—along with everybody else in the darkened theater—stopped stuffing no-butter vegan popcorn into my startled, gaping mouth when a naked Marlon Brando thrust his kinky-haired French girlfriend against the bedroom wall and went at it. *Sweet Jesus! Was this what it was all about?!*

It was all too macho-violent for this dreamy teen romantic and just days later, with decisive gladness, I left crowded, provocative, veal-devouring Paris. Left a roof over my head and any morsel of security, abandoned my need to stay safe and small, and ditched André Gide's *La Porte Étroite* (The Narrow Door), ready to discover, at long last, my own wide-open road to liberation. Into my worn pack I scrunched everything not already clinging to my body: an extra pair of jeans, my fave red-plaid flannel shirt, a ludicrously svelte, white wool jacket (donated by the pitying, recently returned Lasserre: "This is Paris and you have no style!")

plus Kerouac's *On the Road*, my paperback Bible. Even more essential, I took along my shiny new promise to never again touch animal flesh to my now-chaste lips. And somewhere in that satchel I also packed my keen faith that the unknown void into which I was about to leap would shower me with truth and abundance.

Early the next morning, sitting straight-backed and alert amidst all the jostling commuters and blind beggars at Gare de Lyon, an elegant old train station on the north bank of the Seine, I counted my few remaining francs and slowly munched my last flaky croissant, moistening a finger to retrieve any fallen crumbs from my sleeve. Feeling absurdly serene for such an impetuous act, I patiently waited for the next train out of Paris—whatever its destination, whatever its speed— patiently waited for my new life to begin. *Reckless O soul exploring....steer for the deep waters only!* Whitman had proclaimed, and his words drifted in and out of my elated awareness. *Have we not groveled here long enough, eating and drinking like mere brutes?*

What I didn't fully realize at that moment but later came to understand is this: whenever we greet the universe empty of plans or agenda, serendipity unfolds and love abounds. My pack was light, my expectations lighter. I was open to emptiness; I was open to everything. What's more, I was confident my new ethical diet would keep me in good health and good stead. Thus, bag slung across my back and animal rights books safely stowed, for three improbable months—sometimes with the darling Linda, more often alone—I walked, pedaled, trained and hitched through a good chunk of France, Switzerland, Portugal and Spain, all the while sampling a dizzying array of fresh and delectable non-animal cuisine.

That meant, of course, missing out on some classic French dishes, soups, and sauces. There would be no porky, eggy Quiche Lorraine when tramping through Alsace. No frog legs in poulette sauce, thank you very much, while wandering the Loire Valley. As for Strasbourg's famed *foie gras*, fattened goose liver, I'd rather starve than have some greasy, force-fed, veins-plucked animal organ slithering down my supple young throat. Nor would traditional bouillabaisse ever scorch my gullet in Provence, nor even a simple fish soup with leeks and carrots, served everywhere along the Mediterranean and beloved by all who thrive by the salty sea. Certainly I would never savor wild boar from the heathery moorlands of the Midi, its plump cheeks simmered in red wine with sun-ripened pears. *Dégoûtant!* "Why not simmer the luscious pears only, and eat those?" I once asked the locals to vigorous rounds of laughter. Truly, I could not have hand-picked a more meat-loving nation than France to launch my vegetarian career.

HOW MUCH DO THE FRENCH adore their meat? Well, let us consider a pâté de Chartres. The sheer intricacy of its structure, much like the celebrated cathedral, might give even the crankiest vegetarian pause. Blending marinated wild game with pork, veal and liver, a chef mixes the whole disgusting shebang with pricey, subterranean fungi (black truffles with high perfume can fetch up to 4,000 euros per kilo). He then soaks this revolting concoction in fine cognac, fills any remaining space with aspic, wraps the final product in a delicate pastry shell and bakes it to golden perfection. Ah yes, from poultry to pork, fat partridge to lean hare, the healthy French love their meat in every imaginable disguise. This I discovered as soon as I could no longer eat any of it. Instead, like the feral boar, it was the acorns, sweet chestnuts, fruits and roots I was now digging for at every meal, at every outdoor market. And when I had my full, yet found myself still hungry, I'd head over to the town bakery to fill up on my favorite food in all the world: petite, still-warm loaves of crusty bread that slip right into your jacket pocket.

The French revere their bread, *le pain,* perhaps even more than their meat, if that's even possible. With 10 billion skinny baguettes sold in France every year, and 35,000 bakeries flung across the scenic landscape, even the smallest village boasts a charming *boulangerie* backed by centuries of tradition. Starting in the 1400s, bread dough was rolled most often into balls, or *boules*, hence the term, but modern French bread comes in all contours and sizes—from square rustic loaves of whole-grain, to light and fine-spun rolls *aux fines herbes*—and I did my very best to sample every one of them.

But here is an even prettier name in the French language: *la patisserie.* One visit to a French pastry shop and you will wonder if you've stumbled upon a new art form, possibly deserving of its own national museum—not needed, actually, because these exotic confections miraculously reappear every morning in every town, re-created for your lip-smacking satisfaction.

Vegetarians who don't hide from fresh cream and butter will find themselves in the sweetest of paradises at the village patisserie, selecting from highly artistic cakes, tarts, and cream puffs set out in gleaming glass cases like precious jewels. Try the gorgeous tri-colored Le Roussillon: blackcurrant jelly on pistachio pastry, festooned with fresh peaches, strawberry sorbet, and Cointreau ice cream—so lush and spongy it will instantly satisfy your carb or even erotic cravings. And chocolovers, don't you dare miss the Regal Chocolat, a sinfully rich layer-cake seething with dark chocolate mousse and served with raspberry coulis. *O la la!* Who needs a man anyway?

27

Ever leery of sugar, I made visits to pastry shops an infrequent treat, but fresh French bread—so soul-satisfying! It became not only my staff but my sword, my prime defense against a nagging sense of deficit, *an ongoing hunger.** So breakfast in Provence meant pomegranates, hazelnuts and croissants, while lunch in Madrid was a hearty spread of olives, almonds, figs and persimmons—all from open-air bazaars raucous with haggling deep into the night. Dinner in Lisbon meant, of course, saying *nao* again and again to the bounty of local seafood that makes the Portuguese one of Europe's healthiest populations: trout-stuffed crab, charcoal-broiled sardines, even squid cooked in its own dark salty ink. *Yuck!!*

Horrified by what might be swimming in my dinner, I trawled for veggies in every fishy stew and plucked haricot beans out of Porto's most famous dish, tripe. (Intestines are truly relished around here, ever since the townspeople slaughtered their livestock to provision Henry the Navigator's crews, keeping for themselves the entrails.) And beyond warm crusty pão from the bakery next door, every fada-driven Portuguese dinner is escorted by a glass of pale, exquisitely light Sherry, called the wine with 100 souls—although I'd say it's closer to a thousand.

Okay, I don't remember *precisely* what I ate and drank in Lisbon and Madrid, like thirty years ago, would you? I do remember it was fruit, veggie, and fresh bread bliss all across Western Europe. Carbohydrate Heaven! Fat? Why, there was plenty of that in all the nutritious olives and nuts. Protein options at the time? Tofu was available in only a few stores in Paris, plus plentiful beans and lentils everywhere else. Not exactly five-star European fare, but surely all this provided ample protein. I never gave it a second thought. All the vegetarian books avowed (and still do): "There's absolutely no need to worry about getting enough protein on this diet. Just dine on a variety of wholesome plant foods, along with enough calories, and you are guaranteed sufficient protein." Simple enough!

Much to my delight, being a vagabonding veg'n in 1970s Europe was indeed turning out to be easy. Fresh produce was everywhere and farmers' outdoor stalls prospered, not as some nouveau trend but as a continuous part of village life for centuries. Family vineyards and garden plots have long been squeezed into every available quarter-acre, providing Europe's vibrant *plein air* markets with a never-ending glut of local specialties. Grapes once flourished where the Eiffel Tower rises, and Marie Antoinette's rustic hamlet inside Versailles was a working farm with cherry orchards, cultivated fields, and a thriving dairy.

*"I always felt hungry" was the primary health concern cited by ex-vegans in a large survey (Asher et al), followed by worries of not getting "the right nutrients" in their all-plants diet, and "frequent fatigue."

Today's many fine restaurants strewn across France are actually a by-product of the 1789 French Revolution, wherein poor Marie lost more than her beloved little farm. For centuries aristocrats had enjoyed a lock on all the best chefs for their own grand kitchens, but post-guillotine it was the common people who began to enjoy new culinary heights, including animal protein like they'd never seen before and came to depend on. Naturally, when ordering a meatless meal at some village bistro, I didn't come right out and *tell* anyone I was a vegetarian, no way. No one would have believed me anyway, especially in the French countryside where the concept of a no-meat diet is blasphemy. I would have been branded an eccentric, unhealthy, too thin American who led a life of daft deprivation. Take away the meat from all your meals and what do you have, the locals would have asked me. *Rien! Nothing!* Some plant food held together by essential herbs but lacking in complete nourishment and gustatory fulfillment. This is simply not in the natural order of things, they would have declared.

Even their classic bean *cassoulet*, slow-cooked in earthenware pots and a sure bet for vegetarians, or so I thought, is chock full of not only white beans, onions, and thyme but duck legs, ham thighs and buttocks—all in a rich gelatinous broth. Good grief, my youthful self mused, are these French people still living in the Age of Unenlightenment? So why are they eating like wild carnivores, like blood-thirsty barbarians? And why, for all that, does everyone around here look so healthy and happy, especially all those rosy-cheeked children?

In truth, French school children cheerfully sit down to a lunch featuring rabbit, duck, goose, beef, sometimes even offal, an animal's internal organs. ("Awful is right—*gross!!*" American kids would gripe and refuse.) French kids exhibit no such qualms. Their palates are nearly as sophisticated as their parents' and their health is robust. Given their high-fat diet, I was shocked to discover that overweight and obesity rates are quite low among French children (their parents as well), among the lowest in the 34-nation Organization for Economic Cooperation Development. In contrast, today's American children top out at Number One: every third child is overweight or obese. That's not to say America's veg'n kids are likewise unhealthy (a lot more on that later), but merely to recognize that meat and dairy-eating French children are among the healthiest in the world.

THE FRENCH TAKE NUTRITION and the culinary arts quite seriously. They teach it to their offspring as early as nursery school, deeming it a life skill every bit as worthy as science or math. So when it comes to school lunches, the French are kicking our rather wide asses. Instead of sitting down to a meal of pre-packaged mac 'n cheese, or fried chicken fingers doled out with canned peaches, French kids are served a hearty four-course meal of *real food*: fresh and community sourced, organic whenever possible.

It might begin with a leafy green salad and freshly baked bread, followed by a warm main dish of local meat. How about some sautéed chicken simmering in a mushroom crème sauce, or duck Shepherd's Pie garnished with garlic, pepper-corns, and parsley sprigs? Up to four freshly picked vegetables are included in every school lunch—zucchini, radishes, and cucumbers with mint, for example—followed by a cheese course, say Gouda or Camembert, and lastly, seasonal fresh fruit like tart strawberries or sweet, buttery-smooth pears. (Can we order these lunches to go?) Unflavored cow's milk and water accompany each meal, *not* juice or soda pop, and vending machines are banned. Some French schools don't even allow ketchup because of its high-sugar content and fried food is limited to four times per month. *Variety is essential in the French diet as it should be in every-one's, vegans included.* Thus public schools don't repeat a meal for 30 days.

French kids, I also learned, are given an hour and a half for lunch and socializ-ing, a leisurely, civilized pace that encourages conscious, pleasurable eating and proper digestion. Compare that to the 25-30 minutes American kids are allowed to gulp down their highly-sweetened or salted institutional food, trot to the bath-room and then sprint to class. This isn't even enough time to know if you're full or not, let alone exchange meaningful dialogue with your friends.

Yet psychologists and food experts believe that the *way* we eat is every bit as critical for our health as *what* we eat. "It's quite true. What we eat is only half the story of good nutrition," Marc David, director of the Institute for the Psychology of Eating, told me. "The other half is who we are as eaters. Your metabolism is profoundly affected by your thoughts, feelings, and level of stress or relaxation during meals." In an international study of diet beliefs, it was fast-chomping Americans who obsessed the most on buying healthy food but ate with the least enjoyment. The much healthier French, meanwhile, give nary a thought to their health when it comes to mealtime, yet take from it the most pleasure.

Years later, serving my French son-in-law a meal for the first time, it took him so long to finish, I worried he thought it was garbage, barely palatable. But Yohan was simply taking his own sweet time to gnash, digest, and truly savor my brave attempt at spinach-scallion quiche (I'm a lousy cook), while engaging in animated conversation. During self-imposed breaks, he would lean back comfortably in his chair, twine his hands behind his handsome head, and charm us with travel tales. (Compare to Americans eating in cars, mindlessly scarfing lunch while ferociously pecking on smartphones.) The social aspects of French dining are as deeply rewarding as their food. Yohan was as involved with the satisfaction of his palate as he was unaware of the passing of time. And much of that satisfaction, for the French, involves the eating of animals.

So when the national government effectively outlawed vegan meals at public schools starting in 2011—banning food from home and announcing that animals will serve as the primary protein source for all lunches—vegan celebrities like Sir Paul McCartney howled but fewer than 20 Parisians protested. That's because the tally of vegetarians in France is among the lowest in Europe, estimated at less than 2% of the population. (To Spain, however, goes the title of Vegan Hell, with 0.1% of its population claiming no-meat status.) Many French traditionalists still scorn vegetarians, or at least don't understand them, and rural populations remain far less tolerant than their urban counterparts.

EAGER TO AVOID DISCORD and debate while traversing the French countryside, I skipped the meat without explanation and loaded up on all the fantastically fresh carbs. Eyes sated by pastoral beauty, belly temporarily appeased, every evening I sought out a modest guest house or even better, burrowed my body into a mossy hollow beneath spreading oaks just as dusk settled in. Other times, dog-tired from uphill hiking, I would simply crash beneath a fragrant bush in some mountain meadow and enjoy the finest sleep of my life—awakening to the calls of a roving shepherd or the melodic bells of his wayward sheep.

But on the very best nights I sprawled beside plump haystacks in a farmer's fallow field, hands reaching up to touch the night sky before slipping off into easy slumber. In such a heedless, spontaneous manner did I make my nomadic, gastronomic path through Western Europe. I had absolutely no fears to travel this way, alone and unhurried, and quite honestly I don't know why, except to recall the sweet joy of liberation flooding my being with boundless trust and delight. I do know this: my body felt light, my mind free, and I was as wholly devoted as any young person today to my divinely inspired, morally correct, new vegetarian diet.

9.

VEGETARIAN CLASS WARS

Brie the revealing experience, instantaneous and profound.

—Donald Hall

NOT SO VERY LONG after hitting the road, I began my not so secret affair with *le fromage*. I'm talking cheese: notably ripe, oozy, sexy Brie, which the poet calls "the revealing experience" and the French call *formidable*. I'd begun my dietary commitment as what would now be called a vegan, not even realizing this was a distinct class. First coined as a word in 1940s England, veganism was little known in America until the 1980s when it started getting some press and showing up in a few dictionaries. Prior to that time, there were definitely no militant vegans in our collective face. Yet by the end of that decade, People for the Ethical Treatment of Animals (PETA) had vaulted into the national spotlight and the call for strict veganism was gathering force.

Trouble was, eating 100% plants, I was 100% still-hungry almost all the time, unable to function or even think about anything but my next meal, no matter how much delicious and varied plant food I stuffed into my mouth, nor how often. Not a good way to go through life I realized soon enough, but I was determined to never return to my carnivorous roots.

Legumes, grains, veggies, fruit, nuts and seeds, even my miracle loaves of bread—it didn't seem to matter what plant foods I ate or in what combination; the hunger soon returned. Dairy, I eventually discovered, was the only non-fleshy food that filled me up, eradicating my hunger for a reasonable number of hours. The word *complete* comes to mind, having all the necessary components to feel energized and joyously alive. Without dairy, I always felt fractional, my brain half lit, my energy levels in the dumps. I was a slender thing so filling a big gut wasn't the issue. Mine was rather small actually, but always shouting out that something was amiss. It must be a matter of needing additional sources of protein and fat, I reasoned, without a hint of shame or dismay.

Truthfully, I feel incredibly fortunate that strict veganism was largely unheard of during my 20s. My lacto-guilt would have been rampant. As a devout vegan, I would have insisted on no animal nourishment whatsoever, ignoring my wise body's unequivocal messages. I might even be dead by now, or at least fragile-boned and seriously demented, due to the bizarre assumption at the time that plants contain all of the nutrients needed by humans. In addition to vitamins B12, D3 and A (retinol), science continues to discover essential micronutrients found solely in animal sourced food, but who knew?

My first years as a vegetarian, thank God I was still smart enough to listen to my impartial body. Some individuals and ethnic groups have higher protein/fat requirements, I've since learned from the non-biased nutrition literature, and do remarkably well with reasonable amounts of dairy. A wedge of creamy Brie, for example, instantly and miraculously enlivened me, providing a good measure of critical calcium, protein, fat and B12. So yes, a daily slab of farm-fresh cheese was gratefully and intelligently added to my original vegan mix. Although ignorant at the time of genetic and metabolic influences, I did recognize early on that no one should have to sacrifice her health for the plants-or-nothing creed.

TRAVELING THROUGH FRANCE and Switzerland but of course, *bien sûr,* I willingly sampled some of the most superb *fromage* on the planet. Who knew there are more French cheeses than days of the year? All over Frank-Land, indeed much of Europe, a meal is considered incomplete without its cheese course. This would not go over well in America where dairy gets unrelenting bad press as a purveyor of cholesterol and flabby, buttery bodies. Meanwhile, the French stay healthier and slimmer, suffer far less heart disease, and live much longer than we do—all the while enjoying their daily dose (or two or three) of full-fat yogurt, pastured cheese, and rich yellow butter.

Having grown up on Kraft and gooey Velveeta, I was astonished to discover French *crémeries* that overflow with a headrushing diversity of time-honored cheeses from the abundant milk of wandering animals. Soft-ripened cheese with white or red mold, like Camembert or Pont-l'Évêque. Goat's cheese such as Sainte-Maure, hand-rolled and bluish. Or the fatty, fermented sheep's cheese created in the Pyrénées with characteristic grassiness and salty sweetness. And then there's also hard cheese from summertime mountain milk as in the popular Gruyère de Comté, produced by monastery monks since the 12th century and said to possess over 80 aromatic flavors that linger delectably on the palate.

European cheese making is equal parts art and science, requiring dark, dank cellars or caves with the precise temperature and high humidity to ensure proper aging and the sought-after intensity of flavor. Some are washed in salt or spirits, while others are dusted with ash or wrapped in leaves by the skilled *affineur*. Clearly, these are artists in pursuit of masterworks and my French foodie friend, Lasserre, knows it. Gladly will she spend an entire morning making the rounds at an outdoor cheese festival, seeking the perfect round of local shepherd's cheese, perhaps raw-milk Ossau-Iraty—of ancient origins and simultaneously sweet and nutty, hinting of toasted hazelnuts. Pinching off a soft white lump, she'll deftly roll it between her knowing fingers, waft it beneath her cute, discerning French nose and then toss the delicacy atop her discriminating tongue, at which point her already big brown eyes become enormous and squeaks of joy emerge from her ecstatic throat. Ah, the nuanced tastes and textures of curdled sheep's milk.

But such cherished traditions are abhorrent to modern ethical vegans, even if the sheep and goats roam contentedly in high green pastures in the snow-capped Pyrénées or Alps. (A more desirable life, many would agree, than sitting on one's arse all day, facing a blinking, energy-sucking screen in some stuffy, oppressive cubicle, working for the bossman.) Alas, vegans won't go near *any* cheese, even the 100% pastured variety. That's because even this free-roaming animal is being "exploited" to feed humans. Exploitation? What a sad and distorted way to regard our transformative, organic earth. Are humans likewise being "exploited" by plants and animals when our bodies break down into small, easily assimilated nutrition packets in order to serve other life forms?

Yes, we will already be dead, but *somebody* has to be on top of the food chain. Unfortunately for vegans, it happens to be us. No way, of course, was I ready to confront such disquieting realities as an idealistic and naïve vegetarian youth. What I did face up to was the type of rennet used to coagulate the milk. Animal rennet from dead mammalian stomachs was taboo, but cheese makers have been seeking out non-animal sources since the fig juice used in Homer's day—and they are easy to find because plants, fungi, and microbial sources all provide the required active enzymes.

Even today, however, it's all but impossible to banish animal products from one's life. Modern vegans are unwittingly "exploiting" animals nearly every day. Consider cane sugar, found in millions of food products. It's commonly whitened with bovine bone char. Apple juice, alas, is often clarified using crushed shellfish. Love your bagels? Most contain L-cysteine from bird feathers and hog hairs.

34

Paints and adhesives, biodiesel fuels and plastics, even kids' crayons contain animal by-products—hospital gowns of the future will, too.

And if you're really intent on erasing all animals from your consumptive life, get ready to never use an airplane or car, or *any* vehicle that uses hydraulic fluids. Moreover, it's time to give up driving or cycling on asphalt, eating all food grown with commercial fertilizers, and frequenting any building or house constructed with cement blocks—including your own. Even the commercial organic produce preferred by nearly all vegans depends on the soil-amending bones and blood of dead animals. There is no animal-free lunch.

IT'S HARD WORK being a purist. Impossible actually, unless you want to opt out of society and make a dash for the woods. All the vegetarians I knew in my youth included cheese or yogurt in their diet. Those who nibbled the rare or random fish called themselves vegetarians as well and no one even blinked. Today that outrageous claim will get you in a big trouble with the veg'n police. All manner of Pure versus Adulterated diet categories now exist, and woe to anyone who dares to merge them as one!

For some reason—oh let's just call it self-righteousness—applying the correct honor label is crucial for today's plant eaters. For vegans especially, maintaining distinct consumer classes is of utmost importance, functioning something like a caste system, from the purest plants-only diet to the decidedly impure pseudo-vegetarian diets. So if you are a cheesehead, as I certainly was, you are *not* an untarnished vegetarian and must *never* label yourself as such. You are a lacto-vegetarian, one class down from the real deal. Add some eggs to that menu and you descend to lacto-ovo vegetarian. (Eat a bit of chicken now and then and you're what, a cackletarian?) A lacto-ovo veg is thus two entire classes down from the highest, most virtuous form of eating which is, of course, veganism.

Dutiful and unyielding in all lifestyle choices, ethical vegans will not knowingly eat, use or sell animal products of any type or stripe, no matter how faceless or non-fleshy. Exceptionally proud of their top of the class position and (seeming) total abstention, some vegans even refuse to frequent businesses that employ non-vegans. Huh? Oh yes, because their own money would be indirectly supporting humans who ingest or otherwise make use of animals. (The term obsessive-compulsive comes to mind but I will refrain from suggesting my own labels.)

Even if you eat all-plants except the infrequent fish for its health-enhancing omega-3s, you are most definitely a lower class eater and must label yourself a pescatarian (from *piscis*, Latin for fish). And a pesky pescatarian at that, should you dare call yourself a vegetarian in public. *You can't lay claim to our esteemed position,* the pissed-off purists shout. *You are a carnivore, plain and simple!* They love to repeat the old joke that a semi-vegetarian makes about as much sense as a semi-virgin, but I'm not so sure about that analogy. If you had but one meat-eating event in your otherwise virtuous life, even years ago, you can never call yourself a vegetarian according to this standard. Sorry, the damage has been done. Your corporal cells were penetrated by meat molecules and that body memory will persist throughout time. Defiled!

Sorry dude, but when it comes to being a proper vegetarian, you're either on the bus or off the bus. A member of the exclusive club, or kicked out into the mean, meaty streets with the fishmonger and the butcher. (The baker and candlestick maker will be allowed entrance with the proper consumption credentials.) Online contempt for the occasional fish eater is palpable: *Hey, you are NOT vegetarians, people, so GET OVER IT!* The same goes for abstainers who chow on chicken but rarely, for protein's sake. Forget it, declare the classification cops: the word pollo-vegetarian is preposterous and, like pesca-vegetarian, doesn't even belong in the English language.

Ethical vegans are the most stringent regarding who will be allowed entrance into their morally correct society. Most don't even consider themselves a subset of vegetarianism, according to the most recent Gallup poll, but their own separate and, let's just admit it, superior category. Even musician and seafood-eater Alanis Morissette, who calls herself "80% vegan," admits that her V-friends despise her terminology and she feels "a little bit of shame" regarding her recent obsession with oysters. (Lose the shame and listen to your smart body: oysters are rich in zinc, iron and complete protein, harder to obtain from a plant diet.) And when over a dozen Whole Foods Markets accidentally swapped their soy-based curried "chick'n" with real chicken, vegans who inadvertently indulged were both furious at Whole Foods and mortified to have crossed the forbidden border.

All this obsessing on labels strikes many omnivores, including those potentially interested in converting, as nothing more than elitist posturing, especially when vegans in these same blogs use terms like "dumbo" and "dumb-ass" to describe *the stupid carnivores.* "Just because the fish can't reach up, unhook its mouth from your fishing pole, and say OUCH! doesn't mean it can't feel," lectures one plant eater. "Grow a brain, already. VEGANS RULE!"

36

SUCH COMMENTS EMERGE, no doubt, from the churlish mouths of babes, young converts steadfastly pushing their moral agenda in the false belief that they've discovered the holy grail of diets for all human beings. Their surly, often disdainful attitude has not gone unnoticed in blogworld. Writes former purist Lance: "It's ludicrous how hostile vegetarians are to pescatarians." And from Ronnie: "It sounds like you hate us or something....I don't eat farmed fish, only wild-caught, and I only eat them because I can't get essential omega oils in other ways because I'm allergic to plant sources." Kiri elaborates: "The majority of pesca-vegetarians I've spoken to have made the choice to include fish in their diet for health reasons only. Do you find this selfish? Do you find this wrong? By calling themselves a pesca-vegetarian, they're admitting they are not a true vegetarian."

Amidst all the squabbling, Nikki displays the healthiest attitude of all. "I don't really care about labels. I eat fresh-caught fish but nothing with feet. I also don't eat farm-raised fish. I care about animals but really do it for health reasons. I'm trying to maintain an alkaline body to keep diseases like cancer from growing. Call me whatever you want. I don't really care."

Great response, Nikki, but *nothing with feet*? That leaves a whole lot of sliding, swimming, slithering creatures for potential consumption. At one time, the preferred definition of vegetarianism was eating nothing with a face. Of course, that characterization creates its own set of problems. Does a clam feel pain? Does an oyster long to preserve its life? How *do* we know if we're eating an animal that suffers—or eating an animal at all?

10.

THE VEGETARIAN'S DILEMMA

We do not rule the world, despite our conspicuous position in it.

—Elizabeth Thomas

Y OU KNOW WHETHER that stuff in your sushi is animal or plant, right? Then again, maybe not. Consider seaweed, specifically nori. This green-black "wonder food" is believed to contribute to Japanese longevity, but a plant it is not. Rather, it is an amalgam of single-and multi-celled marine organisms now classified in a separate kingdom, distinct from either animals or plants. Sponges, also formerly known as plants, have been determined to be animals—our most distant ancestor actually. (What? You didn't know you evolved from a flagellated eukaryote?) And protozoa—once considered animals—and fungi—once considered plants— are neither. They too merit their own life form classifications.

As if the lines aren't already blurred enough, enter *Elysia chlorotica*, a mythic, emerald-green sea slug that's half-animal, half-plant. Only it's real. A leaf-shaped creature, *E. chlorotica* carries out photosynthesis by harnessing the energy of the sun, exactly like a green plant. Inhabiting salty marshes in New England and Canada, this clever slug apparently robs the appropriate energy-producing genes from the algae it feasts upon, even passing them on to future generations. Thus, chloroplast-blessed, this lucky bloke need never again search for food to acquire energy. Unlike the rest of us stalking or foraging veggies, omnies and carnies, *Elysia chlorotica* simply has to hang out in the noonday sun.

What a splendid life that might be! Especially for those among us who don't especially enjoy shopping for and preparing food, viewing it as mere fuel, a bothersome necessity in the course of an active day. In fact, self-fueling *Elysia* sounds rapturously close to *Elysian,* the field of perfect happiness in Greek mythology. Who knows? The day may yet arrive in this mad scientist, gene-scrambled world, when human DNA will be spliced with chlorophyll, permitting us to pamper ourselves with blissful, noon-time solar naps instead of lunch. The need to recharge will take on a whole new meaning. Among food aficionados, the French would surely put up the fiercest resistance, but at least we could finally toss this divisive, holier-than-thou vegetarian vs. omnivore debate.

For now, however, we remain poles apart from the self-sufficient slug, and each of us must draw our own ethical line between the life forms we will and will not eat when hunger strikes yet again. This task becomes increasingly daunting as our biological knowledge continues to gain in complexity ever since Aristotle split living organisms into two simple categories: Plantae and Animalia. As this strict demarcation between plants and animals shifts and drifts, vegetarians might well give pause before ingesting any plant-like delicacies from the sea. Centuries ago, early veggies likewise considered it fine and dandy to eat cold-blooded, expressionless fish which lack, they assumed, both sense and sensibilities.

But what about the so-called "lower" animals, invertebrates that comprise 95% of the earth's known species? They possess no spine for transmitting electrical signals from the brain. Some have no brain at all. Just 10 neurons comprise a mussel's entire nervous system—compare that to a cat's one billion. Yet dining on marine bivalves such as clams or mussels is strictly taboo for vegans, not because these creatures possess the requisite hardware to feel anything, but merely because they've been placed in the animal kingdom. We are tempted to ask how a living thing so small, simple, and lacking in cognitive capacity can even know that it's being eaten. But should we measure intrinsic value in grams of body weight, in degrees of brain complexity?

Apparently, most humans do. We have a very long history of favoritism toward species that most resemble us in size, shape, and brain size. We revere the wild horse and work hard to rescue it, but give little thought to the wild seahorse, increasingly endangered by coral reef destruction. Nearly everyone honors tigers but detests ticks, most of which do zero harm to humans yet routinely end up ripped apart and doused in gasoline because they die hard, obviously preferring to live. Clearly, all humans—vegetarians included—create hierarchies of preference, albeit unconsciously, as to who shall live and who shall die in the animal kingdom. Even though they vow to never intentionally harm or kill a single critter, we don't see ethical vegans defending hungry ants that swarm kitchen counters by the hundreds (sucking them up with the vacuum doesn't save lives, tried it), nor the bedbugs that snuggle happily into our comforters at night in search of warm, life-sustaining blood—later to be boiled alive in the washing machine.

Almost all of us show partiality toward animals with big brains, big eyes and clearly defined faces, preferably similar to our own human mug shot. We demonstrate far less concern, far less mercy for the slimy, pin-eyed, miserable-looking blobfish than the adorable, wide-eyed panda bear. And most vegans direct the bulk of their energy to preserving ubiquitous soft-eyed cows and sweet-faced pigs rather than, say, the critically endangered Morrow snail whose pinhead-sized eyes are difficult to even discern, or the truly scary-looking naked mole rat being used for cancer research.

I suppose we could call this particular selective tyranny, face-ism. Or perhaps, animal fascism? It's why the World Wildlife Fund enlists the panda and not the blobfish as its international motto, even though both are in danger of extinction. And unless you're an Idaho rancher, or hitched-up with one, the vast majority of Americans passionately support endangered species protection for *Canis lupus,* the grey wolf, but try garnering sponsors and funding for *Sorex nanus*, the dwarf shrew. People will laugh in your face if you try to whip up affection for this snout-elongated, diminutive species—even though both mammals are important players in the ecosystem. In recognition of humanity's overt animal discrimination, the Ugly Animal Preservation Society is dedicated to "raising the profile of some of Mother Nature's more aesthetically challenged children," according to its president, evolutionary biologist Simon Watt. At UAPS events like the Edinburgh Science Fest, crowds are confronted with creatures only a mother could love—like the purple pig-nosed frog—and then asked to love them anyway.

Thankfully, in the relatively short history of animal rights, criteria such as human resemblance and brain power have yielded to the gold standard of sentience. Consciousness is often difficult to ascertain, but pain is usually clearly witnessed. Utilitarian philosopher Jeremy Bentham recognized this in the influential wake of Montaigne and Rousseau, early philosopher-activists who viewed the humane treatment of animals as our duty. In 1789 Bentham famously argued for our moral responsibilities to animals on the grounds of pain perception alone. The question is not *can they reason*? Nor, *can they talk*? Rather, it is this: *can they suffer?* That animals feel pain and suffer, and therefore deserve our protection, is now the primary tenet of every ethical vegetarian, vegan, and animal liberationist.

However eloquent his ideals, Bentham is no poster child for moral veganism. Were he living in this century, PETA might refuse him membership. Himself a meat eater, this father of modern animal rights—and by extension, veganism—avowed that "it ought to be lawful to kill animals, but not to torment them." Our intellectual heroes are human after all, and while Bentham consumed meat for his health or other reasons, he did succeed in dramatically shifting the animal welfare debate from one of brain capacity to pain awareness. (Evidently a swift killing for food constitutes neither torment nor suffering in Bentham's world.)

Two centuries later, an animal's capacity to suffer is still the benchmark for moral consideration. Yet how can we know for certain which animals experience pain and also suffer from it? We cannot. That's why the longstanding "do fish feel pain" debate rages on, fueled by righteous vegans battling defensive anglers tired of being depicted as sadists. For every scientific study that concludes our watery brethren suffer emotionally when pierced by hook or suffocated by net, another study emerges to insist this isn't true.

When behavioral biologist Victoria Braithwaite and her research cohorts from the University of Edinburgh injected rainbow trout with bee venom and observed their subsequent behavior (rocking motions, rubbing the affected area, and temporarily losing interest in food), vegans felt vindicated by her conclusion. Fish do possess specialized pain detectors and exhibit adverse behavior that demonstrates pain awareness, Braithwaite announced in 2003; hence, there exists "no logical reason why we should not extend to fish the same welfare considerations that we currently extend to birds and mammals."

Around this same time, a team of scientists let anglers off the hook, concluding exactly the opposite: pain detection is not the same as suffering and fish cannot suffer, simply because they haven't the brains for it. Suspicious behavior isn't strong enough evidence, asserts lead researcher Dr. James Rose of the University of Wyoming; even microbes flinch when jabbed by a knife. One must examine the actual brain structure of fish to realize they don't have the necessary wiring—nociceptors known as C fibers, along with an evolved neocortex—to emotionally suffer the way higher order animals do. It's a fundamental rule of neurobiology, according to Rose. If the hardware isn't there—and it's not in fish—the sensation can't be there either. Others, like renowned animal behaviorist Temple Grandin, continue to disagree.

A TASTE FOR TARANTULAS

If questions still linger about the suffering capacity of fish, what can we possibly resolve about spineless creatures like insects and spiders? Slugs and grubs? When you poke them with a stick and they promptly curl into a ball, are they expressing physical and psychological pain? Or just an involuntary reflex to outside stimuli?

41

Ethical vegans will be forced to confront this question in the near future as the search for new protein sources becomes ever more imperative on our heated-up, arable-land diminished earth.

Hungry third-world-travelers can already get a taste of this very real scenario. Stop for a delectable treat from Thai street vendors and you may well be handed a simmering plateful of sautéed cockroaches, maybe even a King Scorpion if you hit the right day. Cruising through Cambodia? Smiling villagers will gladly offer you some fried tarantulas, a tradition dating back to the food-scarce days of the Khmer Rouge. Now that citizens have developed a taste for the furry eight-legged arachnids, hundreds are caught, cooked and eaten every day, providing a valuable source of readily available protein.

Disgusted? Revolted? That's understandable in our bug-phobic culture but you better get used to it. In humanity's overpopulated food-scarce future, insects will emerge as a major, inexpensive, ecologically-friendly protein source. Prolific and super-abundant, insects are just about everywhere, offering the possibility of not only substantial nourishment but local empowerment.

The United Nations is seriously looking at insect-based diets as a potent way to eradicate poverty and hunger, reduce child mortality, and improve food availability worldwide. How vegetarians will handle this reality is anybody's guess—although real hunger has a way of making these decisions for us. The best, most environmentally-sane way to secure adequate protein for 7 billion people and counting, a growing number of scientists claim, is to eat much lower on the food chain, i.e. bugs. Along with key vitamins and minerals, insects offer a complete protein source that's high-quality, quickly produced, and more sustainable than almost anything on the planet.

The environmental argument for veganism—that animal-sourced food requires massive amounts of land, water, feed and energy compared to plants—disappears with the emergence of entomophagy: insect dining. Comparing crickets to soy, for instance, let's scrutinize the stats. Raising crickets entails *half* the water of soybeans to produce the same amount of protein—an enormous savings of a fast-dwindling resource. It's also extremely land efficient compared to growing all those legumes because insect farms are built vertically as much as horizontally. Crickets and mealworms actually *prefer* cramped and dark quarters, virtually piled on top of each other, "a concentrated animal feeding operation—without the suffering," as Peter Frick-Wright notes in *Sierra*. Their protein output is profuse, nine pounds for each pound of feed, no chemicals, no GMOs. Insects also possess high reproductive efficiency and, unlike soy and other vegan crops, can speedily convert agricultural waste and other unusable biomass into edible protein. Most significant of all, insects as food curtails the expansion of monocrop agribusiness and thus, greenhouse gas production.

Even beyond protein and caloric density, an insect offers vital nutrients that a plant cannot, such as vitamin B12, vitamin A in its biologically active form, and all the essential amino acids in the correct ratios. But the health benefits of bug gobbling don't stop there. The exoskeleton of insects is rich in prebiotic fiber that ferments in your gut, creating a potent microbiome that increases your overall vigor and mental health, while protecting you from inflammatory bowel diseases (Schmidt; Looijer-van Langen). Moreover, *insect feed for farm animals* improves gut functionality and overall health (Borrelli). This has huge ramifications for animal husbandry, decreasing the use of antibiotics while freeing up potentially millions of acres of grain crops currently fed to livestock.

Furthermore, insect eaters can choose among 2,000+ edible species. Compare that to the repetitive soy regime that many vegans follow, meal after meal, day after day. Yet the way to optimal health is to intake lots of different species! Our human bodies thrive on nutritional variety and the more species we invite inside, the better for our collective health. Worldwide, food diversity also means increased food security.

Ardent vegans, along with bug-adverse omnivores, will undoubtedly resist. The gag reflex will be heard far and wide, yet it's wholly culturally-induced. Modern westerners aside, insects have been part of the human diet for millennia. Early North Americans were especially fond of one salty delicacy: grasshoppers! When archeologist David Madsen discovered the remnants of millions of hoppers in a remote cave on the Great Salt Lake's eastern shore, he found them in nearby dried human feces as well. To this day, the lake collects as many as 10,000 sun-dried grasshoppers *per foot* of shoreline; a single person can scoop up *200 pounds* in just one hour.

At 1,365 calories per pound of hoppers, that translates into a vast amount of food energy per hour of very easy foraging: no killing involved, no ecosystems destroyed, and no processing necessary. To match the calories in that amount of protein-dense grasshoppers, you would need 505 Big Macs or 2,202 soy burgers! (Plus far higher inputs of energy, land, and water.) You can even buy a novel dehydrator to grow and dry grasshoppers in the comfort of your own kitchen. And the taste ain't bad either. Madsen describes dried hoppers as "desert lobster."

Vegans who are sincere about their enviro ethics need to take an honest look at these astounding numbers. Those of you who love chocolate are already ingesting bugs anyway, usually in the form of ground-up cockroaches. Oh, you didn't know that? It happens on the tropical farms, not in factories, so would you rather chew a few insect parts or have tons more pesticides applied to millions of cocoa trees? Currently, the FDA allows 60 "insect fragments" per 100 gram chocolate bar, but roach-rich cocoa isn't the only way vegans are involuntarily eating animals every day. Got pasta? Up to 225 insect parts are allowed per 225 grams, plus 4.5 rodent hairs or excreta. Golden raisins for your afternoon snack? Get ready for 10 whole insects and 35 Drosophila eggs per 8 ounces. (And these are the bags that are actually inspected.) Hops in your beer? How do 2500 aphids per 10 grams sound? Organic makes no difference; basically any grain, nut, seed, nutbutter, dried fruit or spice that you toss in your oral cavity includes a free shot of animal protein. So why not get intentional about it and make insects part of your enviro ethics?

Sorry if I curdled any vegan stomachs with this information. Our ancestors had no such qualms. Beetle larvae were enjoyed by 1st century Romans, and Aristotle instructed Greeks on the fine art of cicada harvesting, recommending females after copulation, full of tasty eggs. The Old Testament advises locusts, while Aboriginal Australians have long had a thing for grubs. And let's not forget modern Japanese foodies who order up fly larvae sautéed in sugar and soy sauce. Across Asia, Africa and Latin America, insect-eating continues to thrive.

It's westerners who are the weirdos for refusing to eat bugs, argues biologist and chef David G. Gordon, who calls termites "the other white meat" and aims to transform our cultural biases via his *Eat a Bug Cookbook.* Meanwhile, Noma of Copenhagen, often cited as the world's best restaurant, is preparing a gastronomic case for gourmet insect-eating, and fringe grocers are already offering cricket-based energy bars for the health conscious and active.

Despite growing optimism, up and coming insect ranchers still face a tough sell, especially among diehard plant eaters. One need only recall customer outrage when Starbucks admitted that the red coloring (no longer) in its Strawberries & Crème Frappuccino comes from crushed cochineal beetles, a common natural dye dating back to the Aztecs. From that vehement reaction, further inflamed by PETA, it's clear that vegetarians and vegans—plus the plain ol' squeamish—will never willingly eat insects, nor tolerate their uncertain suffering.

Yes indeed, exactly which animalia possess awareness and which do not is far from clear, compounding the vegetarian's dilemma. And when science finally confirms, certainly in this century if not the next 30 years, that plants possess not only awareness and intelligence but an irrefutable interest in preserving their own lives, then ethical vegetarians will really be screwed. The evidence, in fact, is mounting that the pain perception system of vascular plants is far more complex than previously assumed; that their selective choices and behaviors are based on sensation, memory, and precise in-the-moment decisions honed by millions of years of evolutionary refinement. If you are looking for signs of intelligence on earth, you would do well to investigate plants.

The new field of plant neurobiology demonstrates how serious this subject has become among respected scientists who study the complex behavioral patterns of plants and their perception and communication capabilities. What's now being published is the rigorous, peer-reviewed research that was altogether missing in the quirky poetic book, *The Secret Life of Plants*, which created a media storm and scientific backlash in 1973. Today a sweeping new plant paradigm is emerging that integrates cutting-edge botanical discoveries with well established areas of research like electrophysiology and molecular biology.

"What unites animals and plants in evolutionary terms is the need to exploit an internal memory that allows organisms to remodel their behavior....to optimize fitness. That points towards shared forms of memory and learning," maintains researcher Francisco Garzon. "Are plants intelligent? Can they compute complex aspects of their environment? The blunt answer is yes," affirms Garzon, part of the new class of brilliant, outside-the-cube scientists who remind us that plants are sophisticated living organisms whose future-predicting abilities and wanna-live, don't wanna-die skills are just beginning to be understood.

Ethical vegans despise the subject of plant awareness and scornfully mock it, refusing to examine with any openness or depth the possibility of consciousness in plants. Any such conclusion, of course, would qualify plants for moral consideration, same as animals. "This crackpot idea is trotted out by meat eaters with guilty consciences," spouts the pompous vegetarian Peter Cox in *You Don't Need Meat*. (Apparently Mr. Cox does not keep up with science: neither botany, nor evolutionary biology.) Actually, the belief in plant intelligence and sentience goes back for centuries, propagated by some of the finest thinkers in history.

Long before modern science discovered the universal ancestor for all plants and animals, Greek philosopher Empedocles recognized our common origin, anticipating the concept of evolution by over 2,000 years. Even more audacious, this early believer firmly concluded that plants experience awareness of pain and pleasure—even sexual pleasure—and that plants, humans, and other animals exist on the same spiritual plane. The "father of botany," Theophrastus, also focused on our vegetal ancestry, penning the voluminous *Enquiry Into Plants* and devoting most of his life to understanding their life processes. And none other than Charles Darwin spent the second half of his career fascinated by active, insect-devouring flowers—and plant perception in general.

In *The Power and Movement of Plants* Darwin delivered what is famously known as "the root-brain hypothesis," concluding that "it is hardly an exaggeration to say that the tip of the radicle thus endowed [with sensitivity] and having the power of directing the movements of the adjoining parts, acts like the brain of one of the lower animals—the brain being situated within the anterior end of the body, receiving impressions from the sense-organs, and directing the several movements." This revolutionary statement and the pioneering beliefs of all these botanical geniuses were largely ignored as Aristotle's hierarchy of superior and inferior beings held sway through the centuries, remaining firmly entrenched in western thought to this day.

What a sham and a shame. As westerners became swept up in the Aristotelian lineage, a sharp line was drawn between ourselves and every other living being, between higher and lower, better and lesser. This narrow, anthropocentric agenda is why, to this day, plants continue to be regarded as passive background material: manipulated, exploited, poisoned, genetically altered, and mass annihilated to serve our human desires. It also allows vegans to eat them without guilt, while heaping immense amounts of shame on omnivores.

Eastern thought followed a far different track than Aristotle's Great Chain of Beings with its glorious gods, angels, and privileged humans (i.e., white men) soaring at the top, and submissive animals and dumb plants scraping the bottom. Sentience is a metaphysical quality inherent to *all* living things, Eastern philosophy teaches. Everything alive is worthy of our respect and full attention. Japanese and Tibetan Buddhists regard plants as sentient beings deserving of our empathy, and indigenous people worldwide have long considered plants to possess spirit and intelligence, communing with them directly to receive wisdom for living and healing. Modern intuitives who live in nature know exactly this.

TODAY'S BOTANICAL researchers are finally catching up with ancient wisdom, unraveling the cellular and molecular reasons that autonomous plants respond to touch, smell and sound, even classical music. Plants communicate via chemical signaling, modern science confirms, impulses that convey "action-potentials" similar to those in animals, allowing individual plants to sense danger and pain. For example, a plant totally knows when it is being eaten by predators and selects precise actions to defend itself and its kin against further threats to their existence.

"They have a specific and fairly extensive vocabulary to convey alarms, health, and a host of other things. We just have sound waves broken down into various languages," Professor Stefano Mancuso told Nicole Martinelli of *Wired*, lamenting that humans and plants will probably never be able to directly communicate with each other. Nonetheless, research continues to unlock their secret lives and the Swiss government has officially declared that all plants, exactly like animals, have the right to dignity and moral consideration "for their own sake." Digest that, ethical vegans.

The history of humanity's moral progress has always been thus: a very slow and begrudged widening of our circle of compassion to include "others" who don't look or act like ourselves. Of course, there have always been those among us who regard plants as *more* evolved and intelligent than humans, certainly more in synch with their environment. Don't we define intelligence as the capacity to acquire knowledge, make good choices, and solve problems? Then plants have much to teach us, according to Mancuso, director of the world's premier lab devoted to plant neurobiology, near Florence, Italy. "Not only are they 'smart' in how they grow, adapt and thrive," he informed Martinelli, "they do it without neuroses." Plants are anything but passive, reflexive life forms.

Ongoing research from plant scientists worldwide is proving just how active and discriminating plants really are: in recognizing self versus non-self; in communicating among their kind; in strategizing solutions with ultra-fast detection systems. Their sophisticated methods for guaranteeing reproductive success are legendary, trading food for sex by luring insects to sticky pollen with complex, directional petal patterns and tantalizing perfumes. Of all living forms, flowers best embody our earth's flamboyant sexuality. All those gorgeous and enticing, color-splattered petals are essentially open vulvas shouting out: *Yoo-hoo! Over here! Come get it here!*

Upon reading the glut of new studies describing plant sensitivity, perception, and decision making ("Plants Can Think and Do Computations," "Plants Perform

47

Molecular Math"), one online commentator predicted the replacement of PETA with PETP, People for the Ethical Treatment of Plants. He openly worried what would be left for ethical vegans to eat. Sterilized dirt and distilled water?

It's true: plants can perform biological light computations. They then use this information to self-immunize against seasonal pathogens. (No doctor's visit, no painful shot, no co-pay—how wonderful would that be?) Plants can also detect gravity, mechanical perturbations, atmospheric concentrations, and magnetic fields. (Can you?) Plants respond to light, human touch, and complex music. (Fields of corn grow faster and denser on the side exposed to Beethoven). They realize when they are being eaten and take action to prevent further harassment (precise chemical volatiles summon insect bodyguards to attack the attacker— quicker and more effective than texting; no clumsy external technology needed).

Plants can make swift decisions based on memories of positive or negative events, enabling them, for instance, to communicate danger to their fellow plants. Let's say an individual is being harassed by a certain hungry animal that wounded it a year ago; it will instantly produce exacting odors to warn its neighbors, who then prepare for the attack with defense chemicals. Plants also speed specific chemicals through their entwined root systems to any ailing members in their community. That's called activated empathy in my book and I wish more humans practiced it.

Just like animals, plants breathe (respire) and most have mitochondria. Just like animals, plants employ cell-surface receptors to detect relevant environmental information: largely protein-linked in animals, enzyme-linked in plants. And exactly like us, plants engage in intracellular communication, called "signaling" in botany lingo. To accomplish this, they utilize many of the same neurotransmitters and coenzymes found in the animal neuron system, including acetylcholine, ATP, GABA, and glutamate receptors. Some botanists conjecture that the chemical signaling of plants may prove to be more complex than the synapses firing of human brains. Moreover, plants understand all the intricate information being communicated among themselves and we do not. As Michael Marder concludes in *Plant Signaling and Behavior:* "What emerges from these discussions is the image of a mind embodied in plant life."

Plants don't have human-like brains, that's quite true—nor human phobias, arrogance, cynicism, obsessive-compulsive behaviors, hysteria, depression, wars, suicides and mass murders. A rose is not confused about its identity or purpose in life, nor is a radish. They fulfill their dharma with enthusiasm and clarity. That's no doubt why we feel so calm and contented in the presence of plants, whether in the home garden or the far fields, while humans can leave us feeling anxious and distraught.

Despite these differences, Mancuso's team chose the controversial term "plant neurobiology" to highlight that the electrophysiology of plants is analogous to our human nervous system. While old-school botanists despise the term and publicly protest, even former skeptics are being swayed due to the precision and scientific rigor of the research.

HUNGRY FOR HIERARCHY

Ethical vegans and animal rightists have not caught up with the new science. They continue to ignore the growing mass of sophisticated evidence, insisting instead on moral status for simple, neuron-deficient animals like oysters. For to acknowledge even the possibility—of plant intelligence, pain perception, and preference-for-life-decision-making—would blow up the entire philosophical edifice vegans have so carefully constructed, the "morally pure" lifestyle they devotedly follow, and the offensive sense of self-righteousness many of them display to "the ignorant meat eaters." As veg scholar Colin Spencer concludes, "Immediately we admit that an organism has preferences, we must admit that it has consciousness, i.e. an awareness of options which necessitate a choice."

Of course, there is no agreed upon definition of consciousness. That's why some scientists are going with the word "cognition" in describing the intentional choices made by plants. It is not their preference, but botanists like Francisco Garzon realize that far too many chain-of-being humans are loathe to bequeath subjective perception to plants, believing it must be brain-generated. And therein lies the problem: it's a conceptual trap to insist that plant intelligence be just like ours, generated by the same kind of hardware. "Intelligence is usually cashed out in animal or anthropocentric terms," writes Garzon, "in such a way that plants plainly fail to meet the conditions for animal or human-like intelligence, for obvious but uninteresting reasons."

The primary uninteresting reason is, of course, human arrogance—our age-old need for hierarchy: to feel a cut above, higher and better than other living beings, whether plants, animals, or the beef-eating human scoundrel living next door. Yet it is neither sensitive nor all that intelligent to assume that plants are insensitive life forms, undeserving of our moral consideration because they don't possess a human-like nervous system. ("Brain chauvinism" one botanist calls it.) Neither do the invertebrates that vegans refuse to eat, although many are far less self-determining than plants. While human evolution depended on specialized brain development, write Kandel and Hawkins in *The Biological Basis of Learning and Individuality*, "the evolution and adaptation of other organisms depended on the development and specialization of various other organs." Such a simple statement of fact. To the enlightened, different is not less.

PLANTS ARE HIGHLY PURPOSEFUL. They pursue their own interests, create the conditions for their own flourishing, and look after their own kind. Do they also suffer? This we cannot know, not in strictly human terms, just as we can't know for fish or invertebrates. But quite clearly plants want to live, *not* be destroyed and end up in Whole Foods salad bar.

And while actively working for their own longevity, plants also continuously contribute to the well-being of humans and the planet in boundless ways, offering oxygen, food, shelter, medicine, essential oils and intrinsic beauty. Meanwhile, ego-centric humans are systematically diminishing, if not decimating, every eco-system we inhabit on earth—and even those we do not: oceans, rivers, wetlands. Intelligent beings? We have some profound lessons to learn from the plants.

Case in point: while *homo sapiens* continue to foolishly wait, waffle, and in some cases outright deny global warming, plants are already acting, marshalling their forces and moving northward; some are already 500 miles further north than just 20 years ago. Yes, as the arctic permafrost melts, smart plants are colonizing it, staking their claim on the right temperature and other environmental conditions for optimal growth, ensuring their future survival. What supreme irony that this unfolding catastrophe is largely human-caused yet despite abundant evidence, we have been sluggish to communally respond, except to persist in pouring mega-tons of carbon and methane into the atmosphere—*not* a sign of higher intelligence by the way. The awareness and responsiveness of plants is decades ahead of the ignorance and lack of action by most humans. Roughly 1.5 billion years ago, when the ancestors of modern plants split off from our shared lineage, perhaps they made the wiser choice?

Plants will survive the folly of *Homo sapiens*, that's for sure, both omnie and veggie. When we big-brained humans are done fouling our own nest, overheating the earth that nourishes us, acidifying the oceans that sustain us, and bombing each other to bits, there may be very few humans left but there will always be

50

clever plants, hiding their offspring and their future in the ground—their tenacious seeds are viable for up to 30,000 years. And whenever cities are obliterated or civilizations burned, whether by fire, volcano or atomic bomb, the plants are always the first life to appear through the mass of smoldering flesh. Their determined green shoots emerging through the fissures of shattered buildings to relish the sun. Their resolute, single-minded roots spreading deep into the earth, sucking up water and sustenance, creating sun-driven energy and global power in ways no human can.

After all, plants have flourished across this planet for over 400 million years, modern *Homo sapiens* a mere 200 thousand. The more you study the intelligence of plants, the more you are forced to admire their ancient shrewdness for survival and proliferation. Their intelligence is systemic: whole organism vs. brain-based. This may well prove to be a more advanced type of intelligence, chemical communication vs. nerve pathways, computing responses at the whole plant level— embodied intelligence, as this generation of enlightened botanists calls it. Humans in the forefront of energetic system studies are investigating the value of this very different kind of intelligence for our own species as well—the intelligence of the body-mind; the intelligence of the colony. Swift perception and decision-making. Existing in exquisite collaboration with one's environment.

Once the systemic intelligence of plants gains wider acceptance—joining fish, insects, and other beings previously considered automatons—vegans will be forced to concede what is already obvious to those who live in nature. Plants are highly sensitive life forms, consciously evolving to ever more efficiently reproduce, prosper in the sun or shade, adapt to human folly, and energetically serve their own and other species.

Plants ruled this planet for millions of years and may well rule again. We can clear-cut them, burn them, ravage them, and in our naïveté and delusional sense of superiority call them lower life forms, but the plants will always, always return and thrive—even if we do not.

11.

THE MEANING OF MEAT

Beneath all our cultural sophistication, we are animals.

—Jule Lorenzen

IF IT'S NOT ALTOGETHER clear which life forms merit our moral consideration, being certain of what's considered "meat" on the menu may be just as tricky. On a recent trip to northern Italy, a friend nervously revealed to her host's vivacious mother, in halting Italian, that she doesn't eat meat. "*Che cosa?*" the hearty lady frowned, perplexed. Then her ruddy face lit up: "I make you mutton stew instead. You love it!"

To the extreme dismay of globe-trotting vegetarians, the planet's diverse food cultures define meat as this, that, and the other. In fact, the more you get around, the more you realize just how multifaceted is this very ordinary word. Apparently you can chow down on sheep flesh in the Mediterranean world and not be eating meat. In Japan, order soup "without meat please" and your waiter will deliver a bowl of miso with delicately sheared, smoked tuna as its principal flavoring. A similar plea in Spain will likely result in a highly-spiced dish jam-packed with juicy chunks of ham. That's because ham is a way of life for the Spanish, many of whom consider vegetarianism a foreign disease. And in the spacious ranching districts of South America's Pampas? Meat emphatically means beef: not pork, poultry, or seafood. When veg'ns tour Patagonia and request non-animal culinary options, according to travel writer Leon Harmon, their guides look at them funny or ask to take their temperature. And don't even try explaining fake meat derived from soy or gluten. A visit to the doctor may be in order.

Commercial meat might even turn into *shmeat* in the not too distant future. Also called *in-vitro* or *frankenmeat*, this is lab food birthed in a bioreactor and nursed by white-cloaked techies. No herds of whole living animals needed, only a few cells harvested from each (non-voluntary) donor cow, pig, or sheep. Millions of now-living domestic food animals can thus be used up, their breeds phased out of existence, exactly as vegans have always proposed for their perfect all-vegan world. Besides ridding the earth of exploited animals, test tube meat offers big environmental advantages, according to proponents—once the technology scales up to feed an expanding population. Not so fast, warns synthetic biologist Christina Agapakis, PhD. "Whenever I hear about industrial scaling as a cure-all, my skeptic alarms start going off," she reveals in *Discover*, "because scaling is the *deus ex machina* of so many scientific proposals, often minimized by scientists (myself included) as simply an engineering problem." To be feasible, shmeat will have to be scaled up to market-ready appearance, flavor, and price. Cell culturing, however, is hideously expensive, resource intensive, and technically thorny.

Basically, the god machine has to do everything the animal now does naturally: attach the cells to some sort of scaffold in place of bone and marrow; keep the cells warm, healthy, and free of contaminants; then provide an artificial perfusion system in place of the heart, blood supply, and fine capillaries that deliver not only critical oxygen to animal muscles but all the necessary nutrients, vitamins, and growth hormones. A system must also be devised to remove all the waste products that are constantly accumulating. Sounds like we need a living body here; what do you think? What's more, minus a moving, growing animal, even if the biotech industry figures out how to economically fabricate three-dimensional muscle hunks—a big *if*—these lab muscles will still require regular exercise by stretching machines to increase their protein and mass, "essentially elaborate meat gyms," as Agapakis calls them. Are you salivating yet?

As far as how to re-create the taste, texture and nutrient density of real meat, that too is unresolved. When the world's first in-vitro burger was served amidst media fanfare in 2013 to a select group of three—a journalist, a nutritionist, and Dutch scientist and creator Mark Post—concerns about disappointing appearance and taste cropped up most often. And this was after egg powder, beet juice, and breadcrumbs had been added to jazz up the original version, described as grayish-yellow and slippery. The bloodless burger also weighed a mere five ounces, yet took five years and $325,000 to produce.

Other conundrums yet to be resolved: how to add real fat to counterfeit muscle (essential for flavor, palpability, and satiation); how to beef up shmeat's scant nutrient profile; how to ensure reliability in the production process; and how to know if pretend meat is even safe for us to eat. Manufacturing flesh for human consumption is unprecedented, and possible negative health consequences are unknown. Let's hope our regulatory authorities conduct long-term human trials before serving this stuff to first graders. Ready to bring back the family farm?

And here's an even more important question: Why are humans in lab coats incessantly eager to replace real food with fake industrial concoctions? Indeed to replace *nature*, the 3.8 billion-year-old biological system that has evolved ever so slowly to complex equilibrium. They're all in such a damn hurry to create new life faster than the speed of life. But earth's unimaginably intricate organic system doesn't work that way, including our own organic bodies. Time is an integral part of our world and even physicists agree we cannot leave time out of the equation, much as we would like to, much as our profit-driven food industries always try to. Everything in the universe gains order and eventually decays (entropy) as part of a natural, time-based process. Our food is no exception. And we mess with this vital truth at our own peril.

That said, I can understand a bioengineer's desire to be creative, to play with techy tools in an attempt to solve human-created problems like over-population and factory farms. Yet critics believe easily replicated meat would *encourage* soaring populations, not curb them: two in-vitro chickens in every pot. We're already projected to hit 11 billion humans by 2100 *if* women in developing nations continue to be educated and fertility rates continue to fall—an inconceivable 27 billion if those assumptions fail. Either way, it doesn't seem to matter to the global Big Ag corporations and biotech labs busy manipulating our food supply while raking in billions annually.

Yet this latest engineered food, shmeat, may be doomed to failure as surely as all the other altered food so readily placed on our grocery shelves in recent years. The long list includes trans fats (implicated in heart disease), artificial sweeteners like Splenda (increased cancer risk), synthetic fats like Olestra (depletes vitamins A, D, E and K while increasing incidence of diarrhea and abdominal cramping), GM food crops (no overall enhanced yield and routinely sprayed with a "probably carcinogenic" herbicide), plus mock veggie-meats (decreased sales growth in the past few years due to unsatisfying taste and suspect additives).

Among the more troubling real food replacements is imitation infant formula, originally developed and constantly lab-tweaked (in vain) to replicate human breast milk, the powerhouse nutritional cocktail designed by nature to meet a baby's every dietary need. At times a substitute is needed, granted. Yet replacing mother's milk is recognized by every major health organization as a significant risk factor for infant disease and mortality, especially in developing countries where commercial formula has been aggressively and immorally marketed as the norm, and to women who can ill afford it. We are, in fact, the only mammal on earth that feeds our babies plant "milk" and thinks mammalian glands are best suited for skin flicks and profit-making.

Or have we simply forgotten that we are mammals? With men shaving their chests and no-risk women scheduling cesareans and forsaking their milky breasts, it's an all too reasonable question. "There is no precedent in nature for feeding young mammals a plant-based protein," proclaims William Sears, MD, who notes that soy protein is not only deficient in taurine and correct amino acid amounts but "does not provide the same growth equivalent as animal protein," nor the enzyme lactase that breaks down lactose, a sugar that aids in calcium absorption and a healthy gut ecology. Replacing human-animal milk with plants and synthetics, the doctor warns, is foolishly messing with nature's ideal recipe.

As for the future of shmeat, even setting aside possible poor health outcomes, do food engineers really think that the world's earthy, rural, meat-loving people in Patagonia, Portugal and Canada—or most city folk for that matter—will willingly eat lab-concocted, animal-absent, earth-deprived, 3D sheets of frankenmeat that spent its brief "life" in a meat gym? This is the same technology used to grow tumors in a lab dish. Social scientists aren't sure which will turn people off faster: the bio-ethics issue or the yuck factor.

The dilemma for ethical vegetarians is even steeper. Animal rights groups generally favor in vitro meat because incorporeal cells can't experience pain like real animals. On the other hand, a lot of vegans are whole food, pro-nature types who find themselves balking at the weird science. Some even publicly opposed PETA's offer of a million dollars to the first company to produce commercially-viable in vitro meat, and that's without even knowing, I suspect, that the growth medium for "donated" animal cells is typically fetal bovine serum, the blood of aborted calves. Removed from pregnant cows right before slaughter, the non-anesthetized fetuses are immediately transferred to a blood collection room where needles are inserted directly into their hearts and their blood vacuumed into sterile collection bags.

According to Humane Research Australia, an estimated half a million liters of raw fetal calf serum (FCS) are collected annually worldwide for human tissue, cell, and organ production, which equates to harvesting, i.e., killing, more than a million bovine fetuses annually. Ethical vegans are repulsed by the thought of possibly using additional FCS for artificial meat and they view PETA's stance as

55

a flagrant capitulation of their "zero animal exploitation" principle. This issue caused "a near civil war in our office," co-founder Ingrid Newkirk told *The New York Times*. "We will have members leave us over this."

SETTING ASIDE, HOPEFULLY FOREVER, this brave and bizarre new world of incorporeal cattle flesh, what's the traditional meaning of this tough yet slippery word, *meat*? "The edible flesh of animals, especially mammals as opposed to fish or poultry" is how most dictionaries define it. Yet the word also means the edible part of a plant, such as a fruit or nut, and "green meat" refers to fresh herbage fed to animals. We're all familiar with its vulgar usage: male/female genitalia and the human body in general as an object of sexual desire. (Oh yes, females objectify hunk-a-meat males, too.) Is it any wonder the word is so loaded and open to interpretation, so fraught with subtext, symbolism, and erotic nuance?

Meat can even refer to the essence of practically anything: the meat of the problem; the meat of the story. It derives from the Middle English, *mete*, meaning general sustenance—meat is nourishment, meat is power—and poets through the ages have made use of this original meaning. As Stephen Crane wrote, "Tradition, thou art for suckling children, but no meat for men is in thee." So the word means a great deal more than chopped hamburger.

It is in many ways an exceptional, versatile word. Certainly not a bad word, except to vegans who revile it and what it represents to them: immorality and cruelty. This signifies a fascinating turnaround because throughout human history "meat," both word and meal, has enjoyed an extremely positive reputation as a symbol of well-being and security. With joyful reverence is how our ancestors greeted the bounty brought home to a hungry family by a hard-working father/hunter. What's more, the ability to provide and share meat has long represented community health and hospitality. Conversely, a good deal of vegetarianism in the world today and centuries past has been involuntary and despised, a function of poverty and drought. As soon as income levels rise, people on plant diets start to seek more essential protein and fat in the form of meat.

By the 18th century, consumption reached its zenith among Western Europe's middle and upper classes. The underprivileged—who died younger back then as surely as they do today—subsisted on bread, milk and root vegetables, with meat a rare nutritional treat. Wealthy landowners, meanwhile, thrived on meals chock-full of animal food: beef and wild duck, giblets and sweetbreads, partridges and blackbirds (and we thought those pie-baked birds existed only in nursery rhymes).

According to *The Historic Foodie,* on a single day, January 29, 1737, an upper-class Scottish family and guests had the following food prepared for them: Cock a Leekie soup with fowl, boiled pork, hare collops and pease pudding, roast turkey and roast mutton, stewed partridge and broiled fish, cold turkey and smoked beef, *plus* (for any whose bellies could hold yet more) hogs' cheeks and eggs.

That's all rather gross in sum, but flesh-heavy meals were thought to reflect the generosity and prowess of the giver, even (his) sexual virility, according to historian Rod Preece, who is among the many veg'n enthusiasts who prefer we use the word "flesh" instead of "meat." What's up with that? Aren't they the same thing? Not at all, they argue; the former is the more inclusive term for the soft tissue of animals and, therefore, the one we should use when referring to "a carnivore's diet." And by the way, that's the human carnivore to which they're referring.

Often have I noticed, with escalating annoyance, that hardcore veg'ns—along with enthused new recruits (my teenage self included)—are enamored of the word "carnivore" to describe humans who incorporate meat into their mixed diet, rather than the behaviorly correct "omnivore." But the word *om*-nivore sounds, you know, rather softer and more flexible than that harsher *ca-ca* sounding word which evokes images of fur-clad, two-legged carnivores violently ripping into bloody animal flesh with fierce canines and dagger-like fingernails.

"Flesh" is also preferred by animal rightists, one must assume, because it is a word charged with human context. We refer to our own children and ancestors as "flesh and blood," certainly never "meat and blood." Flesh belongs to the human realm and so to eat flesh, instead of mere meat, might even conjure up images of cannibalism in the overly-inventive mind. Indeed, scholar Preece insists on the label "flesh-eaters" for non-vegetarians, and in one of his weirder rants points to prehistoric human cannibalism as the likely source of our "imaginary need" and ongoing "lust" for animal food. Furthermore, he claims that it's only our sense of *superiority* over the "lower" animals that allows us to consume animals at all, just as feelings of supremacy allowed for tribal cannibalism in the past. This line of reasoning is quite intriguing because Preece himself repeatedly refers to the moral *superiority* of vegetarians over other humans. Perhaps omnivores in the woods should be looking over their shoulders for, not cougars, but lapsed vegans?

Meat eaters, Preece avows, should follow the lead of ethical eaters who view humans and other animals as equals and then ask themselves how they'd feel "if asked to eat human flesh." Why this man is so fixated on cannibalism, an atypical event in nature, is beyond baffling. Does he really need reminding that animal life

57

on this planet is based upon species consuming other species, not their own? Such a strange argument coming from an otherwise highly intelligent man, albeit one with a blatant, holier-than-thou agenda, for Preece refers to omnivores as sinners in the not-so-subtle title of his book, *Sins of the Flesh.*

WHAT A LOADED WORD, *flesh.* Exactly like meat, it refers to "the soft substance of an animal's body, its muscle and fat," according to the lexicon. Yet the word also means "animals as food, excluding fish and sometimes fowl." So, if it's the word "flesh" they insist upon, veg'ns must take into account this oft-used second definition, which indicates you can nosh on fish (maybe even fowl but let's not go there) and call yourself a vegetarian, as many esteemed men and women throughout history have.

In truth, the origins of western vegetarianism may well have been pescatarian. There is no evidence that the man known as the father of western vegetarianism, Pythagoras, did not eat animal food and a number of respected sources attest that he did. Porphyry, for one, noted that Pythagoras dined on his watery brethren, an entirely reasonable choice since fish was an abundant, reliable source of complete protein in the dry Mediterranean region where he lived out his long and beguiling life. The Pythagorean Diet thus came to mean avoiding the flesh of butchered animals only—allowing dairy, eggs, and fish. *Historically, vegetarianism has always looked very different than the rigid versions being promoted today.*

Many men and women praised as "Vegetarian Celebrities" likewise included fish in their diet and—surprise! Many weren't vegetarians at all. How many times have you heard Rousseau or Emerson quoted in defense of veg'nism? Among the "famous vegetarians" for whom there is no credible evidence to support this label we find: Aristotle, Plato, Socrates, Isaac Newton, Charles Darwin, Charlotte Bronte, Milton, Emerson, Thoreau, Jeremy Bentham, William Blake, Martin Luther, William Wordsworth, Adam Smith, Rousseau, Voltaire, Shakespeare, Schopenhauer and (here's a good one) fox hunter Prince Charles. A hearty thanks to scholar Rod Preece for his honest, impeccable research in compiling this list. There exists no verification that *any* of these famous people were vegetarians, and for most of them, there exists "incontrovertible evidence" that they were not.

Many of those named did in fact *speak* against animal suffering or advocate vegetarianism in theory, but not one of them acted on their lofty principles. They could not bring themselves to give up meat altogether, be it for reasons of health or pleasure we'll never know. French philosopher Rousseau, who popularized the "noble savage" archetype and was the 18th century's champion of vegetarianism, demanded in *Émile*: "How could [anyone] see a poor defenseless animal bled, skinned, and dismembered? How could he endure the sight of quivering flesh?"

Yet profuse written testimony reveals that animal flesh was a regular part of Rousseau's diet. Witnesses to this animal activist's 1764 walking tour reported "a picnic of pâtés, poultry, venison, and a good supply of wine—loaded on the back of a mule." Even Albert Einstein waited until the very last year of his life to give up meat, having written earlier to a friend: "Although I have been prevented by outward circumstances from observing a strictly vegetarian diet, I have long been an adherent to the cause in principle."

Why would all these brainy people publicly renounce suffering for animals, yet return to eating them in private? We could simply assume that they were, in the lingo of animal rightists, self-serving hypocrites driven by meat lust. Alternately, we could assume they made an intelligent choice. Like every human, these men were in need of complete protein, vitamin B12, brain-enhancing long-chain fatty acids, and all other animal-derived nutrients. No doubt, their smart private bodies rebuked their public idealism, clamoring for food which fueled them properly. (*Just like today's subset of "vegans" who admit to sneaking animal food: i.e., they are omnivores. And, of course, we can only guess how many are not publically admitting it.*) Although all these people treasured the idea of not eating animals, they made certain to do exactly that.

Others touted as "Famous Vegetarians" were semi-vegetarians, meaning they weren't vegetarians at all, according to the purists. They munched on fish or even the occasional meat, excuse me, *flesh*. But let's get beyond all this absurd finger-pointing, shall we? Anyone who is truly concerned about animals should warmly affirm all those who have reduced consumption to the minimum they've determined to be essential for their health.

Pleads one anonymous blogger, disgusted by all the rancor: "We can't fight each other like this….it makes others feel that their ethical choices are worthless." What a waste of energy, what a useless self-righteous dispute which gets us no closer to wiping out immoral factory farms. It also fails to address the primary premise of this book: Contrary to the popular myth proliferated by vegans, plants-only is *not* a healthy diet for most of us over the long haul.

HAS IT NEVER ONCE occurred to judgmental vegans that many of us partake of animal-sourced food not out of gluttony and convenience, as they scornfully contend, but to sustain our radiant health? There are indeed many individuals who have found out the long, hard, suffering way that they require, yes *require*, a sufficient amount of whole animal nutrients to maintain their energy and brain power, to realize their full human potential. And be forewarned: *Some of you reading this assertion with contempt will discover this thorny truth for yourself in the difficult years to come.*

Meanwhile, the pressing need to be "100% virtuous" continues among strict vegans, i.e., one-up ethically from the rest of us who are somehow "less than." Is egoism too strong a word? Therefore, to dissolve all elitist distinctions, when referring to both, I've merged vegans and vegetarians into one simple, constructive category: veg'ns. Or, if you prefer, veggies. Most readers have already noted this and some, no doubt, are offended. To which I reply: Get over it.

To be fair, the mellow veg'ns out there don't really care what you call yourself. They're happy whenever someone is making honest strides in reducing meat intake and saying *"no more"* to factory farms. Partial vegetarianism can be an appropriate first step, agrees animal rightist Rod Preece, and advocates should "be wary of being too critical of such impurity." I do appreciate that Mr. Preece acknowledges the validity of step-taking, since he confesses to having eaten flesh while chairman of the Ontario Society for the Prevention of Cruelty to Animals. However, again, his and others' accusations of "impurity" on the part of not-quite vegetarians is condescending and pretentious. Being so pure, rigid, and self-serious really isn't good for one's health. As my hard-working mom always told us kids: "If you can laugh at yourself, you're in good shape."

ALL THIS PURITY-OBSESSING was a complete non-issue for Linda and me as we rambled the beautiful backroads of France and Spain, high on life and plant food. If someone insisted on calling us lactos or cheeseheads, fine. We didn't eat butchered animals—that's what mattered to us. Our ticket to a clear mind and clean body. Redemption and paradise.

12.

EATING AND SLEEPING AS ONE

IF LINDA AND I were vegetarians with a purpose, we were hitchhikers without a plan, not even a map of Europe if I recall. Rendezvousing in late September, we stuck our thumbs into the breeze and read its unambiguous message. *Head south to the mountains*, it murmured, *south to the sea*. And out of that excellent advice emerged our own youthful wisdom: You need to know only two things in life—who your true friends are, and from which direction comes the wind.

Standing on curvy roadsides near mountain-clinging Basque villages, yellow hair flying, we shouted *vive la vie!* to every passing car and hopped with cheerful abandon into plush Audis or tin-can Citroëns as they screeched to a thrilling halt. Amiable, mostly male natives invariably picked us up within five, make that two minutes. Quite apart from Linda's wholesome beauty, hitchhiking around Europe was an easy ride back then, highly recommended for wayfaring 20-somethings. I'd chain my daughter to her desktop before letting her hitchhike two blocks to the mall today, but it was a world *très différent* that Linda and I traversed. Drivers gave us friendly tours of the countryside, offered sweet figs and sun-ripened peaches, then merrily sped us on our southwesterly way.

Naturally, we were totally clueless that some of these same congenial young men were Basque separatists who donned black hoods in neighborhood attics, plotting imminent revolution. Nor did we ever consider that every male specimen, whatever his political persuasion, might not have the purist of intentions. But only once did we have to jump out of a moving 18-wheeler. Approaching his home-land border, our quiet and polite, 40-something Spanish driver suddenly started grinning way too broadly. "You girls from A-MER-ee-ka," he began awkwardly in broken English, "I hear about you." He was offering, not demanding, but as his giant black transporter crawled toward a crowded checkpoint, first Linda and then

61

I took a flying leap from its high silver cab, packs tucked close to our bellies, scraped knees and scuffed palms the sum total of our bodily damage. That night we pitched Linda's pup tent in a zero-star roadside ditch, just north of Spain. Our fetid feet were in each other's face all night long but we woke up laughing in the gray morning rain and once again headed to the side of the road, sticking out cold, competent thumbs in search of a more genteel Rocinante.

Our white steed turned out to be a stripped-down Volkswagen bus loaded with one soft-spoken American and four thistle-tongued Canadians, all in their early twenties, all wannabe vegetarians, all on the joy ride of their lives. Nicole and Tom, ostensibly married, happily sarcastic, owned the aged, mottled vehicle and with it the right to choose who rode along—and who got left in the rain. Quite quickly we realized that our path through Spain was so random, so improvised, the van itself appeared to be leading the way and all onboard had no choice but to follow. American Joe, sandy-haired and mild, a John Denver clone, was a happy slowster who kept to himself. Dark, kinky-haired Razz, stuffed into black jeans, couldn't hold back his sexy crooked grin. And then there was fair Bruce of the shoulder-length tresses. All duded up in US Army camo-gear plastered with red Canadian maple leaves, every night he lovingly brushed his long golden locks and ate bread and olives, nothing but bread and olives.

These old VW vans were straightforward, my friend, a work horse, not some noble stallion. No comfy pop-up bed with double mattress and flannel sheets. No adorable mini-kitchen for boiling brown rice and lentils. Maybe an AM radio if you were lucky. Even luckier if the thing had heat. Its air-cooled, four-cylinder engine is in the rear—all 57 horsepower of it—so it's a mighty inefficient route for any hot air to find your gone-blue toes up front. (One van owner that I knew wore battery-operated warming socks to keep her feet alive.) Its open interior was far roomier than a Porsche, true, but seven veggies in a box on wheels? Oh sure, that was status quo for nomads cruising around Europe with the rear seat flattened into perpetual bed mode, everyone squished together, turned on and sweating, smoking doobies and rapping our anti-meat, anti-war, anti-authoritarian rants.

It was all so peaceful and innocent, our particular arrangement anyway. By day we wandered with no set destination; by night we slept in piney forests near Roma gypsy camps, soft needles for a mattress. And whenever the rain came down in droves, we trotted right back to our metallic horse: three guys crammed head to feet on the makeshift bed above, Linda and I wedged into the wee space below, our heads jammed against the two front seats. There Nicole and Tom slept unbelievably serenely in semi-reclined positions, sweet young mouths hanging open. Now that I'm older and experienced in the miseries of insomnia, I realize you can do basically anything when you're young and still stay healthy and get a good night's sleep: eat carbs all day; drink cognac while standing on your head; and squeeze into a sleep space smaller than your body's total cubic inches.

"I'm ready and hungry for the coast!" Linda sang out one morning and off we headed to nearby Portugal for our usual meatless repast. Bruce? Joe? Razz? You can tell me now: Did every one of you fall madly, deliciously in love with Linda? Did you turn into consummate, duty-bound vegetarians at first sight and sound of her plump, perfect lips waxing ethical/philosophical? I have a feeling that's what converts many of us: some skinny, foxy veg-babe in a yoga class or tofu ad who's obviously in the know. All I knew was this: It was my second month and I was feeling very light and free on my new diet, very buoyant and cleaned out. I was shedding pounds without even trying, exactly as the literature had promised. No longer did I feel weighed down by vile, putrefying animal products, nor with my contribution to the suffering.

Or was it my nouveau life creating such a blissful state? My new sovereignty? Traveling the old, dusty byways with my goofy nomadic buddies, my mind an unsoiled slate, I gazed in awe at the seemingly just created world and it looked nothing like Decatur, Illinois. Delicate pale madonnas graced bulky 12th century Romanesque churches, their stained-glass windows flickering rose and gold behind a hundred votive candles lit by children and lovers, sinners and mourners. Bell-clanging burros patiently plodded ancient uphill paths. And here on the rim of the restless sea: yellow-blue wooden skiffs manned by sun-browned fishermen in baggy trousers, their hand-sewn nets brimming with wet silvery mackerel. Oh dark-eyed man, will you take me home to your burning hearth tonight? Undress me in the twilight hour? Teach me all that I long to know? *And in the early morning light I will cook for you, polenta and tomatoes, over a murmuring fire and I will mend your nets, restore your faith, repair your carnivorous ways.*

Youthful romanticism knows no bounds! But I could already hear Rocinante chug-chugging in the background, impatient to depart in search of some secluded beach-camping by the primal light of the moon. *Obrigada*, my imaginary lover, stripped to nakedness, entwined in fine filament and blazing with wary ardor against the sea-setting sun. *Obrigada!* Thank you! It was the only Portuguese expression I really needed to know in this light-flooded land of inquisitive old women peeking out of darkened windows. And bronzed day laborers dressed in

63

all-white, sauntering down to the sea each night to share bread and politics over chilled bottles of cerveja, shattering our misconceptions. Oh, life is good on the continent's far edge....*muito, muito obrigada.*

IT WAS ON THE PORTUGUESE coast the very next morning, following yet another carbo-packed breakfast of fresh fruit and *torrada*, thick slices of toast swathed in butter, that the irrepressible Linda removed her sturdy leather hiking boots and pink wool socks inside the crowded café. Placing two flawless, apple-smooth feet on the corner of our table, she pulled out shiny metal clippers and proceeded to slowly and sensuously, yes, cut her toe nails—one and then another and yet another. Her impromptu pushing against boundaries never failed to astound me, nor the open-mouthed local men who circled round to watch her every move.

And it was on the Portuguese coast that I slipped away from my comrades, their endless pinto beans and glowing bonfire, to brave December's chilly night air with a mind burning lucid and bright. Simply and suddenly, I knew what I must do: strip down to nothing and plunge headlong into the cold surging waves of the Atlantic. And so I did, in a heightened state of longing. Diving naked and alone into those seven-foot crashing waves by the faint light of a billion nameless stars. Diving again and again as if my very life depended on it, flinging myself into that relentless, booming surf until my body felt pummeled and my lungs screamed out for breath. What was happening to me? From what calm source was all this reckless courage emerging?

Another stormy night in a cheap Portuguese hotel, another steaming pot of beans and rice. And while Tom and Nicole paid for their own separate room, the rest of us—three men, one woman, one almost-woman—pushed three single beds together to sleep as one. Completely non-erotic, unfortunately. Good God, how was I ever going to discover my mysterious sexuality like this? And yet, and yet....utter contentment and body bliss for the first time in my over-intellectual, non-corporal, angst-filled teenage life. The five of us still dressed and sleeping on our sides, backs into bellies, bellies into backs, *ahhhh*, this bodily heat and companionship, this tender touching, this moist breath against my neck....

13.

BRAINS, BLISS, AND PYTHAGORAS

DOES VEGETARIANISM promote spiritual awareness and expansive blissed-out states? What about a clearer mind and brainier brain? Some dedicated veg'ns claim all of the above. As George Bernard Shaw famously declared, "A mind the caliber of mine cannot derive its nutriment from cows." No lack of self-esteem from this unabashed vegetarian crusader, but what about the brain power of the rest of us who abstain from meat?

Benjamin Franklin swore that his meatless diet resulted in "greater clearness of head and quicker apprehension." Others new to the veg regime confirm similar feelings of lightness and clarity upon renouncing what now appears to them as "heavy and greasy" animal food. I certainly felt that way my first year. With plant food the primary theme of my new diet, I was eating far fewer calories day after day. Yes, I felt lighter—15 pounds lighter to be precise. And just look at former President Clinton and the Reverend Al Sharpton. After losing a combined 150 pounds following a vegan diet, they were publicly singing its praises.

Newbie veggies do tend to shed pounds. With online reports of scale-tipping individuals losing half their body weight, it's the latest health and vanity reason for converting. PETA even features before and after photos: chubby girls dropping from size 14 to 4, fat boys morphing into bodybuilders. *Tell us your story!* While it's true that substantial losses will bring health benefits to the obese or overweight, again, watch out if your BMI drops below 18.5, the tipping point for a cascade of serious health issues.

As for the cognitive advantage that Franklin and today's no-meat eaters allege, at least one study suggests that vegetarians *are* more intelligent than their meat-eating friends. University of Southampton researchers explored this intriguing subject by tracking young volunteers for 20 years. At age ten, over 8,000 British boys and girls were given standard IQ tests. When these same children reached age 30, they were asked if they followed a vegetarian diet: approximately 4.5% responded in the affirmative. Scrutinizing this small minority, researchers found that as youngsters they possessed IQs a good five points higher than those who continued to eat meat. They were also more likely to be female, possess a college degree, and work a higher-paying job. Writing in the *British Medical Journal*, study authors say it isn't clear why the vegetarians are slightly brainier but Dr. Catharine Gale notes "the possibility that such a diet might have some beneficial effect on subsequent cognitive performance."

Leaving aside mere speculation, as the research authors certainly should have, here's what their study actually shows: individuals who chose to go vegetarian were somewhat smarter at age ten, *not* that a veg diet made them this way. This makes sense because cognitively sharp people often read more and seek advanced education, increasing their knowledge of health, the environment, and animal welfare issues. Smart people are generally more flexible in experimenting with a non-traditional diet that's received good press. Smart people are also more likely to give up that diet if it isn't working for them over time.

That's why the results would have been much more valuable if researchers had determined how long these individuals had been vegetarian (five weeks? fifteen years?) and continued to track them to determine how many quit, when, and for what reasons. Ben Franklin, for example, turned veggie as a youth, age 16, after reading Thomas Tryon, an early advocate, but only a few years later made a conscious decision to return to eating fish. I doubt any of us need reminding of Franklin's elevated intelligence. And Clinton, no intellectual slouch, consumed fish or eggs weekly as a "vegan" before switching to a paleo-style, low-carb diet.

One of the British study's authors, Professor Ian Deary, tellingly reveals: "As the only member of the research team who has never been a vegetarian, I feel bound to emphasize that the link we have found might not be causal. Becoming vegetarian might be one of a number of more or less arbitrary cultural choices that clever people make, some of which might be beneficial to health, and some not." Thank you, Professor Deary, for your candid and unbiased appraisal.

Unfortunately, author Tino Verducci, who summarized the study for a vegan website, does not highlight in his article, nor indicate in its misleading title, "Vegetarians are More Intelligent," that fully one-third of those classified as "vegetarians" ate fish or fowl, i.e. they were omnivores. Thus, in reality the study points out the modestly higher IQs of veggies who eat dairy/eggs and omnivores who abstain from red meat. The more interesting conclusion here? When it comes to tailoring headline-grabbing research, fish and chicken eaters are more than welcome to call themselves vegetarians, boosting the number of "smart veggies." *Beware vegetarian research conducted or interpreted by vegetarians.* It's a theme we'll see again and again. Vegans, especially, are on a mission to convert and retain. Omnivores have no such agenda.

Although Verducci offers no facts to back up the "eat vegetarian, get smarter" hypothesis, he keeps pushing the theme. "Might the nature of the vegetarians' diet have enhanced their apparently superior brain power?" he posits in *The Future is Vegan.* No doubt Verducci should have presented the study results to a different audience because buried in the middle of his article, without comment, is the fact that vegans scored significantly *lower* in this same study, averaging an IQ of 95.

This is indeed significant. A score of 95 is, in fact, below average intelligence (100 being the average, or 50th percentile). So let's be open-minded and consider this: It is well known that vegans are rigid in their approach to food and lifestyle, refusing to ingest or make use of any animal products whatsoever, to the point of going hungry rather than partake of what is available or freely offered. Might not the research results suggest that the less intelligent persons of those surveyed, i.e., strict vegans, possess less flexible, less adaptable minds—as opposed to what could be called the flexible omnivorous mind—at least when it comes to diet? Instead of remaining open to myriad possibilities in food selection, they possess a fixed, ideological mindset that refuses to adapt to shifts in availability, fluctuating circumstances, and real body-based dietary needs which vary considerably among individuals and change over time.

After all, behavioral adaptability is the key to our human evolution and brain growth. We modern humans wouldn't even be around if our ancestors had not been open to all manner of new foods, both plant and animal-sourced, when they scrambled out of the trees. Choosing to be omnivores has allowed us to survive every climatic and environmental condition presented through the eons, and in the coming century, drastic changes may be on the way. Thus, if our future is indeed strict, unbending veganism, our species may be in trouble.

IN STUDY AFTER STUDY, higher IQs are positively correlated with increased longevity. Same idea: enhanced intelligence allows these individuals to be more perceptive and flexible in their behavioral responses to unpredictable challenges, thus increasing their lifespan. So where does this leave vegans who scored below average on the British IQ tests? Does a ten point difference even matter to quality of life? Well, yes it could, if these same vegans fail to respond to any possible future stress signals that a plants-only diet isn't working for them as the years build up. *If they refuse to modify their austere diet in response to explicit bodily signals, their health and even their lifespan may indeed be altered.*

Of course, these IQ statistics are averages from one study and most of us know some very intelligent vegans. Some may continue to thrive on their diet, and some will know when it is time to get out. Others, inflexible in their ideology, may come to regret the unbending nature of their beliefs. For it is brain plasticity, not rigidity, that allows individual brains to change and "get smarter." It's called cortical remapping. When we positively adapt to new information—*this food makes me tired within an hour; this other food gives me long-lasting abundant energy*— our brain physically changes, forging new neural pathways and enhancing our odds of enjoying a long, healthy, successful life.

So will those higher IQ, more flexible vegetarians who ate eggs and dairy in the British study—along with the "vegetarians" who dined on fish and poultry— live longer on average than their strict vegan cohorts? The enormous problem in answering such a pivotal question is this: there has never been one credible study that follows life-long vegans into old age. This phenomenon is simply too new amongst the masses and, hence, unproven over time. This is indeed unfortunate for all the young vegans betting their life-long health, indeed their very lives, on this restrictive diet. And if you're shouting *The China Study!* right now, forget it. That over-promoted "vegan" research didn't even study vegans. More on that important topic later, but for now let's just note that the authors of *Vegan for Life* refused to incorporate statistics from *The China Study* into their book—they found them unconvincing and irrelevant to their purposes.

OPEN-MOUTHED BUT UNDETERRED, wanna-convert-U veg'ns will trot out the Seventh-day Adventist studies instead. Rock-solid proof, they argue, that they're above and beyond the rest of us on the health and longevity track. So let's take a judicious look at this oft-quoted research, conducted on members of a Protestant denomination that emphasizes a conservative lifestyle and recommends, but does not insist on, vegetarianism.

From 1976-1988 the National Institutes of Health funded research on 34,000 Adventists living in southern California and determined they live 4-7 years longer than most of us, making them one of America's longest-living populations. A diet high in plants was determined to be just one factor in a multitude of healthy life-style choices that contribute to this truly amazing statistic. Moreover, the lower disease risk found in Adventists is likely *not* due to meat abstention, researchers openly admit, but to their higher intakes of nuts, legumes, and fresh produce. "Upon multivariate analysis, the latter often appeared to be the case," concedes respected researcher Dr. Gary Fraser.

How often do we hear veg'ns claiming that meat eating causes colon cancer? The Adventist study showed only a possible association between the two and that was seen only in the meat eaters who didn't eat legumes, *not in the meat eaters who did.* The lesson here? You can eat sensible amounts of non-processed meat and be healthy (Micha et al), but you gotta eat your veggies, fruits, nuts and beans as well. Sounds like an omnivore's diet to me, what do you think?

Now back to that ever slippery definition of vegetarian. A more recent look at these well-scrutinized Adventists, a 2007-2013 study by Loma Linda University (an Adventist-run college by the way, i.e., an inside job), continues the tradition of including a broad spectrum of eaters in its definition of "vegetarian," all but guaranteeing riveting headlines like this one in *Science Times*: "Vegetarians Live Longer Than Meat-Eaters, Study Finds." Too bad such skewed headlines—which far too many people instantly believe—can't offer more discerning and truthful infor-mation. Same goes for the study authors' brief, oft-quoted conclusion: "These results demonstrate an overall association of vegetarian dietary patterns with lower mor-tality compared with the nonvegetarian dietary pattern."

Again, we must ask that all-important questions: What exactly is a vegetarian according to this study? You have to do a bit of digging to realize the researchers define "vegetarian" as everyone from strict vegan, to regular dairy and egg eaters, to regular fish eaters, to those who consume red meat and/or poultry once a week and are suddenly and miraculously recognized as honorable vegetarians for the purposes of this study. Once again, you can only conclude what you include.

"This study's results don't prove that eliminating meat from one's diet is a recipe for a longer and healthier life," writes long-time veg and journalist Susan Perry. A more honest headline—and conclusion—would have been "Fish Eaters Live Longest Lives of All, Study Finds." Of the 70,000 people studied over six years, fish eaters had the lowest risk of death from any cause in all categories. But since fish eaters were lumped with the other so-called vegetarians—a definition many veggies abhor because it's actually describing an omnivore—the researchers were able to declare an association between "vegetarianism" and a longer life.

69

That's a *huge* problem with this entire body of research: the wide-ranging definition of vegetarianism employed to this day. In a 2014 meta-analysis of veggies and blood pressure, the components of a so-called "vegetarian diet" varied with the country and the individual and, once again, could include fish and small amounts of red meat (Yokoyama). Until all these studies employ *the exact same definition* and disallow all fish and meat, they are essentially useless as a body of evidence that supports a "vegetarian" diet—let alone a vegan one.

If only veg'ns examined actual research results themselves, instead of relying on biased veg books and blogs! Many of these sources are still comparing veggie health statistics with those of SAD Americans and their really dreadful processed-meat, high-sugar habits—but we're on to that deceit. When true vegetarians (zero meat or fish) are more honestly compared to health-conscious omnivores, there are *zero* significant differences in disease risk or mortality.

As researcher C.T. McEvoy points out, "The health benefits of vegetarian diets are not unique." Indeed, a rich body of research indicates health advantages to omnivores who incorporate fish and limited amounts of pastured meat and dairy into plant-rich diets, such as found in the much lauded Mediterranean Diet. In an unprecedented move, a large, rigorous study on the Med Diet was halted early, in 2013, because the health paybacks from eating ample olive oil, fresh fish, nuts and veggies were so overwhelming that it was considered unethical to deprive the control group (Estruch).

Besides Mediterranean dwellers, plenty of other healthy populations—who live even longer than Seventh-day Adventists—aren't even remotely vegetarian, certainly not vegan. On the island of Okinawa, Japan, you'll find some of the longest living people on earth, fish-eaters all. And in isolated mountain villages of Sardinia, hardy sheep herders reach 100 years at an astonishing rate, all the while feasting on plentiful dairy, plus pastured sheep and calves they raise and slaughter themselves. What *is* common among all these long-lived people is a plethora of intelligent choices that bring health, joy, and meaning to their lives: real, whole food eaten with gratitude; a love of their daily work; regular exercise that reduces stress; strong social networks and lifelong family ties.

What these extraordinarily healthy populations choose to leave out may be just as critical: processed food; constant snacking; sitting long hours before the altars of technology; risky sexual behavior; living alone; a self-centered life. We can also look at wise choices like the Adventists' abstention from smoking, alcohol, and drugs to get the idea of a higher than average IQ at work here. Choosing to

70

refrain from unhealthy lifestyle habits not only extends one's years but is in itself an act of elevated intelligence.*

CLEANSE ME! FREE ME!

I don't know what my IQ measured as a teen, but I do know that as a nouveau vegetarian I experienced blissful altered states. What's more, the less food eaten and the fewer calories consumed, the more soul enhancing and intense the event. At times this brought me close to fasting, an intentional experience with a long tradition of inducing spiritual awareness.

For millennia, indigenous people have gone into nature to strip down, abstain, and pray for life-guiding visions. Ancient shamans altered their consciousness to gain hidden knowledge via impassioned drumming and fasting—and modern shamans do the same. Today nearly every religious discipline still sponsors an occasional abstention from food. The Christian Bible refers to fasting repeatedly, while the Qur'an states: *For to fast is better for you—if you only knew.*

Wandering wraithlike through the drizzly, wintry woods of Massachusetts, Inanna Arthen is a fast-aficionado. She'll stay out in the weather for days on end, subsisting on water only, her body wet and cold, her mind and soul profoundly altered. "Around me Spirit is immanent," she pens in *FireHeart*, "and I am keenly aware of it. Everything I see takes my breath away with wonder, and the sound of water, dripping, trickling, bubbling, rushing, fills the air with a constant song."

Clearly, this spry, pixie-haired woman is a self-taught authority on pushing boundaries via safe, conscious fasting, confronting our deepest hungers and fears so that we can grow inwardly via radical new perceptions. "Fasting is one of the most primal of the challenges we can set to ourselves," Arthen affirms. "It sharply outlines the limitations of our own self-control and demonstrates the degree to which we are slaves to our own appetites and unconscious of our eating habits."

Anyone who has stopped eating for even a day or two knows what this woman is talking about. It's hard work, your body is crying out, your mind is shutting down, and all you want to do is stuff your face with bagels and bananas— anything to stop the hunger and self-pity, the perception of pain and lack. "To fast is to recognize the fragility of our life," admits Arthen, who believes it changes us emotionally and spiritually—forcing us to confront our weaknesses and mortality.

*The world's "Blue Zones" of longevity do not include Vilcabamba, Ecuador, as often cited by vegans. This myth has been debunked by scientists, due to age exaggeration and lack of birth records. The 5 longest-living populations hail from 1) Sardinia, Italy; 2) Okinawa, Japan; 3) Nicoya, Costa Rica; 4) Loma Linda, CA USA; 5) Ikaria, Greece. None of these populations are vegan and 4/5 are not vegetarian.

By breaking through our everyday, repetitive food habits, we open a doorway that leads to self-transformation. Like a ravenous fire, we burn through all the layers that are not true.

When you finally break a fast, you find yourself eating slowly and reverently, with intense presence. Perhaps for the first time in decades, you are deeply aware of the life force—be it plant or animal—that flows through your food and through your body like a gift, like a sacred offering. It's a powerful experience that most first-time fasters never forget and may choose to repeat.

Intensifying our appreciation of the life forms that nourish us was never the intention of religious fasts in the western tradition, including meat abstention, a mild form of the practice. Fasting and abstention served as a counterbalance and apology for the revelry and occasional pig-out by the common people. The first western vegetarians were self-mortifying ascetics, *not* animal lovers or health fanatics. They were men, they were patriarchal and they were into purification, isolation, and sexless self-denial. They certainly weren't teenagers trudging off to high school every morning and staying late for soccer practice. These early meat-abstainers shunned society and lightened their food load for just one overriding reason: to purify their despicable earthly bodies and get closer to the gods.

Centuries later, Christian saints likewise isolated themselves and practiced meat abstinence and, occasionally, prolonged fasting that bordered on starvation. "Sometimes the starving saints broke their fasts and were found at midnight raiding the convent larder," writes Hilary Mantel in "Holy Disorders." How did their mother superiors explain this humiliating lapse? "They simply said that, while Sister X snoozed celestially in her cell, the devil assumed her form and shape, tucked his tail under a habit, crept downstairs and ate all the pies."

Even more startling, a number of these female saints from the Middle Ages were more than likely anorexic, according to modern scholars, reminding us that this unhealthy, life-threatening practice did not originate in today's skinny-model world after all.

These holy abstainers didn't choose to suffer in order to look as gaunt as their adored, crucified Lord. They did it to attain "total purity" of body and soul, a self-sacrificing motive that couldn't be more different than the anxiety and pride driving today's anorexics, many of whom become veg'ns as a socially acceptable way to eliminate entire food categories, i.e., "bad foods" they fear might make them fat and unbeautiful. Women with eating disorders in this country are four times more likely to be vegan or vegetarian than other females. Their primary motive?

"Pride is the besetting sin of the anorexic. Pride in her self-denial, in her thin body, in her superiority," confesses Kate Chisholm in *My Hungry Hell*.

Bony or fleshy, male or female, the overriding goal of early western meat-abstainers was not to glorify a thin body but to *free* themselves of the body—and attain ecstatic union with God. Not long into my own vegetarian diet, I too was ready to unite with God. Having had zero luck merging with men, I figured the Almighty would be a terrific back-up for experiencing mindless ecstasy. So I sought out my very first yoga teacher as an ad hoc spiritual guide and the human that I settled on, definitely had that luminous, otherworldly look in his shiny, coffee-colored eyes.

Contrary to the popular "noodle yoga" of the day, wherein students flopped into soft plows or half-ass warrior poses, Robert practiced what we affectionately dubbed "military yoga" due to its severity, intensity, and obligatory use of macho props like thick gnarly ropes and metal folding chairs. More than once, this thin, ethereal young man commenced the class with standing backbends, immediately shooting me into another world alright, a world of truncated mind babble and expanded body pain. He was testing our self-induced limitations, Robert explained, and young fool that I was, I believed everything he told me, including the suitability of everyone on the planet to be a strict vegetarian, exactly like himself.

I'd been attending class just a couple weeks when our venerated teacher began encouraging all of us to experiment with three-day fasts, consisting of water and apples only. For those of us who followed our guru's every suggestion like goofy sheep, it didn't take long to realize the power of this stripped-down, one-fruit diet. Swiftly, wondrously, it freed my right brain from the tyranny of my word-drenched, ego-infested, analytical left. By the end of the third day—two gallons of tap water and five Golden Delicious apples into the journey—my mind erupted into a visual feast of scintillating mandalas, spontaneously arising one after the other: geometric and finely detailed, complex and beautiful beyond words. It was all I could do not to meander into rush-hour traffic as I paused, hypnotized on a honking, frenetic Paris street corner, watching for God knows how long—time no longer existed—as the kaleidoscopic, color saturated, 3D cosmic artistry unfolded inside and outside my brain, blasting me into open-mouthed Nirvana.

What was private esoteric experimentation back then is all the public rage today. Juice and other partial fasts clog the veggie health blogs, with actresses like Gwyneth Paltrow co-branding a 21-day cleanse and other celebrities starting fancy new juice lines. *Cleanse! Cleanse!* is the new female mantra. And while it's true that intermittent fasting can train overweight bodies to burn fat instead of sugar, most of the "cleansers" I know are already skinny and their intention, once again, seems to be as prosaic as getting even skinnier—not painful abstention, soul searching, and altered consciousness. *Every day in every single way, my hips and ass are getting thinner!*

Moreover, none of the sensational health claims made for juice fasts have been proven, and many health professionals consider them little more than a marketing ploy or, worse, another possible tool for concealing an eating disorder. Still, vegans are flocking to online fasting communities, sharing weight loss numbers and bathroom clean-out stories. But are they cleansing themselves of fat cells or self-disgust? Gaining confidence or a snootiness complex?

SEX, BEANS, AND OTHER ALTERED STATES

Meat abstention is not true fasting and it didn't originate for health *or* ethical reasons, let alone female fat cell removal. Yes indeed, vegetarianism has its roots in religious atonement: apology and self-punishment for one's sins. For millennia it's been an act of penance observed by strict religious societies, and to this day devoted Hindis refuse beef year-round. Similarly, Muslims won't eat pork; Jews who keep kosher are banned from eating certain animals; and staunch Catholics practice "meatless" Fridays, devouring fish instead, a boon to the global fishing industry and the reason McDonald's invented Filet-o-Fish. Recently, some local bishops have relaxed the Friday rule, calling for even tougher forms of abstinence one day a week, like *no texting.*

Early Egyptians avoided eating animals for more practical reasons; they didn't want to consume their father, mother, grandparents, aunts and uncles. Along with aboriginal societies, Egyptians were among the first to believe in the doctrine of metempsychosis, or soul migration, wherein the spirit of a dying person migrates into the body of another human, animal, or even a tough old plant. Thus, when Egyptians abstained from meat and fish, it was not out of compassion for animals. They wanted to avoid the guesswork and guilt of not knowing who they were eating for dinner.

Belief in soul transmigration was taken up by that wiry Ionian, Pythagoras. Recall that he is among the first western promoters of vegetarianism; so if you're a veggie of any stripe—total, semi, or pseudo—you should definitely get to know this charismatic guy, dead now for about 2,600 years. You probably recognize his name from the mathematical theorem you had to memorize in middle school, but during his lifetime Pythagoras was a renowned spiritual teacher with a faithful following of thousands. He was also the first Greek to disseminate a belief system regarding the soul's existence.

It goes something like this: since human souls are immortal, capable of never-ending transformations—somersaulting into new life forms between each death and birth—other creatures are literally our kin. Thus, to kill any animal for food was to murder and then eat, quite possibly, your brother or best friend. This belief in transmigrating souls does *not* imply an equality of species such as practiced by contemporary animal rightists. It's more like a person-trapped-in-an-animal-body ethic.

Yet even honoring soul-voyaging ancestors was secondary to these early veggies' main objective: to purify their coarse, vulgar, unwanted physical bodies through acts of extreme asceticism, thereby freeing themselves from our brutish animalism and, if the winds of fate were with them, joining up with the gods. The human body as something to loathe. Everyday life as something to escape.

Wandering the Mediterranean region for over 45 years, Pythagoras did indeed pursue feats of asceticism in his search for godlike truth. While in Egypt to study priestly purifications, he undertook a five-year vow of silence and in Babylon he sought out the sage Zaratas, hoping to psych himself into mind-zapping altered realities. From Mr. Z, Pythagoras learned "secret Magician rites which involved ritual cleansing through drugs and herbs," according to historian Colin Spencer, "the use of hallucinatory drugs from plants being the preparation for mystic union with the gods." *(Why did our middle school teachers leave out all the good stuff?)* Fasting as needed, Pythag spent years hanging out in caves in deep meditation, a sure-fire formula for bending reality and receiving divine truths. This severe style of meditation was later emulated by sects like the Essenes, Gnostic and Christian hermits, and Egypt's monastic Desert Fathers. (There were also Desert Mothers, by the way.)

Still flourishing during his lifetime, the Orphic religious cult also influenced Pythagoras, as well as subsequent meat-resisters through the centuries, right on down to today's preachy, activist vegans. It's good to know one's roots. Orphics took their name from the Greek mythical hero Orpheus, he who soothed the wild beasts with his rapturous lyre, turning them from vicious predators into the most docile of plant nibblers—surely a vegan vision of paradise. For the Orphics and Pythagoras there was but one way to free ourselves from our animal nature and all those annoying reincarnations into physical form: follow a life of poverty and austerities, including the renouncing of all animal flesh.

Fascinating, isn't it, that all these restrictions and purifications didn't preclude using hallucinogens? They were, in fact, frequently and enthusiastically ingested by participants in the Eleusinian Mysteries, Orphic religious ceremonies held in honor of Demeter and the annual harvest of the grains. Ever take a close look at depictions of this earth goddess? Those are opium poppies crowning her lovely wreathed head.

In one splendid image, a bare-breasted Demeter rises from a black fertile earth, snakes coiled around her slender white arms and capsules of opium in her outstretched, beckoning hands. All those 1970s brownie eaters had nothing on early Greeks, who were well versed in the psychoactive use of opium. Their ancient medical literature lists it as an essential element, a *theriaca,* or antidote, and calls for 24 ounces of opium to be added with sacred herbs to exactly 960 ounces of raw honey. Besides banishing all sorrow and depression, this magic elixir was known to deliver deep sleep, prophetic dreams, and enchanted encounters with the spiritual world.

Traveling to Eleusis for the Mysteries, the father of vegetarianism most likely joined other Greeks for a purifying wash in the sea before entering the cave-like shrines of the gods for their all-night rites and drug fests. A special vegan dish attributed to Pythag and designed to stimulate hallucinations—a delectable cross between a hash cake and a bowl of muesli—was served to all comers according to Colin Spencer, who informs us that "the drugs induced a sense of timelessness and unreality where fantasies would appear and the celebrants would hardly know whether they were awake or dreaming."

Leaving the wild Orphics behind, a more sober Pythagoras voyaged to southern Italy where he founded a highly respected school at Croton. His devout followers were of two classes and, pay attention here, each was prescribed a completely different diet regime than the other. The *mathematikoi*, Pythag's elite inner circle of contemplatives, lived on-site, abstained from flesh, drank no wine, and ate all their meals in silence. Pythag's outer circle of believers, the *akousmatikoi*, or "the people," lived and labored in ordinary society, just like you and I do. Instructed to help themselves to animal flesh on certain days only, they abstained on others.

When "the people" did consume meat, they were absolutely forbidden to eat the marrow—the soft, living, innermost part of the bone—because "messages from the gods" were concealed there, a prophetic precursor to DNA sequencing perhaps, and the many secrets there revealed. (Encouraging his people to periodically eat animals, no doubt sped up this memo-from-the-gods retrieval process.) Just as important, the high-density nutrition of meat allowed them to continue as hard-working farmers and laborers, contributing to the greater society. Pythag's own son-in-law, Milo of Croton, was one such active citizen, and stories abound of this intrepid war hero saving his city from annihilation. Such dynamic physical work demands an enormous caloric and protein load, and Milos was known far and wide as a massive meat eater who could put away an entire bull in one sitting.

Pythagoras and his inner circle of vegetarians, please note, were *not* working class people with jobs, families, and societal obligations. They were not raising children or protecting the citizenry, building roads or harvesting fields. Nor were they commuting long distances, toiling 8-5, attending classes, preparing three meals a day, doing endless laundry, chasing kids or having vigorous sex. They weren't having sex at all. In stillness and contemplation is how they spent most of their days, requiring far less protein and calories than the norm. In their free time they sought out aromatic herbs like asphodel and mallow, considered miracle foods because, much like today's stimulant-packed espresso, they were fantastic at suppressing the body's natural hunger.

SO BESIDES LIVING OFF appetite-smothering herbs and fresh coastal oxygen, what the heck did the first western vegetarian and his circle of ascetics actually chow down on? Well, it wasn't beans, a dietary mainstay for modern vegans. This guy absolutely hated beans and forbade his followers to eat them, anytime, anywhere. Despite the substantial nutrition they offer, Pythagoras was even more adamant about abstention from beans than he was about meat.

As I sit here in my bountiful green garden on a simmering July day, munching scrumptious, just-snapped Kentucky bush beans, I can't help but wonder *why*?? Turns out that Pythag, Egyptian priests, and other such godly men intensely disliked both the sound and smell of their impure bodily emanations. As the authors of *Food: The Gift of Osiris* suggest, a priest's pride would be blown apart if he were to suffer the indignity of farting in the middle of a holy rite. Other scholars believe the bean ban started in old Egypt due to favism, an inability to digest fava beans by (mostly) males with an enzyme deficiency. There's a symbolic explanation as well because *iwryt*, Egyptian for bean, is similar to the word *iwr*, which means to conceive, as in the creative act of conception, as in sex. Scholar Colin

Spencer takes the visuals even further: "I would also suggest that fava beans, squinted at sideways, bear a resemblance to female pudenda." The story goes, no joke, that when Pythagoras first buried some beans in a muddy spot and later dug them up, they had transformed into the shape of a woman's vagina.

Whew! Okay then! In addition to foregoing all unseemly farts, let's just forget altogether about dem sexy beans and their captivating vulvas, certainly an unholy distraction for ascetics and priests. (Do historians actually get paid to contemplate the female pudenda of legumes?) For bean-deprived Pythagoras and his disciples, that basically left grains, honey, fruits and vegetables—all carbohydrates and not all that dissimilar to the diet of many contemporary vegans. Despite the precarious low-protein, low-fat content of this diet (no wonder he gobbled fish from time to time), Pythagoras believed his food regime to be healthy. Apparently it worked for him. Some historians describe Pythag as mountain-goat frisky well into old age, scampering about the rocky Greek terrain in search of the divine. Of course, this is all conjecture; no one *really* knows how long the father of modern vegetarianism lived, nor his health condition—because nothing was recorded at the time. Everything we know about this influential man, or think we know, was written at least 700 years after he died.

Beyond health benefits, Pythagoras believed vegetarianism thwarts anger and other strong emotions while promoting passivity. The whole idea of the pacifist veg'n may have begun with Pythag for the legends tell us the man was never seen to laugh or cry, express joy or even sorrow. Serenity, yes, it's a superb state but to never laugh in glee at the delights of life? Never chortle at the absurdities of our all-too-human condition? Nor cry out in anguish at the death of a loved one? Who among us, vegetarian or otherwise, would choose to never feel or share these deep-seated sentiments, no matter how peaceful and centered at the core? Rising above all such passions, as some extreme meditators and yogis advocate, is surely not quite human. God-imitating, yes, and that's exactly what the father of western vegetarianism and his inner circle of unmarried, childless, appetite-suppressing, hallucinogen-ingesting ascetics sought: escape from imprisonment in the human body and ascension to the gods.

"THE CRACK BETWEEN THE WORLDS"

Indeed, the man acquired a Christ-like reputation as people came to believe that Pythagoras possessed supernatural powers: healing the sick, walking on water, flying through air, even appearing in two different locales at the same time, just like Carlos Castaneda's Don Juan and his wild cast of inscrutable sorcerers (a phenom recently validated by quantum physicists who proved an electron really can be in two places at once). This early vegetarian also claimed awareness of his own pre-existence and firmly believed that each one of us, by abstaining from meat, will be able to: *refine our consciousness, regain lost memories, and clearly recall our previous lives.*

I nearly choked mid-quaff of my morning coffee upon reading these words, jolted awake by long-forgotten memories of my own eerie past-life experience. Wasn't it late autumn in the Midwest? The season of falling leaves and goblin moons? Ah yes, I remember…an introspective 20-year-old, one year into her new diet and supremely confident after a solo trek through Europe. It's coming back to me now….a hushed October evening slowly dissolving into dusk, the time of day Castaneda calls "the crack between the worlds" and which the French describe as *entre le chien et le loup*: between the dog and the wolf. As the room began to darken by imperceptible degrees, I found myself staring for long moments, and for no particular reason, into a large oval mirror on the bedroom wall. My eyes and mind were unfocused, a blank slate in hazy shades of shadow and gray.

I used to do this often when younger, this letting go of the verbal brain, this gazing into nothingness: the way all children do when they suddenly stop talking. Mesmerized as they stare into the vacuum of space; oblivious as you call out their names and slowly wave your hands in front of their their far-away eyes. Their brain waves have shifted into theta, seeing something which we cannot see and which they cannot explain upon return to consensus reality. The voice of theta is silent, visionary, and profoundly creative. As adults we have mostly lost, and sadly so, our capacity to instinctively enter this trance-like state that synthesizes and resolves dual-time experiences.

In this dusky state, this fissure between the worlds, without effort or warning there arrived before my eyes, stunningly clear visions of humans, many dozens of them appearing sequentially in the mirror, male and female, adolescent to elderly: some jovial, some quite somber. Unlike with the riotous Orphics, no drugs were involved, none, swear to Demeter. I hadn't indulged since Paris, over a year prior. I was, in fact, squeaky clean, totally sober, and utterly serene as my own 20th century face vanished into the glass, replaced by a living, incandescent canvas of benevolent men and women of wildly varied countenance, period dress, and demeanor. Each leisurely arranged him or herself before me, looked me straight in the eye—often with a whimsical smile—then gradually disappeared like so many glimmering pixels, only to slowly reappear in a different human form. How long this went on I have no idea. Two minutes? Two hours? Time as we know it had no meaning.

Were these images from my past, or merely the creative conjuring of an overly inventive mind, freed to participate, like the meat-abstaining Orphics, in some timeless parallel universe? Electrons dancing here; electrons dancing there. Take your pick, but at some point—the end of your life if not sooner—you too will find yourself dancing between the two worlds. At the time, I knew nothing about so-called past lives; yet zero doubt arose regarding these manifestations. I was, in fact, remarkably calm, completely knowing, and all-accepting of my own trans-formations through time. Gradually the room grew too dark to see anything and within a few days, telling no one, I forgot all about it.

ON THE FAR EDGE of southwest Portugal a monster wall of rock rises out of the sea. Called Sagres today, it was known in antiquity as the End of the World. In 1420 Prince Henry the Navigator established his famous school for explorers and shipbuilders on this rugged, windswept point. Magellan, da Gama, Columbus and Dias are all said to have studied here before pushing off into a sea of darkness and the unknown. Named Sacred Promontory by the Romans, it was the kind of awe-inspiring place that called out far and wide to pilgrims in search of rapture, in search of the gods.

But unremitting Atlantic storms had turned too riotous for even this aquatic, bliss-seeking vegetarian. So when a shimmering afternoon sun finally material-ized out of the misty ether, my fellow van travelers and I likewise emerged from our cozy dive-hotel, our waterlogged fatigue, our communal cuddle, and headed in rumpled three-day old clothes for the craggy cliffs of Sagres, in search of some holy mischief. We were bonded now, the seven of us, and exhilarated by the fresh westerly winds, we bounced around the high outcropping like jubilant children just let out of school, shouting to the welcoming sky, to no god in particular: *erleikda! erleikda! lighten up!!*

I was wrapped like the Michelin Man in Linda's big-tubed, goose down jacket, warm to my fiery core (and reassured by my compassionate friend that no geese had been killed in the making). As I took leave of my companions to perch like a mindful gull on a nearby jutting rock, the sky smeared itself blood-red and the sun sank slowly into a dark, still-churning sea.

Wasn't it Thales, the first Greek philosopher, who boldly announced over 2500 years ago that all life comes from the sea, that everything is full of gods? Chanting *hum* with my in-breath and *sah* with my out-breath, my mind dissolved into sacred silence. Was it vegetarianism, or meditation, creating my new clarity of mind and expanded states? Human touch or the mighty, purifying sea? Surely this moment of non-duality would go on forever! But whatever the source of human euphoria, it never lasts. And like too many sailors who pushed off from this same rocky shore, I was about to crash and drown.

14.

MARTINE ON THE ROCKS

Only the vine reveals to us what is the real taste of the earth.

—Collette

IT WAS ONE of those unforgettable days in the City of Lights—dreary gray and thickly polluted—when I was smacked down by a turning-twenty, existential breakdown. There I was, back in Paris, roaming the gritty backstreets, solo and miserable, all but surrounded by clinging and clutching, tongue-sucking French couples. If I had known the stats, at least I would have been prepared. In America, I've since learned, pairs touch on average only twice an hour, but here in France it's 110 hot feels in those same sixty minutes. Zero for me and the poor Brits.

Amidst all that frenzied, funneled passion, I found myself mucking around the smoky industrial outskirts of the drizzly city, my raincoat long and unkempt, my hair tousled and dirty. And into my wretched, upturned collar I was mumbling a tune to my absent angel....*no money, no man, and sure as hell no satisfaction,* when suddenly I realized, like an agonizing seizure, like a fist slammed into my heart, how much I lived alone inside my head and how much I desperately wanted to get out, to free myself from this self-saturated, ludicrously analytical mind.

How I longed to kiss the raw earth, my own tender naked body, a man's secret parts, longed to embrace the elements—wind, waves and stars—and fly madly around the flaming night sky like Saint-Exupéry. How I urgently, yes, *urgently* needed to feel my earthy origins, harvest my own life, grow my own food, reap my own nourishment and share the rich bounty. But how could I fully realize this emergent life quickening inside of me, aching to be born? Where could I run to glisten in the sun, lick purple juice off the sticky fruit, suck vital nutrients straight out of the rich black soil? *Where! Where!*

And then *zaaap* out of nowhere....l'épiphanie. Thank God for the brilliant shooting-star epiphanies that blaze without warning during the vacant deserts of our lives. What better place to celebrate the soil and the harvest, it abruptly dawned on me, than the ancient, storied vineyards of wine-drunk, love-drunk France? I started singing ridiculously loud, right there in the middle of the street, like some old char woman gone loony. Nobody cared. Everyone was still gazing like goners into the eyes of their lovers. Without thinking (ah, that's the ticket— good woman!) I did a little hop and a joyful skip, something I hadn't done in, what, a decade? Since I was ten and still living in my body? But your body knows when you're on the path, when you've finally got it right. Look for the skip, the song, the spontaneous howl, the deep melodious sigh. *I know something that you don't know, oh talking mind, oh words on the page!*

So it was with sublime patience that I rode the métro to a work service office in the shadow of the Eiffel Tower and stood in line with a hundred other students, nearly all of them French, to sign up for the fast-approaching harvest. By the next morning over thirty of us were tightly packed on a school bus, speeding toward Vergisson and other small villages in the Rhône-Alpes, a region of limestone hills and alkaline soils not far from the Swiss border. Here I was to live with a family of grape growers and join them in the fields.

There was no turning back now, and when the vividly orange vehicle rolled in after sunset, apprehensive locals were milling around the town square, anxiously awaiting their much-needed crews. I happened to be the sole worker assigned to my family, a middle-aged couple with the handsome, roughened faces of farmers who labor every day of their lives in the sun, wind, and rain. And when our last names were called out as a match, I saw them light up with surprise as a solitary female stepped forward. *Et vous êtes américaine!* they exclaimed, pumping my shy hand in welcome.

My daily routine on the 8-hectare, 20-plot vineyard was promptly established. Every morning in the inky blackness, earlier than I had ever risen in my life, I got up for farm work, reluctantly shedding thick piles of warm quilts to pee in the enamel pot placed in a far, frigid corner of the spare room. The stone farmhouse had no central heat, no plumbed bathroom, and I quickly surmised that beyond nighttime pissing, everyone was to use the well-ventilated outhouse set not nearly far enough away from the main quarters. Here, neatly torn pieces of *Le Progrès* and other old newspapers were stacked beside the yawning black hole, serving a far more valuable purpose than mere reading material.

Suddenly, *I* was the distinctive one: the crazy lemon-haired American girl who traveled alone and declined to eat meat—*mon dieu!*—no one could fathom it. Every noontime and nighttime, the tireless, red-headed martyr-mother served dish after generous dish in the classic farmhouse tradition, all of them centered around animals: wild rabbit, mutton, duck, goose, beef, pork and even, to my horror, horse. Better to feed many people from a mare turned out to pasture, they kindly reassured me, than to let her body waste away, used for nothing but glue. On one hand I had to agree but on the other, I dearly wish she'd been left to die naturally in that same verdant pasture. *Had they never read Black Beauty?!*

Differences in French and American food attitudes are stark but the gulf is perhaps widest when it comes to equine dining. The French ingest over 25,000 metric tons of horse meat annually, Americans officially zero. And when a 2013 food scandal sent ripples of disgust throughout the US and Britain—unlabeled horse meat was discovered in European processed food, including Ikea's Swedish meatballs—the French just shrugged. After all, they have been eating horses for centuries during times of war and famine and have come to rather like the taste; some even prefer it to beef. It's also higher in protein, lower in calories and fat, and noticeably cheaper. During World War II, American housewives hid horse-meat in their casseroles due to beef shortages and until 1985 the Harvard Faculty Club served a very popular equine steak, but Americans never took to it like the French. Veg'ns might say this separates us from the pagans, the presumed reason Pope Gregory III banned horsemeat across Europe in the 8th century. A number of scholars, though, believe he *really* did it to preserve horses for warfare.

Whatever the original reasons, cultural food preferences and taboos are deeply entrenched, from the forbidden dog meat of Muslims (while allowing camel flesh) to the poached puppies favored by Koreans. In agreeing what is acceptable eating behavior and what is not, we define ourselves as a society and cohesive group. Equally as important, we define ourselves in opposition to others, creating our unique identity. And when it comes to the food they allow or disallow, vegans possess a formidable and near unbreakable identity—and so do the French.

Both love animals. However, Francos seem not to mind the idea of horses or hogs becoming part of their own bodies. And Icelanders have no issue with in-corporating rams' testicles into their corporal cells. Nor Togo natives with forest rats. "Food is often the subject of taboo or disgust because it is internalized," maintains ethnographer Carole Counihan. "Any revulsion we have for the food is magnified by the thought it will become part of us." Vegans, undeniably, want no animal bodies as part of their own. "Just the thought of eating meat makes me want to puke," I've heard many a veg'n proclaim. Their greatest desire appears to be abolishing not only meat, but all earthly suffering and death, while the French face these inevitabilities head-on.

Living in the duck-rich district of Gers, my French friend Marie has witnessed the slaughtering of local fowl, but still likes to eat them for what she considers robust good health. Now and then she even contemplates her own death (something Americans are loathe to do) and decided long ago she doesn't want to end up in a dank, dark box visited by hungry worms and centipedes—not the right image for her sensibilities. (Evidently, humans are very picky not only about what we will eat, but what will eat *us*.) Many years after my youthful trip to France, as mature adults, Marie took me on a pilgrimage to her final destination, not far from the village where she was born. Walking along a high, stone embankment in Biarritz on France's stormy western shore, we gazed down into the wildly crashing, no-mercy Atlantic, which Marie calls "my fierce origins, my true home" and where she wishes to return for sea burial at the end—full of good Burgundy, ripe camembert, and duck au confit. No doubt the hungry fish will internalize all that is offered, and with no qualms whatsoever. Surely we are the only species on earth that agonizes over what we eat.

THE FRENCH, NOT SO MUCH. Not only do they adore their wine and pastries with no apologies, they love their domestic animals, many of them still raised with care and affection on small family farms—backyard poultry owners number in the hundreds of thousands. Yet when it comes time for the animals to serve as food, these people have no taboos or aversions that I've discovered. They don't believe in wasting one part: livers of chickens, shoulders of beef, intestines of calves (fried in thick goose fat), and most proudly for the inhabitants of Alsace: *cervelas*, originally the brains of mature pigs and now simply shoulder meat and bacon mixed with port, pistachios and chopped truffles, stuffed into the thinnest of skins and hung out to dry. OMG, that had to be the single most revolting meal any teen would pray not to encounter in her young vegetarian life.

Yes, landing in picturesque little Vergisson with all the other students, I had once again stumbled into carnivore paradise. The district's capital city of Lyon— a vibrant trade center for food and spices since Roman times—is considered one of Europe's finest centers of the butcher's art. "It is the respect paid to the less glamorous parts of the animal, such as the head, trotters and chitterlings, which has formed the basis of Lyon's tradition of high-quality cuisine," extols author André Dominé, noting that anyone who can transform mere entrails into first-class sausages "must be able to create masterpieces from more noble ingredients."

Whipping up one animal plate after another, the perpetually moving, persistently laboring French *maman* was clearly worried about me. After every meal, finally plopping down to eat only after all the men had finished their four courses (signaling their approval with a resounding group belch), this domestic diva in a floral apron would then begin to cluck at me. *Cluckity, cluck!* How can you possibly survive without meat? You are too thin! *Mangez la viande!* Eat your meat! But when frog appendages in hot dripping butter were unceremoniously offered (surely I could not resist such a delicacy, full of protein and easy to digest), I once again expressed how happy I was with my recent dietary decision.

And the family, it turned out, was happy with me, especially my work ethic and obvious admiration for their simple rural life—and the exceptional products we were creating. The vigorous purple Gamay grapes I was snipping hour after hour into the basket slung around my sore, throbbing neck would later emerge as a respectable Beaujolais, the world's most popular red wine: zesty, fruity, and low in tannins. As the old saying goes: *There's a third river that flows through Lyon besides the Rhône* and the *Saône—it's the Beaujolais!*

Yes, the wines of this valley are known far and wide. For the lustrous green-skinned grapes picked earlier were Chardonnay, perfectly suited to the clay and limestone soils of this region and destined to become Pouilly-Fuissé: dry and delicate with subtle touches of oak and pear. Expressing the truth of the Chardonnay grape and each individual plot—different in slope, soil composition and sun exposure—that's what motivates the vintners in this region to this day. And they are passionate about fulfilling their duties. "It is about precision and sensitivity," local winemaker Audrey Braccini explained to my favorite wine connoisseur, Tom Cannavan. "My task is to listen to the vineyard, to be invisible."

And then there was Martine. How to explain my growing love for the untamed *Mar-teeen*, even to myself? The daughter-in-law, she arrived with the eldest son and their pair of plump, fair-haired toddlers the day after I showed up. Not much older than myself, she was long of tooth and bulge-eyed as a fish, mouthy and tart as wild cherries, sassy and sharp as the serrated shears that constantly pricked me in the fields. Yet as the days unfolded I began to find her inexplicably beautiful. How could this possibly be? Gradually I realized it was Martine's agile body, her bright, quick mind and joyous self-assurance that consumed me, and I began to observe her every move. She possessed ten times more radiance and energy than this pale, dawdling vegetarian. Martine zipping down the long rows yakking and laughing, snipping grapes faster than any man, even as I labored and lumbered. Martine gleefully scarfing down mutton, pork, and tiny boiled potatoes. Martine in the kitchen. Martine in the vineyards. Martine on the rocks, balancing on large boulders at the meadow's green edge, striking a dancer's pose. I wanted to imbibe her brilliant essence and laugh at life the way she did! But all I could do was gawk in wide-eyed adoration.

During our customary two-hour lunches, nursing backaches from the constant bending, all thoughts of laboring in the vineyard would instantly flee with those first pleasing sips of *vin rouge*. Same thing during our late, leisurely dinners, occasionally preceded by a rowdy stomping of juicy grapes in ancient oak vats, still wearing our work trousers and muddy rubber boots. As the weeks passed, I began to sense an unhurried but perceptible internal shift. I wasn't quite sure if it was my new vegetarian diet and lightness of body bringing it on, or the immense satisfaction of physically working the earth, hands eagerly searching among the tough old vines for luminous orbs of fruit beneath a fresh, wind-scattered sky.

It was late October and the sun was both radiant and mellow, turning my fair skin a golden hue. My arms, heavily scratched and cut, were becoming strong. My legs gripped the earth more solidly. My head was clear. My heart torn open. When hunger struck, which was often, I picked fresh fruit and walnuts straight off the nearby trees. Our food came from the soil we walked on. It came from local fields, backyards, and family dairies: herbs and greens, thick butter and cream, hardy goats and ducks—their open-air bodies rubbed by dirt and splattered with sun and rain. No doubt about it, I was falling in love with this simple agrarian lifestyle and the profoundly real and earthy people who inhabited it. My new, more natural way of living and eating was bestowing me with greater clarity, a surge in heartiness and health. Gone was the social inhibition, the ungrounded intellect, the constantly yapping brain.

And so to all pale geeks, be you veggie or omnie, with your head stuck in a tablet or book: may you come to the Rhône valley and rub your very own lovely body in its fertile soils beneath the noble Mont de Fuissé. May you bloom *wildly* in the lush countryside while vine-scratched solar-kissed women feed you scented almonds and succulent purple grapes. And may you forever flourish, in your own inimitable way, beneath the dazzling French sun.

15.

THE KINSHIP OF CUISINE

They will say you are on the wrong road if it is your own.

—Antonio Porchia

RETURNING TO AMERICA after four months of lust and wandering, the reserved, pork-chomping teen was gone. The hopeful innocent who had escaped to Europe with a handful of twenty-dollar bills shoved in her pocket had finally come home: to herself. In place of that tidy, timid nerd strode *MOI*, a confident young woman with a feral new look and stripped-down diet the likes of which my family had never seen.

If my friends seemed puzzled, my parents were outright baffled: "Good Lord, what happened over there!" First, the flashy gold ring in my left ear, something only gay men and pirates wore at the time: so asymmetrical, so slacker bohemian. Ugh! They just didn't get it. Nor the bleached-out jeans with gaping holes in the butt, nor the tie-dyed sleeveless man's undershirt that clung like cellophane to my pale skin and was nearly as transparent. Eeek! My faultless older sister, president of her sorority, had worn pleated plaid skirts with matching baby-blue cashmere sweaters. My mother cried—*cried*—when she discovered that I no longer owned a dress.

But it was what lay beneath that really set off their cuckoo alarms, for under those tight, ultra-thin male undershirts lay—nothing. That's right, nothing at all but two lovely liberated breasts. The idea of not wearing a bra, and *so obviously,* turned my traditionalist mother into a quivering mass of peach jelly, still sweet but temporarily disturbed. And my upright, respectable father was beside himself with my dark unshaven legs and equally hirsute armpits—animalistic! "We are not living in Communist Europe you know. And last time I checked, you weren't a timber wolf!"

Even more renegade was my blasphemous new diet. How could I ever hope to reconcile my devout vegetarianism with my mom's love of family-style cooking, her prized meat dish the gustatory lynchpin of every meal? Choice tender beef cuts simmering in a baby carrot/red potato stew; chopped liver and onions sautéed in soft, leftover beef grease; and our incomparable after-church supper: Grandma Maggie's hand-rolled egg dumplings tossed into the big ol' family cooking pot alongside a juicy, stewing, fat golden chicken. Though my mind had shut down to all such indulgences, each Sunday afternoon my chops would start spontaneously salivating around that last one, likewise when the poor chicken morphed into the crunchy fried version for family celebrations, accompanied by spankin' hot corn fritters and buttery mashed potatoes.

Intellectually and philosophically, I had absolutely no desire to eat any of this stewed, crisped, or poached animal flesh. As for my body's intuitive response? I had no control over that. Unlike some vegetarians who condition themselves to practically retch at the mere smell of cooked meat, having not done so as a child I saw no reason to begin now. My body, after all, was entirely separate from my moral mind, which now understood that cooking and eating animals, even when lovingly prepared in my family homestead, was just plain wrong if not sinful. Yes, my corporal reaction had been radically different at the Paris meat market but *that* was visual, visceral, and first-time shocking; *this* was my own mother's beloved canteen, no severed heads or bloody entrails in sight. Thus, on certain cooking days, in order to circumvent my new mind/body schism—highly righteous thoughts negating my body's instinctive affirmative response—I simply stopped hanging out in our warm, alluring, aromatic kitchen.

Yet my mom was a fine cook and nurturing her husband and five children with healthy, delicious meals every day of the year was more than a matter of pride. It practically defined her being. In many ways these common meals also defined our life as a family, the seven of us ritually gathering every evening in a pre-dinner prayer of thankfulness as, night after night, we bonded in communal food sharing and lively conversation. Such collective food traditions reach *way* further back than our parents and their parents. They harken back to our great-great granddads and mums who landed on America's shores from Italy and Ireland, Poland and Romania, Kenya and Japan, and to the special cuisines, recipes, and dining traditions that arrived with them. Family foods play a tremendous role in our ethnic identity, Canadian Dan Haran correctly notes, and "no self-respecting Acadian could pass on rapture pie, which Anglos accurately nicknamed Frenchman's glue.

Gooey-grated potatoes pressed of their juices, baked in a chicken stock—Yum!" Be it fish on Fridays, kosher or halal, all ethnic and religious groups impose their own customs and contracts concerning food. Transgressions, Haran testifies, will often alienate you from your family or faith community.

The truth is this: where you grew up, with whom, and the food you shared with your relatives and friends will forever be stamped on your conscious and unconscious identity. (According to the Humane Research Council, nearly 60% of veg'ns who quit "did not see veganism/vegetarianism as part of my identity.") Furthermore, your ethnic/genetic heritage determines, in part, which foods work best for your unique body. So even if you are largely unaware of your dietary roots and crave pseudo soy sausages, each one of us is the beneficiary of a long line of ancestral cuisines and eating traditions, a huge majority of which celebrate meat as our primary sustenance. And there I was, breaking that communal food chain for the first time in centuries, maybe even millenniums. I mean, really, how many veggie ancestors did you or I have in 4th century Gaul? Or 15th century England for that matter? None, I would venture, not by choice anyway. Poverty and scarcity have forced humans to take up a meatless diet from time to time, including in today's poor or drought-scarred regions, but vegetarianism didn't emerge in the West as a full-fledged, conscious movement until the turn of the 19th century. And even then the numbers were puny.

Did I now risk alienating myself from my beloved family, my ancestral traditions, and the entire communal dining ritual that practically defines civilization as we know it? Sneaking a peanut butter and sprouts sandwich in the kitchen, while 24 family members gather as one at the jovial dining table to feast on roast turkey and giblets, is not exactly socially integrative. British philosopher Roger Scruton makes a persuasive case for the civilizing nature of human dining rites, as opposed to eating by and for oneself. It's essential, he insists, to emphasize the integrative aspects of family and social dining, the critical bonding and affirming that occur in the midst of communal food sharing.

Since prehistory, any offering of meat was proudly shared with the entire community, but the same wasn't true of hand-gathered plants which our hunting-foraging relatives ate right away or shared only with the nuclear family. It was the scarcer, revered meat protein which bound a community tightly together. Gathering around the post-hunt cooking fire emerged as a pivotal social event, much as today's dinner guests instinctively drift as one unit into the oven-warmed, gravy-scented kitchen. Shared meat unified the community beyond one's immediate family; it became a symbol of the group's identity, health, and strength. Animal protein, however, was in no way guaranteed to our ancestors. They endured long periods without and treated its appearance as a true gift, an occasion of collective thanksgiving for the essential nourishment provided.

So there I was. A stand-alone. An odd-ball really, in my enormous, extended, meat-eating, Scotch-Irish-German-Dutch family that spans the continents and the centuries. Flesh-eaters all. I am quite certain I would have heard mention of an eccentric Great Aunt Tilly who had scandalously declared herself a vegetarian, refusing the esteemed succulence of Grundy County-raised pork or Marshall County-shot duck. So how did that make me feel, to openly break and defy such a powerful and enduring chain of animal-eating ancestors? Honestly? I was thrilled.

16.

RENEGADES! A BRIEF HISTORY OF VEG'NISM IN THE WEST

VEGETARIANS ARE CULTURAL rebels, no way around it, and we've rarely had an easy go of it. Throughout western history we have been mistreated and mis-understood, persecuted as dissidents, forced to eat separately or even beat it out of town. Quick: how many heroes or heroines can you name from western literature or mythology who were vegetarians?

Heroic warriors in *The Odyssey* dined on meat and more meat, rewarded for their hardship and courage with sumptuous banquets. As Homer penned, "Hunger is the sorriest way to die." Moreover, to the most honorable warriors went the choicest cuts, like "the chine's portion of the white-toothed pig" presented to Odysseus. In Shakespeare's *Julius Caesar,* an angry Cassius demands, "Upon what meat doth this our Caesar feed, that he is grown so great?" And in Joyce's *Ulysses*, everyman Leopold Bloom begins his whacky, adventurous, redemptive day by heading to the butcher's to buy a fresh mutton kidney for breakfast.

Yes, entire cultures are defined by their food traditions and to choose non-participation in the communal diet is to risk suspicion, if not out-and-out hostility. For early Greeks, cultural participation meant the classic Mediterranean diet: fish, olives, barley, wheat, fresh produce and wine. (Too bad they're not still doing that; Greek children are becoming obese, eating the media-promoted global diet of junk carbs.) Animal flesh beyond fish was greatly valued by early Greeks but eaten sparingly, mostly during festivities or to honor the gods. And woe to those who chose not to join in the community meat-sharing! They were castigated as outsiders and obliged to create a new identity outside the mainstream culture.

Ancient Greek public life also meant animal sacrifice, a god-appeasing ritual whose bloody roots are lost in antiquity. After an animal's vitals were offered to the deities, its flesh was boiled and distributed to everyone in the community, its entrails made into thick puddings. The social group thus expressed "its solidarity, and a rare opportunity to eat meat was enjoyed," declared John Wilkins in *Public and Private Eating in Greece, 450-300 BC.* "Solidarity was important, as now in the meat-eating codes of the Jewish and Muslim communities....Anyone who was a vegetarian was not taking part and was in a sense opting out of society."

Today's veg'ns would applaud: hell yes! But early vegetarians often hid their status from public view for fear of harsh retribution. First century Stoic philosopher Seneca may have practiced abstinence in private but indisputably consumed meat in public, attempting to dodge imperial condemnation. Living about the same time, fellow Roman Ovid also apparently lied about the vegetarianism he discreetly followed at home. Centuries later, French poet Alphonse de Lamartine wrote feverishly about his terrifying childhood experience in a slaughterhouse, praised vegetarianism, and converted many to its cause. Yet he too confessed to the habit of eating flesh when dining in public due to "the necessity of conforming to the customs of society."

That's why the openly anti-social attitudes of meat-abstaining Pythagoreans— skinny, long-haired, barefoot-shambling ascetics who taught and begged throughout the countryside—pissed off a lot of Romans, who either condemned them or banished them outright. And although less cruel, Greek comics of the era were known for lampooning the "wretched vegetarians," none more broadly than the wit Antiphanes. Fragments from his popular 4th century BC plays remain: "A devotee of Pythagoras, he eats nothing that has life, but takes a sooty piece of barley-cake, the largest possible for a ha'penny and chews that....So help me Zeus, good sir, that is the finest 'meat' there is!" Much of the public simply could not tolerate their frugality, their holier-than-thou godliness. "Just set before them fish or meat; if they don't eat them up and their own fingers too, I am willing to be strung up a dozen times!"

As for the Orphics, who practiced a dissident religion and meatless diet as far back as the sixth century BC, Aristophanes writes in *The Frogs*: "Orpheus taught men to abstain from murders." These early veggies certainly did believe that meat-eating was tantamount to murder, that to eat an animal was to implicate oneself in the original pitiless deed. However, they refused to participate at great political risk. "The so-called Orphic way of life is not reducible to an insipid vegetarianism," proclaims Marcel Detienne in *Dionysos Slain*. He proceeds to label meat abstention in the ancient Greek citystate "a highly subversive act" because to alter one's diet was "to throw into doubt the relationship between gods, men, and beasts upon which the whole politico-religious system of the city rests."

However perilous, the Orphics remained committed to their rigid dietary code and other acts of purification, aspiring to free themselves from the shackles of the human body. Yet how tremendously ironic that this ascetic vegetarian sect arose out of the riotous cult of Dionysus, whose radical female worshippers—the Maenads or "mad ones"—swilled copious wine while roaming the Greek countryside smashed out of their gourds. Dancing themselves into orgasmic frenzies, they experienced ecstatic states that the rational mind cannot grasp. Upon reaching a zenith of primal and sexual ecstasy, they would tear into live animals and devour them raw. For animals contain the god spark, they fervently believed, and by bodily merging with them, a holy union with both gods and beasts was possible.

"They escape the human condition by way of bestiality, taking the lower route among the animals," explains Detienne, "while Orphism proposes the same escape on the divine side, taking the upper route by refusing the meat diet that spills the blood of living beings and eating only perfectly pure food."

Has anything changed, really, as these contending belief systems continue their reach through the centuries? Today we have the austere, ethereal vegans—philosophical descendants of frugal monastic types and still very much a micro-minority—firmly believing that to eat animals is not only unnecessary and impure but against nature's sacred, peaceful plan. Pitted against them are the earthy and exuberant flesh-eaters. Most now cook their meat, true—occasionally in ritualistic barbeque-style out on the back deck—yet in a very primordial way, they are the descendants of both Dionysus and our ancient hunting ancestors: humans who believed that animals are nourishment provided by the gods, that they embody the mystical life force and to join our flesh with theirs is a most natural deed, an act of communion with the universal spirit of nature. And while it's true that most of today's meat eaters would be incapable of articulating why they act as they do, the word "enthusiasm" definitely comes to mind as we watch them rip into juicy ribs of beef or gnaw on succulent, blood-tinged pork chops with open-mouthed gusto and elation. *Enthusiasm*, in fact, derives from the Greek *enthousiasmos,* whose archaic meaning is "extravagant religious emotion."

What's more, historians continue to be captivated by the striking similarities between the flesh sacrifices of Dionysian rituals and those of Jesus, as reenacted in the Christian communion. For true believers, the god Dionysus actually existed in the wine and flesh consumed with such wild passion and reverence. Likewise for stalwart Christians: the body and blood of Christ are truly present in the communion bread and wine: *Take, eat; this is my body; do this in remembrance of me….Drink….for this is my blood of the covenant, which is poured out for many for the forgiveness of sins.* Note the uncanny resemblance between Christ's words and those from the Mithraic mystery religion practiced in Rome during this same era, whose primary icon was the god Mithra slaughtering a bull: *He who will not eat of my body and drink of my blood, so that he will be made one with me and I with him, the same shall not know salvation.*

EVENTUALLY THE VEG ORPHICS blended with the veg Pythags and what came to be known as the Pythagorean Diet or "vegetable regime" largely went underground as Christianity swelled in scope and influence. Officially recognized by Constantine in AD 313, this new Jesus-reigns religion had a disastrous effect on the West's nascent animal rights movement. Because Christianity heavily promoted human supremacy over all other living creatures, meat abstention was seen as a defiant act against God. Vegetarians were reviled and persecuted, and Saint Augustine's famous 4th century statement on animals, echoing Aristotle—"they are meant for our use, dead or alive"—set the mandate for the next 2,000 years.

The Catholic Church, expanding in power century by century, did sponsor meatless days but this had nothing to do with ethics, not animal ethics anyway. In a manner that apparently only celibate male priests can understand and preach, an excess of meat was believed to stimulate carnal lust and dampen humility. (Fish was fine because it wasn't considered "meat" and was equated with Jesus and piety.) Besides lust-control, cost-cutting was another big factor in these no-meat days, as animal flesh was becoming increasingly scarce and expensive. By the Middle Ages, average blokes who were fortunate enough to own a few livestock practically slept with their animals—flies, feces, and all—and didn't look at them as sensitive, sentient creatures to be petted and coddled but, rather, as essential protein for their family. They were slaughtered to feed hungry children. But as the price of livestock and animal flesh kept rising, meat emerged as the province of the wealthy, often in disgusting excess.

By the early Renaissance, a few nonconformists—notably the Dutch humanist Erasmus and French essayist Montaigne—began to bravely speak out against the lavish gluttony of the flesh-eating upper classes, as well as the "blood sport" of hunting (echoed in England's popular 2004 ban on fox hunting). Yet, however forcefully and emotively these mavericks campaigned against the mistreatment of animals, guess what? Not one gave up eating them. Two centuries later, Rousseau declared, "Humans, be humane! It is your first duty." And the French humanist Voltaire wrote vociferously against cruelty to animals and the "frightful inconsistency to believe that animals feel and at the same time to cause them to suffer." Inconsistency is right. Exactly like Rousseau, this wanna-be animal liberationist continued to enjoy his choice-cut beef and mutton in private. Of all the so-called veg-celebs of the 15-18th centuries, Leonardo da Vinci probably came closest to being vegetarian in both word and deed, vowing to never allow his body become "a tomb for other animals, an inn of the dead.....a container of corruption."

The most influential vegetarian you've probably never heard of was a pugnacious Englishman named Joseph Ritson (1752-1803), the first to extend the idea of "rights" to animals. Ritson avidly proclaimed that all life has value and mustn't be exploited or destroyed. He insisted that flesh-eating is unnatural to human physiology, that a diet of blood coarsens the mind and "disposes men to cruel and ferocious actions," a belief echoed in the meat-creates-lust-and-violence fallacy that, although bogus and unproven, persists among today's peace-loving vegans.

"Meat Eating Makes You a Violent Sex Criminal!" a veg blog screams. Yet if the alternative encourages a peaceful disposition, what then shall we make of the murderous Roman gladiators, superstar athletes who dined on leeks and barley? Or the brutal Roman legions, likewise vegetarians according to historians, who conquered the world while eating coarse wheat porridge. (And for a scholarly review of Nazi vegetarianism, read Boria Sax's *Animals in the Third Reich*.) Evidently, just like some of today's vegans, Ritson didn't know his world history all that well, when he asserted that flesh-eating disposes humans to vicious acts: "a fact to which the experience of ages gives ample testimony." Hmm. Was the Buddha cruel? Was Jesus ferocious? How about the saintly and selfless Mother Teresa who regularly and gratefully partook of meat? Or the benevolent Lamas of Tibet who do the same? Let's finally bury this fallacious argument. Human beings—their physiology and psychology—are infinitely more complex than vegans want them to be.

SINCE SO MUCH EARLY ADVOCACY involved preaching without real practicing, vegetarianism didn't arrive as an authentic social movement until the turn of the 19th century, largely due to the influence of radical atheist, militant socialist, and sublime Romantic poet (*sigh*) Percy Bysshe Shelley. Though his poetry has much to do with nature, art, beauty and the prophetic tormented poet—and very little to do with animals—it was the handsome, idealistic Shelley who breathed new life into a floundering movement and greatly influenced succeeding generations of ethical vegetarians and vegans.

In *A Vindication of Natural Diet,* Shelley feverishly argued that vegetarianism is humanity's natural food regime, advancing health and long life while freeing animals from suffering. (Unfortunately, he wasn't able to self-test his longevity theory, drowning at age 29.) Pre-dating today's raw foodists, Shelley blamed Prometheus and the discovery of fire for our fallen nature: "It is only by softening and disguising dead flesh by culinary preparation….that the sight of its bloody juices and raw horror does not excite intolerable loathing and disgust. Let the advocate of animal food force himself to a decisive experiment on its fitness and, as Plutarch recommends, tear a living lamb with his teeth, and plunging his head into its vitals, slake his thirst with the steaming blood."

Many consider Shelley's over the top essay the best-ever written argument for abstention and if George Bernard Shaw had gotten his way, we'd all be calling vegetarianism "Shelleyism" to this day. This would have proven a very peculiar tribute to a man who supped on "bread and raisins" while home in England but is known to have indulged in flesh-eating while traveling abroad. *Ironically, Shelley himself might be one of the best-ever arguments for following an omnivorous diet.* Suffering from poor health and serious depression for nearly all of his adult (vegetarian) life, Shelley was so exhausted after a rowing trip, he broke down and gorged on three mutton chops one after the other. Following a second boating trip and plentiful meat, an accompanying friend testified that the poet demonstrated "renewed enjoyment in life," according to historian Rod Preece. So was Shelley a loathsome hypocrite and sloth, as animal rightists love to call turncoats? Or just another fat-and-protein starved vegetarian?

Fortunately, Shaw never got his wish and the Pythagorean diet officially became "vegetarianism" at an 1847 meeting of the soon-to-be-birthed Vegetarian Society in Ramsgate, England. Health, animal welfare and, rather surprisingly, the environment were discussed at the Society's inaugural meeting, attended by 140 brave citizens. "Animal flesh is both unnecessary and unhealthy" emerged as the society's primary message; humans, animals, and the land are much better served by vegetable production. If not overtly hostile, the public was certainly skeptical of these eccentrics on the outskirts of England's meat and potatoes diet.

Not exactly going gangbusters, the Vegetarian Society's membership sank to 125 by 1870. It didn't help that the Society's first president, James Simpson, died a mere 12 years after its founding at the relatively young age of 48. The fledgling Society couldn't have dreamed up worse publicity for its cause. *The Manchester City News* described Simpson in pitiful terms: "of a weakly and delicate constitution.....a poor specimen of humanity." And although Simpson always insisted that his diet had nothing to do with his illness, the public thought otherwise—regularly supping on hearty beef broth would surely have saved him.

Yet the movement persevered and by the turn of the century membership had ascended to 3,000, with an amazing 30 vegetarian restaurants thriving in greater London (still a hub for veg'n eateries), with bucolic names like The Garden and The Apple Tree. Many were frequented by single women who felt unwelcome elsewhere (a woman dining alone in public in 1900 possessed "questionable" morals). Vegetarianism was finally making its way into the urban middle class and, exactly like today, bold young females comprised its advance guard.

By this time, acclaimed literary figures like Leo Tolstoy and George Bernard Shaw were moving western vegetarianism ever closer to respectability. An ardent socialist and self-proclaimed misfit, Shaw turned out to be a mixed blessing for the animal rights cause. Though he was fond of labeling meat-eating "cannibalism with its heroic dish omitted," Shaw's printed hand-out on vegetarianism very clearly stated: "If we do not kill animals they will kill us.....rabbits, tigers, cobras, locusts, white ants, rats, mosquitoes, fleas and deer must be continuously slain even to extermination by vegetarians, as ruthlessly as by meat-eaters." What's been biting you in the deep, dark middle of the night, George?

A DECIDEDLY DISSIDENT movement at the start of the 20th century, western vegetarianism remained a faction of distrusted outsiders for another 100 years. In many rural and cultural enclaves, it still is. Dan Haran knows how it feels to be ridiculed as a societal outsider. He cites "a very high social cost" as the reason he abandoned the meatless lifestyle after enlisting at age 20 for environmental and health reasons. Dan is not alone. In a *Psychology Today* survey, social stigma was cited as the second leading cause, after poor health, for giving up all forms of vegetarianism (Herzog). And it's not only the eye-rolling and tongue-clucking that might greet a new plant-eater in a meat-loving family; these can be tolerated. It's the ensuing, often unspoken alienation that "will often do [veg'ns] more harm than the food they would consume to keep the peace," writes Haran. "I'm not just thinking the occasional Thanksgiving lapse to please the parental units. There's also the job interview, dates, sales calls and everyday social engagements [and] refusing food from someone who cooked it surely is horrible karma."

While the public has become much more accepting of vegetarians, and even vegans, in recent years due to an upsurge of well-crafted marketing, the movement will never swallow up mainstream society. It will fail in this ambitious goal not because it is an injurious diet for some and too difficult a diet for others—both of which are true—but because it is too anti-culture. Across the globe, loyalty to kin and kind, to our ethnic traditions, is deeply ingrained in the human psyche. And along with these behavioral factors, come genetic and metabolic determinants as well.

Sea-blessed Sicilians will never willingly give up their anchovies and calamari, nor Louisianans their ham and shrimp jambalaya. And you won't find West Africans exchanging their *kansiyé*, a rich lamb or beef stew, for mock chili concocted from processed soy. Cast off these family and tribal traditions and, as the Orphics, Pythagoreans, Essenes and Dan Haran experienced, you are swiftly an outsider, one with little real chance of convincing the other 97% to mutiny their cultural diet. Yet try telling that to a passionate new vegan. They are as deaf to familial admonishments, as potentially blind to their own body's metabolic reality as I once was. Young and idealistic, we are renegades with a righteous cause and none shall dissuade us!

17.

TO KILL OR NOT TO KILL

Who killed the pork chops? What price bananas? Are you my Angel?

—Allen Ginsberg

WITH MY NEWLY ACQUIRED, albeit unadmired vegetarian status, the rebel in me came full circle. First memory, age two: leaping out of the bathtub to run doe naked through our staid, middle-class neighborhood, hollering mom in full chase. Not for the sake of angering my parents did I do this, but because it felt so good and so right! And that's why most of us choose to break our meaty traditions: not as some defiant anti-authoritarian gesture but because it feels good and right to do whatever we can, in whatever small way, to prevent the suffering of animals.

What turns one bacon-loving kid into a vegetarian but not her classmate? Why will one child gently toss an unassuming beetle out the window, while another will mirthfully stomp it to smithereens? For many it's the innate, often spiritual connection we feel with non-human animals. We love hanging out with them and, simply put, regard them as our kin. Not in the Pythagorean sense of human souls suddenly plopping into animal bodies, but in a real-time, biological sense. As co-inhabitants on this earth, we are all deserving of respect. Evolution binds us even tighter. Although far from noble as relations go, every living being now on earth descended from a single-celled LUA, last universal ancestor, alive 3.5 billion years ago. Proof from science of the kinship we instinctively feel.

Just like da Vinci, who sneakily released birds from market cages, or Shelley, who purchased crawfish only to throw them back into the river, most pre-veggies start out quite young in their quest to liberate animals from pain and constraint. Dashing onto highways to grab plodding turtles. Releasing frantic mice from no-kill traps and pedaling them to grassy fields far, far away (only to be replaced by a dozen more). In third grade I ratted on Johnny Sandman for ripping earthworms

100

in half during recess, shoving them down his throat to impress all the screeching girls with his afternoon snack (strange kid). To be free and fully alive in nature was my own wild, true desire and I realized that all animals—at least those not thoroughly dulled by domestication—keenly desire this too.

Concern for non-human animals includes the small and the scorned. If bees, butterflies, or even gnats lie water-slogged on the surface of a swimming pool, we will cautiously set them back on dry land and with our own warm breath, blow life and flight back into their fragile bodies, into their wet delicate wings. Some vegans won't even kill a fly, no matter how many pathogens they're carrying. Mosquitoes, though, really test one's critter ethics. They are mini-vampires, indiscriminately sucking blood, right? Actually, they're after your jamba juice so they can lay healthy eggs and perpetuate the species, following nature's dictum. But they do carry deadly viruses and even the most moral vegan, one can only hope, would squash a skeeter hovering over a human baby.

Disease carriers and vampires excepted, you either try to preserve the life all around you or you just don't care. It's not nearly so glamorous or heart-stopping, but interspecies respect has existed alongside cock fights, bullfights, and blood-splattered gladiator dens throughout human history. Our western animal rights movement didn't appear out of nowhere. A high regard for animals, even animal worship, commenced far back in prehistory. Ancient Egyptians celebrated the fighting spirit of the bull, while early societies in the Indus Valley honored tigers and elephants. And by the time the Rig Vega was written, circa 1200 BC, the cow had emerged as the most sacred animal for Hindis, "the mother of all life."

For Native Americans, wild animals have long been allies and guardians, and medieval artists created *bestiaries*, finely illustrated compendiums of beasts, both native and imaginary, with each animal representing a different Christian virtue. Kindness to animals is legendary among the medieval saints, especially Saint Francis of Assisi, whom biographer Thomas of Celano described as a man of "great tenderness toward lower and irrational creatures; he called all creatures *brother*." Today, feisty members of PETA risk jail time to ambush board meetings and G-20 international summits. They go undercover at research labs and factory farms to document abuse, slamming corporations and universities with lawsuits that allege "unspeakable suffering" and "corporate denial."

From pre-history to PETA, it all sounds so virtuous and admirable, doesn't it? In reality, human-animal relations are often paradoxical and complex. For many of these cultural groups, respect for animal life was not applied equally to all species, nor did it necessarily exclude consuming an esteemed animal for dinner. Totemism and its reverence for all life hasn't stopped tribal warring, and India's precious cow, idealized for its life-sustaining milk, is often treated quite poorly (stolen from the streets and sold to illegal butchers). Because she can feed us even after her life ends, not just the first few years, even Gandhi believed that "Mother cow is in many ways better than the mother who gave us birth….Mother cow is as useful dead as alive" (Jha). And while Native Americans venerated all bison, they also quite happily devoured them. Even gentle Francis gladly ate the meat of his animal brothers, abstaining only on compulsory fast days, and contemporary Franciscans are not vegetarians. In nearly every case, it's not only cultural beliefs and traditions but honest protein hunger that determines if, when, and which animals will be eaten.

Only the latter day PETA-type vegans have radically split from their cultural base to not simply revere all animals, but to refuse to ever eat or utilize any part of them. In this way they follow in the footsteps of—hardly anybody. Who they most closely resemble are those historically tiny, scattered enclaves of religious zealots who broke with societal norms, risking alienation and condemnation (the disdain heaped upon the PETA crowd is well documented) in order to forge a daring new path on the fringes of the cultural mainstream.

Despite my own unswayable decision to break with tradition, *of course* I sat down to supper with my flesh-eating family. I just skipped the gross meat and greasy gravy and chowed down on everything green, rooty and fruity, especially those scrumptious coconut-cream pies. Back then, nothing special was planned for any veggies who dined with omnivorous relatives. We simply hoped to find enough alternative nourishment on the table.

Because I knew in my heart I was participating in the healthiest, most ethical diet on the planet, it annoyed me to no end that my mother worried out loud I wasn't getting proper sustenance and variety in my new diet—enough calories, protein, and good fat. Crazy how often our moms turn out to be right.

18.

WHAT ARE VEGANS EATING, *REALLY?*

DINNER MENU FOR THE EVENING

Vegetable soup, brown bread and rice, vegetarian pie, potatoes, cauliflower with white sauce, stewed gooseberries, stewed rhubarb & sago pudding

A CHIC VEGAN BANQUET in 21st century America? Actually, no, it's the three course meal sponsored in 1876 by one of London's first vegetarian restaurants, the People's Café Company on Farringdon Road. This "experimental dinner" cost a bit over a shilling—about thirty cents—and is notable for its sheer abundance of carbohydrates and near total exclusion of protein and fat. Witnesses commented on both the skinny bodies and huge appetites of the vegetarians in attendance, all of whom happily gorged on this nutritionally imbalanced feast.

Flash forward to 2016 and a fashionable new restaurant serving house-brewed ale just west of Denver. The vegetarians at my table are once again indulging in— CARB HEAVEN! Has anything really changed in over 140 years? Perhaps not. The last vegan I ate out with, just days ago, ordered a kale salad and French fries for dinner. (He has a PhD but obviously not in nutrition.) Earlier I met friends for lunch at a trendy, health-conscious, fill-your-own-bowl kind of cantina. All the omnivores tanked up on fresh greens, red quinoa, chopped veggies and sensible portions of chicken or fish. Everyone that is except Tiffany, a vegan who brought her own meal: dark chocolate and a pear. Yes, that was her dinner. Sadly, I was reminded of Tolstoy's vegetarian regime: fruit jellies, porridge, and preserves.

Hoping this was an arrant aberration, I decided to shadow vegans for several months at my home town's healthiest hotspots. I wanted to answer one burning question: Are today's plant eaters, by and large, still ingesting carbo-loaded, fat and protein-deficient fare? I'm not aware of any individual or organization that's gathered first-hand, reliable field data on this important subject, although the

USDA, T. Colin Campbell, or someone's mother certainly should. Hopefully, my own telling observations will get somebody cooking on this vital research project.

Since empirical evidence begins with clear-eyed observation, for decades now I've been secretly scrutinizing what my veggie friends put in their mouths, and the results are not pretty. To be truthful, as I gained in nutritional knowledge over time, I became more and more aghast at their food choices. Thus, my decision to widen my investigation and discover if today's new crop of devout vegans are still stick-thin, packing in the carbs, and incessantly hungry the way I always was, the way those 1876 diners apparently were. Staking out non-animal eaters in public dining places, I surreptitiously recorded their actual meal intakes, *something researchers rarely if ever do*. Fortunately, I live in the ideal town for veggie voyeurism.

So right now I'm sitting at my frequent lunch stop, the crowded deli café at Boulder's Whole Foods Market. Guarding my little table like a pit bull is more like it. I was lucky to even find one, nabbing it with some embarrassment while two sporty-looking women in lightweight running shoes were still gathering up their compostable bowls, before sprinting off to some nearby mountain trails. Unless you've been living in a cave in Kashmir, you know that Whole Foods sells more organic victuals in its 360-plus stores than any other retailer on the planet, raking in $15 billion annually. Its overflowing food bars offer oodles more vegan fare than carnivore dishes (although paleo is fast making inroads around here). Thus, it's the perfect location for my discreet, whole-meal observations.

While engaged in veggie-tracking missions, I am able to record only the easily spied upon, i.e., plant eaters who sit nearby, their food choices clearly visible. Early on, I decided not to don trench coat and low-slung cap and turn into a table-wandering voyeur, sashaying bug-eyed past peopled tables, obnoxious notebook in hand. No, I was discreet and polite but did emerge a master of the sidelong glance and enigmatic smile. So here are my noon hour observations on this brisk autumn day: a pale young woman dining on broccoli and sweet potatoes (only); an energetic young man digging into his lunch of raw greens, yellow peppers, and cauliflower; a middle-aged mom slurping potato-leek soup (hefty hoard of wheat rolls on the side); a bored child playing ring-toss with her macaroni and cheese; and two impossibly leggy teenagers nibbling on blue chips and coleslaw. Granted these people may not be strict vegans but they *are* consuming strictly non-animal meals that contain a lopsided amount of carbs, including, for many of them, juice blends with sky-high natural sugar loads: up to 45 grams per 12-ounce bottle.

Now I'm off to record veg lunches at Alfalfa's, a top-notch independent grocer just down the hill from the U of Colorado campus. It too caters to the young and health-wise, two of whom are seated near me at this round communal table. The beautiful, doe-eyed 20s female is eating rice and cucumber sushi while chatting about meditation's simplicity. Meanwhile, the beautiful, strong-jawed 40s male right beside her is elucidating esoteric astrology while dining on dried seaweed and four varieties of fresh fruit, swished down with steaming Tulsi tea. (Boulder has a lot of beautiful people who eat seaweed and sushi.) That's the extent of their meals. Where's the fat and protein? Now hold on, you say, surely they obtained these essential macronutrients during breakfast. Possibly. Yet breakfast for every vegan I've ever known is cereal or granola with a splash of soy or almond milk, often just a bagel with coffee or juice. No significant protein. No significant fat. Carb City.

Okay, I've just spotted another plant eater, a slim female with long raven hair, around 30, wickedly attractive. Here's her chosen meal: vegetable minestrone soup, a loaf of artisan whole-grain bread (dispatched by the fistful), a raspberry filled pastry of considerable dimensions, and blueberry-pomegranate iced tea (25 grams of sugar per can). I ladle up some of that minestrone soup to check for protein and find just a few dozen white beans swimming in the entire enormous pot. So altogether we're looking at an estimated 130 grams of carbs and astonishingly little protein or fat in this particular vegan meal. (I didn't stick around to see if she consumed the entire loaf of bread, half-demolished when I left.) Other no-animal eaters cunningly observed at Alfalfa's: three college-age friends wolfing down mushroom pesto pizza; two chatty females enjoying apple-pecan arugula salads and creamy pumpkin soup; a quiet, middle-aged twosome quaffing more of that few-beans soup (along with chocolate chip cookies as wide as your face); plus an older gent eating white rice, black olives and....what?? Popcorn. I did spot one no-meater tossing edamame beans into her open mouth. Protein—yes!

Next, a pit-stop at Julia's Kitchen, a minimalist gluten-free café that advertises "raw cashew-coconut macaroons, raw fig bars, sourdough bread, and sprouted grain crackers." Hmm, what have we here in the front dining room? (Excuse me while I yawn and put away my magnifying glass.) Yep, basically the same thing all over again. The plant eaters I'm close enough to monitor are tanking out on carbs. Granted, these people may not be vegans; nor can we extrapolate any firm conclusions from the limited number of individuals presented here. (Although I've read published vegan "research" on as few as six people, seriously, and most studies collect no data on specific meals eaten.) But I've been conducting these observations for years and always come up with the same result: Carb Overload. Nutritionist Nadia Petrova of *Daily Raw* offers similar testimony about her vegan clients: "The truth is that for the past years I have seen them make so many mistakes that it's hard to say some of them eat healthy at all." So take a good look around for yourself and report back to me.

While scrupulously recording actual vegan food choices does not a scientific study make, nobody else seems to be doing it—or *any* substantial research exclusively on plant eaters and their life-long health results. Even pro-veg Dr. Winston Craig admits that too few studies exist on too few people for any definitive conclusions about vegan health and disease outcomes. So yes, *please,* let's launch that respected cohort study on 30,000 vegans followed for 30 years, so young people taking up this dicey new diet will understand what they're up against.

CARBOHYDRATES ARE SUGAR. Whether you are taking in simple or complex carbs, high-glycemic or low, your body doesn't discriminate when it breaks them down into simple glucose in your digestive tract where it's absorbed into your bloodstream. That's why eating excessively high-carb meals day after day, year after year, is a sure way to consistently raise blood sugar levels, impacting your glucose metabolism and paving the way to possible insulin resistance down the metabolic road. With this condition, your body is no longer able to properly unload sugar from the bloodstream, creating havoc with your health.

It's true that low-glycemic carbs don't raise blood sugar levels as fast, but it's crucial to understand that although the extent and timing varies, *all* carbs except pure dietary fiber will elevate your blood sugar, stimulating insulin production. Therefore, *the total amount of carbohydrates* eaten per meal or snack is just as important as glycemic index in determining blood glucose levels and insulin response. (Dietary fat and protein help keep levels stable.) Together, carb quality *and* quantity determine your *glycemic load*, and that's why carbohydrate awareness at every meal is essential.

The nastiest culprit is highly concentrated fructose—avoid it like the metabolic devil it is. While glucose is used by every cell in your body, fructose goes straight to the liver where an excess has been implicated in hypertension, higher insulin response, and increased risk for heart disease. High-fructose corn syrup is 55% fructose, but agave syrup, heavily marketed as a health food for vegans, is up to

106

90% fructose. Oh, you didn't know that? Hoping to find a safe sugar substitute, the Glycemic Research Institute conducted trials using agave but had to cut them short due to severe side effects in diabetics: one group passed out after ingestion and had to be rushed to the hospital. The Institute has now de-listed and outright banned agave, and companies who produce it or use it in their products are legally liable for any negative health results. Vegans, beware Madison Avenue.

Don't get me wrong. You need carbs, your body's preferred energy source, but for proper metabolism you need not only the right kind but the right amount, not an overload. So even if you forego those nasty media-pushed foods in favor of fruits, veggies and whole grains, a high carb diet carries health risks. And those 100% juices you think are so healthy? Most are bomb-loaded with natural sugar but with zero fiber to buffer a sharp glycemic spike. Any vitamins or antioxidants they offer don't begin to make up for their high fructose content, sometimes more than a can of blood-sugar-crashing soda.

If followed for years, excess daily carb consumption not only trashes your metabolism, it will accelerate the aging of your immune and hormonal systems. "Sugar interferes with the use of nutrients and damages your metabolism on a cellular level," warns Dr. Diane Schwarzbein. "Eating an excess of carbohydrates can cause cancer by increasing insulin levels and other potent growth hormones while at the same time damaging cellular DNA faster because excess sugar is an oxidant." Think of iron rusting and disintegrating. That's oxidative stress and it damages protein and fat as well as DNA, and damaged DNA can lead to cancer. An explosion of new research confirms the link between high-carb/high glycemic loads and increased risk for breast, pancreatic, and other cancers. Meanwhile, a *low-carb* diet that includes enough vegetables was found to be protective (Fung).

You might also start losing your mind, literally, with excess carb consumption. Research confirms that atrophy in the brain's memory center, the hippocampus, is associated with the elevated fasting glucose levels created by high grain and sugar intake (Cherbuin). Your brain actually begins to shrink when you eat too much of this stuff. Not a pretty picture—especially if you are no longer able to conjure it. And fasting glucose levels don't even have to be that high to affect brain cells, prompting study authors to state that the concept of normal blood glucose levels may need to be reevaluated, along with the definition of diabetes.

High glucose levels also increase your susceptibility to a destructive process called glycation, the bonding of amino acids to sugar molecules. These abnormal proteins can wreak havoc to the collagen in your skin. It's called wrinkles and high-carb eaters may be shocked how damn early they start to show up. Glycation also contributes to the onset of dementia, assert the authors of "Nutrition and Alzheimer's Disease: the detrimental role of a high carbohydrate diet" (Seneff). Individuals who follow a high-carb diet are *four times* more likely to develop cognitive impairment, a precursor to Alzheimer's. Proteins and good fats offer important protection; individuals who get plentiful amounts of both in their daily meals are less likely to suffer cognitive decline and dementia (Roberts). David Perlmutter, MD, calls a high-carb diet "among the most prominent stimulators of inflammation pathways that reach the brain."

SO WHY ARE VEGANS chomping so many carbs? For several not so great reasons. First, without animal food, their protein-dense sources are much more limited, ditto their hunger-satiating fat sources. This leaves ubiquitous carbs to fill the hunger and nutritional void. And unlike with protein and fat, wherein your body signals satiation early-on, there is no such biofeedback mechanism with carbs. They move quickly out of your stomach and have to complete the entire digestion/absorption process before your brain finally stops sending its anxious *feed me now!* signals. By then you've inhaled an entire bag of chili corn chips. What's more, research implicates carbohydrates with addictive eating patterns. Processed carbs in particular stimulate the same craving and reward center of the brain that lights up in alcoholics and crack addicts.

But you can be eating whole grains, especially wheat, and still be a carb addict. That's because modern wheat—including whole-wheat, organic, and sprouted—is an opiate that stimulates your appetite and cravings for *more, more, more*—hence my numerous Whole Loaf observations of vegan eating patterns. Go a few hours without wheat and an addict will become "nervous, foggy, tremulous, and start desperately seeking out another hit of crackers, bagels or bread, even if it's the few stale 3-month old crackers at the bottom of the box," warns cardiologist Dr. William Davis, who calls today's modified whole grains "destructive genetic monsters." Genetic engineering is an inexact science at best and when the protein gliadin was inadvertently altered by geneticists trying to increase wheat yield, this increased the appetite-stimulating properties of wheat as well. So now we have gazillions of humans, including every vegetarian and vegan I personally know, addicted to this powerful eat-me-now modern grain that raises blood sugar levels higher than Hershey's Kisses.

108

Yet vegan authors and activists continue to praise a high-carbohydrate diet, noting that government nutrition guidelines since 1980 have swung in their favor, emphasizing more veggies, fruits, grains and plant oils. (*While failing to note that during this same period, the prevalence of stroke and heart failure increased dramatically; rates of new cases of all cancers rose; and diabetes rates tripled.*) These same activists point to vegan dieticians' advice that 55-75% of our daily calories should derive from carbs, a higher amount than the Institute of Medicine recommends. Meanwhile, some raw vegans and athletes are pushing an ultra-high carb regime, 80-10-10, created by chiropractor and banana lover Doug Graham: 80% fruits and vegetables, 10% protein, and 10% fat. Adherents love to argue about the value of achieving such an extreme ratio and exactly how to do it. "You can generally accomplish this with two or three large fruit meals during the day," counsels Dr. Graham, "plus a large salad in the evening."

Excuse me? Cutting down on grains is a good idea but just the thought of consuming that much fructose, glucose and fruity fiber sends my blood sugar soaring, pancreas pumping, and anus protesting. *Yech!!* (Or, as one practitioner described it: "OMG, all I do all day is eat, drink, pee and poo. No time for dating!") Moreover, modern hybridized fruits are far bigger and sweeter than their wild versions, perpetuating a metabolic state dependent on sugars, according to Dr. Peter Havel, who has been studying the effects of sugar in its various forms for over 20 years. Fructose leads to fat accumulation around our internal organs, Havel discovered, a key risk factor for insulin resistance and chronic diseases like type 2 diabetes.

ONLY TIME WILL REVEAL the long-term health results of today's high-carb, high-plants diets; however, once-vocal supporters have already bailed. "For years I advocated a plant-based diet as the healthiest," confesses an ex-vegan on *Open Mind Required*. "I am coming to believe that a high-carbohydrate diet is harmful over the long haul, and a high-fruit diet is possibly the worst....It's disconcerting to find that what I've believed the past five years might be way off base."

Meanwhile, historically tested diets call for moderation: 40-60% carbs along with sufficient intake of protein and fat for your lifestyle and unique needs (you are not Doug Graham; you are not Martina Navratilova). Endorsing an anti-inflammatory diet, Dr. Andrew Weil advises that just 40-50% of your calories derive from carbs, low or moderate on the glycemic index. Furthermore, you should start every day with a well-balanced mix of all three macronutrients, *not* a bowl of granola and bananas.

Not only breakfast, all your meals should be a balance of high-quality protein and fat, plus complex carbohydrates. Even your snacks shouldn't be stand-alone carbs—eat hummus or cheese with that Gala apple to prevent a blood sugar spike. When eaten alongside carbs, dietary fat slows glucose absorption and the protein augments insulin release, increasing the clearance of glucose from your blood and promoting the uptake of amino acids. And while I've read articles by vegans who claim they plan every day's meals to obtain all the nutrients needed to function at optimal levels, most seem to be doing what my friends and I did—winging it. They figure they're eating healthy organic food all day long, so why worry?

And often they *are* eating healthy food, just too much of the same thing. As my ongoing veggie voyeurism confirms, mountains of creamy carrot muffins are being ravaged out there in Veg World, as well as fudge pecan cookies and pasta primavera. These are obvious culprits, but what about quinoa casserole with corn and zucchini, or simple brown rice and beans? Don't be misled: rice, quinoa, corn, even beans and almost all legumes are first and foremost carb foods. Veg'n sponsors who call grains and non-soy legumes primarily protein foods are misleading a bunch of folks.

Beans are, in fact, very high in carbs—pinto beans have a whooping 45 grams per cooked cup, three times its protein content. It's a mildly inflammatory food that raises your blood sugar. Medium-grain brown rice is higher still: 46 grams of carbs per cup with a mere 5 grams of protein, a 9 to 1 ratio. Even quinoa delivers 39 carb grams per cooked cup to just 8 grams of protein, a 5 to 1 ratio. Sure, there's essential protein and fiber in the aforementioned fare but the vast majority of grams belong to one food group. Always remember: *If it raises your blood sugar, it's a carb.*

Carbo-inhalers or pastatarians, as they've been aptly dubbed, don't seem to be counting their daily protein and fat intake. And that's a problem. And the greater problem is a lot of them don't seem to know there's a problem....until 15 or 20 years down the metabolic road and they're staring down a protein or fat deficit, along with other possible deleterious consequences from an imbalanced diet.

WHAT'S FANTASTIC IS that you *can* lower your carb intake on a vegetarian or vegan diet, *if* your choices are conscious and smart. Whether it's Ann Arbor, Middlebury or Santa Cruz, veg'ns tend to live in progressive college towns teeming with alternative markets. But step out of Whole Foods Village and it's not always so easy to find abundant and varied choices.

110

Beyond my own Boulder Bubble—"25 square miles surrounded by reality"—it can still be downright tricky to find wholesome veg meals, and forget organic. I'm talking road romps through South Dakota, annual trips to your Jewish in-laws for a Passover Seder, and summer stopovers at Aunt Jenn and Uncle Bill's during an impromptu pig roast. Many a starving vegetarian has dined on green bean casserole and honeyed yams during the high holidays, or succumbed to past-prime Pizza Hut salad bars while motoring through southern Kansas. I love traveling the gravelly backroads in my dinged-up Chevy S-10 but dining out in rural Wyoming or Oklahoma is *not* conducive to securing well-balanced veg'n meals.

Their pleasant but teensy grocery stores invariably feature last week's grapes, mottled head lettuce, and a half-dozen shrunken green peppers harboring suspect lesions. Searching for protein options can be even more painful. When I inquired after the missing tofu at a village market, the sturdy, pork-fed stockboy frowned, squinted at me suspiciously, then went right back to stocking Hungry Man frozen dinners.

Hoping to find a reasonably nutritious café in central Nebraska, I ambled into the only business on Main Street showing signs of life, the Bullet Hole Bar, and politely asked where the nearest restaurant might be that catered to vegetarians. The very ample, white-aproned proprietor looked my skinny self up and down—as if she wouldn't mind putting that bullet hole through me herself—then scornfully pointed east. What's over there? I innocently asked. "New York City," she said, pokerfaced. "If you leave right now, you can get there by daybreak."

19.

LIEBIG AND 15 CUPS OF RICE

ARE YOU TOO FINDING it difficult to be a 24/7 honest, healthy veg'n? Trust me, it could be far worse. Imagine yourself surrounded by never-ending corn fields and giant stinky pig farms. It's late 70s central Illinois, bastion of conservatism, and you're galaxies away from the cultural sophistication of Chicago, light-years from the radicalizing influence of Madison. Yet even in that liberal Wisconsin city, you'd have been hard pressed to find the kind of veggie fare we now take for granted. Unless you had access to the rare oriental market, soy products were just about non-existent. My own prairie state produced 300 million bushels of soybeans annually at the time, yet most Illinois natives couldn't fathom joining the cattle, chickens, and voracious hogs in actually eating them.

So go ahead and close your eyes and try to picture this: no tofu, no tempeh, no soy cheese, no soy milk. And no almond, hazelnut, or coconut milk either. Zero soy-saturated energy bars to pull you through that late afternoon work fizzle. Zilch powdered supplements from the highly sought-after hemp plant, and forget about green smoothies whipped up with chlorella. Scratch rice and pea protein supplements. Amaranth, millet, chickpea or quinoa? Nope, not in my town. Ditto for mock meat sizzling on the outdoor grill. We ate real food where I grew up. *Vegetable burgers, ha ha ha! What kind of sick joke is that?* So what was a loyal plant-eater to do?

Back in Champaign-Urbana, my vegetarian options creaked open by way of Strawberry Fields, an unassuming clapboard farmhouse turned health food store. Its quintessential prairie-porch overflowed with local produce, and its bulk bins exploded with—brain-boggling at the time—five varieties of granola! Tucked next to a U of I practice football field, it was two blocks from the 7/11 and the only veg game in town. It was here, and only here, that a few hundred wannabe hippies scored our organic brown rice (white rice was detestable, for the ignorant masses), along with our snap beans, summer squash, and luscious fat tomatoes— as only the hot, sweaty Midwest can create them.

Home was a rundown brick mansion on Green Street, filled with eclectic art students and moody poet-drifters. I shared the third floor with Ramona—a wild and sagacious Scotch-drinking dancer with ice-blue fiery eyes and a penchant for black jazz musicians—along with two brilliant, gleeful, large-breasted lesbians. One of whom tried to convince me I'd make a good butch. *Wrong.* (The fact that I carried a comb in my jeans' back pocket turned her on, and yes, I am fascinated by voluptuous Rubenesque women of any sexual orientation, myself being any-thing but.) These were big women, big meat eaters who got a hoot out of vegetar-ians and an even bigger hoot out of a room full of westerners standing on their heads. I was both veggie and yogi at the time but I fell in love with them anyway: platonically, emotionally, intellectually. They were the dark, unshaved, man-forsaking counterparts to flaxen-haired Linda and I adored their vivid minds, their avant-garde paintings, the downed tree branches and other bizarre found-art they hauled in from unlit back alleys, the pretty elfin women they brought back to their rooms to love behind closed doors.

Ramona, though, was like me: a man-crazy, passionate vegetarian. Together we sought out any non-fleshy food even remotely fit for human consumption, including ten pounds of Illinois' finest soybeans. We had no recipe and no idea what we were doing—knew only that soy was the new manna for no-meat eaters. But it took us all night to soak 'em and half the next day to boil out their stub-born, toxic resistance. Throw in some explosive spices and we ended up with a red-hot gooey gumbo that stuck to the roofs of our ravenous veggie mouths. Good God, the gray scummy froth those tough little beans put out—and the hellacious gas my poor little body discharged. Pythagoras would have wagged his god-like finger in my pained, distorted face: *Fool, I warned you!* Ramona, for reasons I couldn't fathom at the time, fared just fine on those same evil legumes.

When we weren't dancing up a midwestern storm to John Mayall (*not* John Mayer—we are talking raw sexy blues here), Ramona and I were busy devouring *Diet for a Small Planet.* Revolutionary at the time, Frances Moore Lappé's big bestseller sounded the original alarm against modern grain-fed meat production, proclaiming it unhealthy, environmentally wasteful, and a primary contributor to global food scarcity and hunger. Her book outlined basic rules for eating a plant-based diet and liberated early veggies from the prevailing high-meat paradigm, empowering us with the insight that our food choices really do make a difference. In many ways, today's food-politics authors are merely reiterating what Lappé put forth over 40 years ago in her classic manifesto.

"When my mom became a vegetarian in the early 90s, she read *Diet For A Small Planet*," writes Laurel in her *Goodreads* review of the book. "I remember thinking 'wah wah wah, my mom is such a boring loser moron head.' I pitied her for picking up a book with the words 'diet' and 'small planet' on the cover—and a pile of grains, to top it all off. This was around the time I hid all the 'Now Serving Veggie Burgers!' pamphlets from our favorite diner because I didn't want that nasty crap on our table. But mom was onto something...."

Recognizing that beef-pounding westerners were inherently mistrustful of a vegetarian diet, leery of both its taste appeal and ability to supply sufficient protein, Lappé sought to reassure the public on both counts. Her book introduced a wealth of tasty meatless dishes, along with the theory of protein combining. The idea that veg'ns need to combine plant proteins within the same meal to ensure complete amino acids has since been disproved (and recanted in a later edition of the book). Turns out you just need to eat complimentary plant proteins throughout the course of a single day. Yet Lappé's protein-combining theory served early vegetarians quite well. Without it, I doubt any of us would have given even the slightest thought to amino acid completeness.

AT LEAST RAMONA and I were aware of the differences between animal and plant protein. Members of the original Vegetarian Society didn't even know that. Their leaders declared that absolutely no difference existed and insisted they had the scientific proof, a confident claim that certainly encouraged membership. Alas, these early veggies were overly influenced by the 19th century German chemist Justus Liebig, who boldly asserted (or lied big) that plant and animal protein are "exactly and simply" the same.

Today, of course, we know that Liebig and the Veg Society were "exactly and simply" wrong. While animal protein contains all nine essential amino acids in perfect balance for an adult human's daily needs (essential to eat because your body can't produce them), plants have deficient amounts of one or more. This means that every plant food is incomplete, i.e., too low in one or more amino acid to support proper biological function. Lacking even one of these will, over time, affect your physical and mental health.

114

Grains, for instance, are low in lysine while legumes are low in methionine, including the revered soybean. Jack Norris, RD, himself a vegan, admits that it's "very hard" for vegans who don't workout every day to meet daily lysine needs. They're simply not consuming the amount of calories necessary to obtain enough lysine from plants alone. (Small or naturally slender vegans have an even tougher time intaking adequate calories to meet requirements.) Norris labels lysine "the limiting amino acid" in a vegan diet, meaning protein synthesis will be limited, i.e., inadequate, whenever there are insufficient amounts.

The amino acid methionine is also much lower in plant versus animal-sourced food, five to ten times lower, and deficiencies have been found in vegans. That's why plant eaters need to pay close attention to this sulfur-containing amino acid as well—vital for nerve function and immune cell production.

Contrary to the upfront Mr. Norris, most advocates are quick to assure vegans that it's "really, really easy" to get sufficient quantities of all the essential amino acids. In "Protein in the Vegan Diet," Reed Mangels, RD, suggests four foods, which if "eaten in the amount specified, would provide the recommended [daily] amounts of all essential amino acids for an adult male": 15½ cups cooked brown rice OR 12¾ cups cooked corn OR 2½ cups of tofu OR 8 large potatoes. *Fifteen cups of rice, anyone?* Even though Mangels admits the obvious—that this "would be a very monotonous way to dine and you might miss out on other nutrients"—is it any wonder a great many vegans remain confused on this important subject and keep insisting that plant protein is complete and equal to that of animals?

Before it recently became non-PC to tell the truth, animal sourced food was called *primary protein* because it offers the highest biological value. Plant food was *secondary protein*. Period. There's an excellent reason for this distinction: "If just one essential amino acid is low or missing," writes Mary Enig, PhD, "the body is unable to synthesize the other proteins it needs even when overall protein intake is high." If vegans don't want to believe Dr. Enig, perhaps they'll believe their hero Dr. T. Colin Campbell, author of *The China Study,* who confirms that "amino acids derived from animal based proteins are more readily available for our own protein synthesizing reactions which allows them to operate at full tilt." He calls plant proteins "compromised by their limitation of one or more amino acid." That's why protein awareness is essential for every plants-only consumer. Yet how many are monitoring their protein intake for daily completeness? I don't know a single one.

HEY, NO WORRIES! There's protein in nearly everything—just eat enough calories and you're good to go! That is still the rallying cry in nearly every veg'n book out there, but my own honest body told me straight-up I was coming up short. When you dine on large meals of diverse and healthy foods, you shouldn't be hungry in an hour or two. And you shouldn't lack the energy to complete your daily tasks.

Naturally, this doesn't happen to everyone who embarks on the veg'n path. I would never be so presumptuous to assume that our individual bodies metabolize every food in exactly the same way, that my diet should be your diet. Even some strict vegans zoom around with energy, at least in the initial years. Yet it became more and more clear as the years piled up that an animal-restricted diet wasn't working for me—for a whole bunch of us. Ever since that fateful day in Paris when I took my sacred vow, I never missed the taste of meat, not once. What I did miss was the after-meal sensation of being energized and well nourished.

Meat was taboo but whenever I went even one day without dairy and its high protein/fat content and critical B12, my energy levels plummeted and my brain fuzzed-out. As an omnivore I'd always been a healthy and focused, high-energy kid—full-steam ahead! And I desperately wanted that feel-good energy back. So Ramona and I started making our own thick, cultured yogurt in the communal kitchen, slowly warming and congealing it in clear glass jars. Oh what joy to slice our spoons into that firm, tart, beatific whiteness! Valiantly I would attempt to consume just one yogurt per day, licking up every last delectable dribble with an eager tongue, but most days I plowed through all four jars just to sate my overwhelming protein/fat hunger.

Some things never change—and for good reasons. In spite of today's immense variety of processed plant proteins and enzyme-charged raw protein powders, my slender vegetarian niece eats "an astounding amount of yogurt, *tons* of yogurt," according to her father, his voiced tinged with awe and disbelief.

20.

HUNGER, CAFFEINE & SEATTLE'S NAKED BEAUTY

FOUR WORDS ARE SCRAWLED across two pages of an 8x10 journal kept at age twenty: *I am so HUNGRY!!* One year into my honorable vegetarian diet, I was convinced this burning message concerned, not my protein and fat intake, but my newly awakened, insatiable sexual appetite. Federico was ten years older—from Chile, not Scandinavia. He read me steamy Latin American poetry at dawn and together we worked that king-size waterbed in the middle of his living room from midnight 'til first light. Only quick showers to cool off could tear us away from that colossal, spongy love-bed that swallowed up all inhibition.

Eventually though, my love thirst quenched, I had to admit I was just plain nearly always *hungry* no matter how much delicious sex I was finally enjoying, no matter how many proper veggie meals I was consuming. Even creamy yogurt wasn't turning out to be enough. I was like a foraging grizzly in late September, always eating berries, greens, grains, nuts and seeds and always looking for more. I didn't quite match an ursine diet of 35,000 chokecherries a day, but surely felt capable. No matter how much plant food I polished off, the gnawing hunger soon returned. I chalked it up to the vegetarian way, just part of the pain and sacrifice that comes when you're on the righteous moral path, when you're doing the right thing.

Maybe it was my 15 years of obligatory Sunday School, Disciples of Christ style, that made me so adept at selflessness and veg martyrdom, of accepting my suffering for others, in this case our animal brethren. Maybe it was my youthful zeal and unwavering devotion to a just cause: animal rights merging with environmental salvation. Whichever, whatever, I simply couldn't keep eating all this

117

constipating dairy to stave off my near constant craving—a raw animal hunger that a steady supply of healthy plant food could scarcely diminish.

Voila, my salvation: coffee! Yes, I said, yes I will—*yes!* Living among other student addicts in Champaign-Urbana, I took up the caffeine habit and excitedly observed that coffee *instantly* eased my incessant between-meal appetite and sent my lagging energy soaring. Witnessing this astonishing transformation, my newly secured boyfriend audaciously announced that without a doubt, if discovered today, caffeine would be tightly regulated by the FDA, just like any other drug. And whenever I missed my two strong morning cups and endured debilitating Grouch Mama headaches from withdrawal, unable to lucidly think or speak, I was forced to admit he was right.

What's baffling is that all prescription meds are *required* to list any caffeine because it's a central nervous system stimulant, but easily acquired soda pop and energy drinks sucked down by ten-year-olds? Nope. A doctor-prescribed Fiorinal capsule contains just 40 mg of caffeine while a bottle of Jolt delivers 290. Turbo Shots from Dunkin' Donuts pack a whopping 436 mg, whereas a 4-ounce serving of Bang!! Caffeinated Ice Cream injects a more modest but still loaded 125. The prize goes to Crackheads Hyper. Each 1.3-ounce box of choco-drenched espresso beans punches out an outlandish 600 mg of caffeine, a yummy and perfectly legal way to give yourself a buzz. My brainy boyfriend was right. With caffeine now in everything from chewing gum to sunflower seeds, the FDA is finally giving this popular public drug a good look-over.

Yes, caffeine is one powerful stimulant, the most frequently ingested, psycho-active substance on earth and I couldn't resist it back then any more than college students can today. Since caffeine occurs naturally in over 60 plants worldwide, it's likely our longest-used drug as well—our ancestors were getting high all the way back to the Stone Age. Today, Americans gulp down half the world's coffee and 50% of us claim we'd give up our cell phone before our daily java bounce.

Caffeine is also one heck of an appetite suppressant, abolishing hunger and fatigue within minutes of that first addictive morning slurp. That's what central nervous system stimulants do: arouse our adrenal glands to produce extra cortisol, in effect disguising our tiredness and hunger by jolting us with a short-term lift in energy and alertness. Not unlike their omnie peers, most veg'ns I know can't get through their day without that cup of joe or other well-caffeinated beverage, be it Brazilian yerba mate or Matcha Japanese green tea. All of these brews are great for skipping breakfast, losing weight, and getting close to zero macronutrients for half a day. But at what cost? Especially to already slim vegetarians? Here's Susan Bourette describing her first of three noble attempts to abandon meat during her undergraduate years at the University of Toronto:

> I was barely living proof that mere rejection of meat won't make you the picture of health. If a doctor had examined me, he would have rushed me to the hospital for tests. My raccoon eyes, my lethargy hinted that something was amiss. I was so tired I couldn't lift a pencil, let alone write an essay. But the tests would have defied diagnosis. All the physician had to do was probe into my diet. A muffin for breakfast. Green peas and rice for dinner. Oh, yes, I was drinking about twelve cups of coffee a day.

An exaggerated case perhaps (although I know one vegan who bolts this much jitter juice). The point is caffeine does indeed inhibit appetite for most of us. And here's the problem with no longer hungering for a hearty breakfast or lunch as a plant eater. Just one skipped meal represents a lost opportunity to boost that day's calorie and protein intake. Vegans especially are known for their low intake of both, as well as their low-body weight, compared to same-age omnivores. So consider the health consequences of replacing a substantial protein-based breakfast with caffeine (and perhaps some carbs) multiplied by 365, on and on through the years. Moreover, *diets too low in protein bring on a low-serotonin state of fatigue and apathy*, which feeds this cycle of craving stimulants like caffeine and carbs in the first place.

When you consume stimulants, insulin levels rise quickly, creating a rush of serotonin from your brain that is rapidly used up. Other neurotransmitters are affected but serotonin is the one that creates that sudden, enchanting feeling of well-being, even euphoria. So you feel incredible, totally revved after that early morning zap of joe or chai. You're practically moon-walking down the sidewalk! You're on planet high! Yet you've eaten hardly anything; you're not hungry in the least. But when serotonin levels abruptly drop a couple hours later, you start to feel tired, strung out, usually craving more caffeine. The same thing happens when you eat a load of carbs. You get a nice high; your mood sinks; you want more. Depending how caffeine or carb-sensitive your body is (genetically determined, by the way), this drop in serotonin can feel more like a mind-numbing crash, followed by depression. Either way, this is the pattern of an addict. And one stimulant often leads to another, like craving caffeine and carbs together.

Vegetarians are far from alone in this. Our national addiction to carbs, sugar, and caffeine has a lot to do with the low-serotonin levels in our collective brain. Over time, if not adequately nourished, your brain will stop producing and storing enough serotonin to keep your energy and moods stable. If you're a veggie and this sounds like you, here's what has to be done to rid your brain of stimulant craving: *eat sufficient daily protein.* That's because serotonin is derived from the essential amino acid tryptophan, which comes from the proteins you eat. Nine of the top-ten, high-quality food sources for tryptophan are animal-based (soy is the exception) so vegans need to be especially vigilant in getting plentiful protein on a regular basis. If you don't, your brain cannot synthesize enough serotonin and you will continue to crave stimulants in the form of carbs and/or caffeine. If inadequate tryptophan from skipped meals and insufficient protein persists over time, you'll eventually experience low energy, irritability, ongoing depression, insomnia and, quite possibly, a maddening inability to concentrate.

With coffee as my newest plant staple, I definitely lost my constant *feed me now!* hunger pains. Unfortunately, I also lost weight from my already slender frame, lost track of when I last ate, and had absolutely no concept of protein completeness. Truthfully, I became pretty spacey on my plants-and-caffeine diet or, as my friends kindly noted, "ever more delightful but ungrounded." Pumped up on my carbo-charged fruit, grains and coffee breakfast, I was known to smack head-first into the occasional giant white oak while drifting around campus reading Proust. Or I'd be strolling through traffic, head-writing an 18th century fantasy wherein I time-traveled into the body of William Blake's wife—sassy, fleshy counterpart to Will's ultra-illumined brain—anywhere and everywhere but here and now, grounded in my very own protein-depleted, caffeine-ripped body.

If you think coffee doesn't put most of us in our heads and outside our bodies, whose nutritional and other smart messages we then ignore, try this experiment sometime. Assuming you currently have a bed partner, make love with him or her after several days of abstaining from coffee. Take in the unbelievably luscious sensuality of this whole-body experience. (That is, if you're not out of action due to severe withdrawal headaches.) Continue this noble experiment a few days later by making love with this same person 30-60 minutes after drinking a cup or two or three (your usual) of highly caffeinated java. Notice the body disconnect as your mind rambles on and on, analyzing every move and every thrust, evaluating, judging and effectively removing you from a direct and fabulous body experience in the present moment, replacing it with.....caffeinated brain babble.

This is the very reason writers so love their coffee! It puts them smack in the middle of the talking, discursive Broca area of their brain's left hemisphere, that part of the frontal lobe responsible for language. It's also the reason that coffee houses originated in 15th century Europe as the adored domain of authors and intellectuals. Because caffeine moves easily through the blood-brain barrier, it radically speeds up neurotransmitters, delivering increased energy and a faster, clearer flow of thoughts for banging out that masterpiece.

COFFEE WAS DISCOVERED, or so the legend goes, when an Ethiopian goat herder observed his animals erupting into crazy cavortings after munching the berries of a coffee tree. He joined them in the dance! Not surprisingly, therefore, when the first-ever coffee shop materialized on the streets of Constantinople in 1475, this mind-altering substance swiftly endeared itself to the citizenry. (Staid opponents promptly branded it "the bitter invention of Satan.") So valued was this new brew that a Turkish woman could legally divorce her husband if he didn't supply her with enough mocha mojo. When invading Turks introduced this same dynamic tonic to Vienna—whose citizens added filtration, milk, and sugar to mitigate the harshness—it soon became all the rage and spread to London, whose first coffee houses opened in 1652. Eventually every European city boasted these literally stimulating hubs of business dealings, scholarly debate, and poetic exchange. Author Steven Johnson even makes the claim that our early coffee houses were the creative breeding ground for the Age of Enlightenment. In a statement that surely includes today's LinkedIn, cappuccino-guzzling crowd, he concludes that "chance favors the connected mind." Even more, chance favors the caffeine-buzzed connected mind.

Caffeine gets those neural connections zipping alright. It shifts your brain into fifth gear, then overdrive, then overspill. Words and ideas suddenly start cracking, cackling, cascading all over the pixilated page. Take away coffee and all other sources of caffeine from the world's writers and I wager 90% of them will want to kill you because they cannot write without it. Or, more fairly, can't write the same without their caffeine, with such sweaty, passionate profusion.

As a vegetarian, I cherished coffee not only for its mental stimulation but because it bulldozed my hunger the way nothing else could, certainly no food I had found in the plant kingdom. Indeed, I *needed* coffee to stay true to my ethics of ecology and compassion, lest I run to the deli and rapaciously clamp my canines into some forbidden animal food. Unfortunately, in detaching me from my natural hunger, caffeine also distanced me from my body and its healthy yearnings. In sum, my body's messages—for more varied and abundant protein and good fat—were being squelched. Beyond contributing zero nutrition, caffeine also interferes with the body's absorption of vitamin B12, iron and zinc, critical neuro-nutrients that are already more difficult to derive from a plant diet.

By age 22, my hunger-suppressing fix meant a daily trip to Sambo's cozy booths with gal pal and fellow veg Ramona. Yes, Sambo's, the decidedly non-PC restaurant chain started by two white men in Santa Barbara. There we could drink endless cups of java for fifty cents and get just as good a caffeine fix as today's five-bucks caramel mocha latte. Better: no sugar or cream to staunch the powerful acidic effect. As for taste, we'd spit out that same coffee today, but who knew? We were beyond happy. Enveloped in blaring red plastic, imbibing that serotonin-arousing black brew with deep girl-sighs, Ramona and I would linger over steamy mugs of joe for hours, discussing world religions, animal rights, and which uber-smart professors we wanted to lay. Back then, smart *way* pre-empted cute.

And yet, much as I loved my caff-addicted pals and solid midwestern roots, unquenchable wanderlust kept nudging my restless spirit onward. Though no job, friend or even acquaintance awaited me, after a spring graduation I jumped into my salt-rusted van and headed west through nascent fields of corn and soy to God knows where. Going to the Promised Land, that's all I knew, all I dreamed about, and more than I even told my parents, who assumed I was still in Champaign-Urbana, come to my culinary senses at last, and chowing down on real burgers with the best of them. By the time I arrived in drizzly, hyper-green Seattle—not even close to being the next coffee capital of the world—something was up with my three-year-old diet. No longer a subversive, solitary vegetarian, a food weirdo among straights, a lone herbivore amongst the ignorant carnivores, in Seattle's progressive milieu I finally fit in.

BY THE LATE 70s a few no-meat restaurants were taking a chance in Seattle, like Sunshine Café in the Roosevelt District, still dishing out sautéed vegetable tofu to this day. Local health food stores were springing up, pulling in curious customers; organic was happening; and vibrant Pike Place Market, overlooking serene Elliott Bay, drew me like a sucker fish to its bright, multi-colored lures.

Sauntering happily out of Left Bank Books one blue-sky June day, Bloomsday it was, I fell madly in love with a tall, lanky street musician strumming his steel guitar. Only to discover, far too late for my eager heart, that he had "all the best girlfriends all over town." (Oh yeah, and one pregnant wife.) What a bozo of a hayseed I was, what a Midwest innocent, alone in that big coastal metropolis of five floating bridges, seven lofty hills, and one kooky Space Needle. What an idealistic, quixotic, loser-dreamer! You might as well have strapped me to the stillpoint of a moving windmill, my few remaining dollars falling out of upside-down pockets, people grabbing and laughing and running off, and I would have sweetly responded, "They know not what they do." Because at 23, I actually believed that a man loved you if he said he did, actually believed that when you opened your soft naked body to a man, he would call you the next day and offer his hand for a stroll, his mind for your discovery, his whole world for the sharing.

It took me a very long time to let go of that particular lean, mean, blue-eyed musician and my naïve fantasy because every free day (which is basically *every* day when you're young and jobless) I cycled back there, back to lively, citrus and patchouli-scented Pike Market—whose hawkers, herbalists, fish peddlers, fortune tellers and free-spirited women in flowing blue velvet and Mid-East sandals, I found irresistibly romantic. Someone on the corner was always selling consciousness and beads, some new male bard in purple floral wailing in the background, fiddle in hand, ready to fly. And I would stand spellbound next to bountiful heaps of shiny red Washington apples for long timeless moments, bewitched by all the bustling, transitory beauty.

Then one rainy afternoon at the Market, a quiet winter's day, I wandered into an inconspicuous shop with a very strange name, Starbucks, that sold coffee, ceramic mugs, and little else. Definitely someone's very first, bare-bones startup and not all that inviting: a few wooden tables and chairs crammed between open barrels of greasy coffee beans. No one seemed to stick around very long—I wondered if the place would even make it. But I loved to linger and sniff every stout metal-hooped cask, inhaling deeply of those heady, robust smells that fueled my appetite-smothering addiction. If I drank enough of this buckaroo's rip-roaring coffee by late afternoon, I could stay a steady course on my veg diet and rid myself of all those annoying hunger pangs, day after rainy day.

It was 1979 and Seattle was already a gorgeous, green and growing city, abounding in art galleries and terrific small bookstores. And with great fanfare, a couple of yoga studios and massage classes were starting up, right out there on the alternative fringes! In all innocence, I signed up for the latter, an extension course offered through the University of Washington which met every Tuesday evening for twelve weeks at a professional massage therapist's house. Free vegan

123

snacks were part of the offering. That's all the incentive I needed—my kind of clan! So when I showed up one warm May evening at a charming bungalow in the Wallingford District and was greeted in the lilac-fringed backyard by another student—a thin, bearded, very naked man—I sucked in sharply and thought: OK, cool, lean veg gal, you've come a long way since your buttoned-down-collar days in corn country but let's get real: you were undeniably *not* expecting this.

Turns out all the classes in Carol's warm, low-light, pastel-painted basement were conducted in the nude. And everybody was completely in-the-know and nonchalant about this unpublished fact except, apparently, little 'ol dense me. Naturally, I didn't let on to a single soul—and already there were ten beautiful male/female bodies and souls in attendance. Almost all were steadfast vegetarians in tauntingly fantastic shape, and everyone was so at ease, so wonderfully genial and uninhibited, I slowly began to release my rigid, up-tight musculature and feel right at home. Overcoming my midwestern modesty with remarkable speed, I tossed my glasses, tore off my clothes, and leaped into the naked mêlée.

The weekly ritual was set. First step: everybody crowded into the large wood-burning sauna in Carol's basement for a sweaty, searingly hot purge of any toxic nasties our bodies might be harboring from pollution, stress, junk food, or rotting animal flesh. Just like today's still-mistaken vegans, we firmly believed that any-thing as disgusting and foreign to the human body as dead animals surely took days if not weeks to break down in our way-too-long-to-be-a-carnivore digestive tract. To accelerate this highly unnatural process and avoid putrification, massage coupled with blistering heat was just the ticket.

To this day I can still smell that evocative, aromatic wood smoke, the tinctures of eucalyptus, the dripping human sweat—all tangled up with the intoxicating cedar fragrance of Carol's well-used, well-loved sauna. Once seated inside, no one spoke, not a word. Shoulders touching, thighs brushing, ten unadorned bare bodies jammed juicily together as we listened to the rhythmic communal sound of our quiet exhalations. I can still hear those same cadenced breaths, still hear the water slowly trickling from a porcelain cup, striking the woodstove with a fiery sizzle—still feel the fast-gathering steam as it hits my naked chest and rises to inflame my wide-eyed, sweat-soaked face. And now I see the incessant Northwest rain lashing against the sauna's miniature window, pouring down into the empty streets, into the open arms of trees.

You stayed on and on in that searing, silent, meditative cave for as long as your body could bloody take it, your corporeal being slowly melting into clammy liquid goo, your mind evaporating into the ether. Second step: Out you dashed into the dark fresh night for your final purge, a shocking plunge in Carol's frigid pool. Last step: Pull yourself out into the forty degree air, shrieking, whole again. Shaking off glistening water beads like some wild exuberant mongrel. By January our sleek animal bodies were diving through thin layers of ice, breaking back through with high, piercing yelps on the pool's far side.

Raw celery, carrots, and cucumbers were offered after our ritual cleanse, right before the real work began: massage instruction on the floor of a very warm and thickly carpeted room, accompanied by low lights and plentiful heated towels. Everything was completely non-sexual (really). Even sexual innuendo wasn't tolerated, although gazing sweetly at all the naked beauty was certainly allowed. Long strokes up and down the spine, percussive movements, gentle effleurage. We practiced as the Swedes have for centuries. Joint manipulation, belly spirals, neck work, breath work, intense openings of the heart.

An artist and master masseuse, Carol was a delightful, super fit, 38-year-old dynamo with one exceedingly lucky boyfriend, a good ten years younger. She asked us to work in alternating pairs, sometimes women together, sometimes men—and sometimes five or more people working in sync on one extremely blessed and blissed-out human being. *O la la, forget the afterlife.* There is heaven on earth indeed. Right here, right now, in Carol's warm, womb-like, hands-on, clothes-off, tranquil Wallingford basement.

With hair gone limp, soggy linguine for a body, and a dazed smile still playing on my moist, plumped-up lips, every Tuesday night I rode my bicycle back home from Carol's—right through the center of Seattle's north side. Week after sauna-blessed week, I rode up, over, down and around the hills of the U District and Ravenna, pedaling back to my rented room on an ecstatic wave of inner silence. Who needs food? Who needs coffee? All hunger satiated, all thirst quenched, I rode and rode into that muggy darkness until the black unseen clouds descended close and then closer, bursting open yet again. And the lights of the clapboard houses flickered brightly as the everlasting water flowed down and down into the liquid Seattle of our dreams.

21.

DIGGING IN AND GETTING HIGH

YET THE HUNGER always returned, doubly so after our torrid nights of sweating and near fasting. So off I would go for my daily jolt of caffeine, right after my plants-only breakfast that never seemed to do the satiation trick. As for how many calories and how much protein I was consuming in the course of a day, I hadn't a bloody clue. I was staying skinny and true to my moral and political philosophy, and few things hold more importance to an idealistic 20-something.

All winter long Seattle stayed verdant and vibrant but lovely as this Emerald City was, and still is, by springtime I was again longing for the pastoral: the soil and the source. Big cities, with their raucous streets and yakking sidewalks, eventually start to unnerve me. So instead of all this grating noise, where could I wake up to simple silence? To the sweet smell of wet hay and the fallow? And every bit as urgent, where could I grow the kind of good veg'n food I was eating and start sharing it with others? If some kind of organic farm or freewheeling commune didn't come to my attention soon, I was determined to just start walking until I found one: trek through north Seattle's cat-haven back alleys and follow its covert creeks into the hinterlands. That was my latest madcap plan. Anything to get back to the earth, anything to get back to the loamy dirt and wide-open wind.

Just as I was contemplating my most auspicious direction via the I Ching, the answer magically appeared in the *Times* classifieds instead: *Naturist Vegetarians: Come live, love, and labor with us! Cooperative farm on the scenic Skykomish. 206-754-8773.* Perfecto! But how far left of normal was this setup going to be? Would everyone be traipsing around in the buff, grazing on sprouts? When I phoned for more information, the cheery young woman on the other end didn't mess around: she asked first for my birth date and *then* my name. I could hear the astro-calculations whirring. Oh yes, co-op founders Jane and Thom chose only astrologically compatible live-ins who foreswore all meat. So to mess with their heads, I gave the wrong birth year—but they must have liked whatever that made me because right away I was in the running to join their revered inner circle.

All brave souls who passed the star-crossed phone screening received a written invitation to the 120-acre farm, only to experience an equally bizarre mode of interviewing upon arrival. Did Thom and Jane inquire about our previous farm experience? Our dedication to organics and the vegetarian way? No way. They sat us down in front of their mystical, medieval Rider-Waite tarot cards to have our past lives revealed and our auras sensitively read. Two major arcane cards turned up again and again for this vagabond veg'n traveler in search of the divine: The World—symbolized by a euphoric, scantily-dressed woman prancing through the clouds—and even more fittingly, The Fool. Striding forward with white rose in hand, a dashing youth gazes heavenward with naïve optimism as, totally clueless, he's about to step off a cliff.

This agrarian-aquarian couple—30ish, impish, a few missing teeth—claimed to see both in-person and television auras. (Mine turned out to be rose while auras of high-ranking Washington Republicans, they swore, were ominously black.) Any revelations that emerged from these inimitable interviews were for purposes of energetic and sexual attunement, I was to later learn, because following this Northwest farm venture the pair already had their next grand scheme in place: to gather up the best, brightest, most procreative among us and start a new human race on the eastern slope of the Rockies. The Blue Race, they called it, and eventually we'd transition from living on plants, to water and sun energy only, exactly as higher dimensional beings had revealed to them in meditative dreams. So yeah, despite their excellent taste in Thai buds, Van Morrison and vegan cuisine, I did realize from the get-go that Jane and Thom were more than a little whacked.

Honestly though, while living on the farm with the playful Skykomish River whooshing by and the rich soil constantly birthing new life, I existed in a heightened realm of awareness. This sensitive state had very little to do with the infrequent reefer smoked and almost everything to do with my constant immersion in nature. And surely my light, clean, mostly-plants diet was assisting in this very obvious shift. Every evening, walking home after working the fields beneath an open, giving sky, I felt deeply calm and reverent. Though still clothed in the same familiar body, having spent all day, every day, kneeling in the fertile dirt of our ancestors, my spirit had undergone radical transformation. I distinctly remember

127

entering the modest white farmhouse one late afternoon and finding it strangely empty and quiet. It was the end of the work week. The boisterous gang had already departed for the big city, and I breathed in big mouthfuls of sweet, affable silence. Heat radiated off the vacated chairs, and languid flecks of dust—stirred up by the living bodies of my just-departed comrades—danced in golden streams of window light.

Out of nowhere a sudden knowing jolted my consciousness and with a sharp cry I stumbled to the floor. A knowing, you understand, not cognition. A potent knowing that within my soul I carried all women throughout all time who have ever walked upon, seeded, harvested or bent down to touch the soil. The sowers and the gatherers, the warriors and the nurturers—all converging in one universal feminine spirit. Getting up slowly, stepping out into the warm twilight, I bathed my being in this powerful field of connection as long as possible, but oh so predictably, it disintegrated within the hour as the dim-witted ego once again began babbling its song of separation and denial.

What is it about working on your hands and knees in the soil, like a prayer, like shameless gratitude, that so alters one's awareness? Another late spring evening, another revelation on the farm. Having just weeded a row of tender radish sprouts by hand, I came in from the lilac-scented night, moist dirt still clinging to my forearms, and floated to the bedroom ceiling, leaving body and mind behind. Swiftly I apprehended that you and I—yes that would be *you,* that would be *I*— were the Buddha, and *you* and *you* and *you.* Why that moment? It had been years since I'd read Siddhartha or even consciously thought about the guy. Not that I was *the* Buddha, of course, but one and the same in essence. That we are all Buddha Boy and Buddha Girl, just insanely unaware of our boundless true nature, draped in a fog of self-illusion and self-importance. I must have floated in that celestial awareness for what? Half the night? Time has no meaning in that altered state, but by the next morning I was just me again, walking the long green rows, checking for aphids and beetles, shooing away pesky flies.

THE SKYKOMISH FARM had been planned as an exclusively organic, hands-on, non-mechanized venture, and that first season we tilled the acreage with a hand-pushed wooden plow. Good God, it was hideously hard work. I felt just like Bessie the Ox—awkward and achingly slow—like I'd been beamed back to the 18th century as a poky, clumsy farm animal. Thomas Gray's rough ploughman could not have felt more miserable, he who "homeward plods his weary way/

128

And leaves the world to darkness and to me." After too many grueling weeks of this not very noble-looking attempt, Thom took stock of the long hours needed to press even one crooked line into the stony dirt, then drove clear to Granite Falls and bought a small green and yellow beauty of a tractor: a used John Deere 4030 that turned the soil cleanly and ploughed it straight.

We did, however, continue to sow acres and acres of vegetables and greens by hand, employing a spinning mechanism that dispersed organic seeds hither and yon. And when our shallots and radishes miraculously materialized in the mid-spring mud, we manually harvested them in the pale morning light, filled recycled wooden crates and hoisted them into my trusty van. Then I drove the hour to Pike Market all by myself. Oh lucky, lucky me! Most bounteous blessings! Working in that lively open-air market, immersed in fresh tulips and ripening fruit, was immensely pleasurable, the best life has to offer. Friendly Italian farmers offered marketing advice; pretty young women in lace and hiking boots played angelic flutes; and the outsized smells of Puget Sound wafted up from the waterfront below, enveloping us all in a fishy, fecund haze.

Everybody else on the farm longed for this task—a dozen of us altogether, young and starry-eyed—but I was the chosen one. Why? Because Jane and Thom instinctively knew my "don't fence me in" Sagittarian spirit wouldn't last even one summer unless they gave it ample roaming space. Pity the poor home-loving Cancerians! They had to stay in the kitchen all morning and chop vegetables.

Massive quantities of raw produce routinely graced our plates and we hunted down our own wild mushrooms. Rain-slick cow patties yielded prized psilocybin; Doug firs the very best chanterelles. Surely I was eating the finest nourishment on the planet! So what if I felt ungrounded on my veg diet, even beyond-this-world at times? Those precious departures from consensus reality were fast becoming part of my persona. I treasured them and still do. And what did it matter if the words "fat" and "protein" were never part of our group consciousness? Since we had renounced all animal flesh (the devil's food) and ate all-organic plant fare (manna from heaven), we were 100% assured to be consuming the most superior diet known to humankind. And, of course, anyone with any brains and a heart should be doing exactly the same thing.

Ah, the over-confidence, the cheerful idealism, the conceit, the smugness, the swagger of youth.

22.

ANNOYING ATTITUDES/
DUBIOUS RESEARCH

The ego is a tyrant that must be dethroned.

—Carlos Castaneda

OKAY, IT DOES SEEM a bit edgy to attribute some of the intrepid vegan attitudes I've encountered over the years to egoism, at least in part. After all, this is the same group of people sacrificing their ethnic heritage and easy protein pickings in order to rescue animals, possibly even the environment. Upon deep and honest reflection, however, I have to admit this is often the case, my own youthful attitude included, because egoism is the elitist attitude that refuses to look into the depth and complexities of an issue, insisting instead that my way is right and your way is flat-out wrong.

With our final Skykomish harvest gathered and sold at market, it was time for my annual trek to Corn Nation. By now my Illinois family's initial distress had vanished in the time tractor's dust and my parents, siblings, and entire extended family—loving to the core—fully embraced my vegetarian lifestyle and never again questioned me. Ah, but each time I paid them a visit, something inside of me subtly, silently questioned them.

Secretly I began to feel, dare I say it, a tad bit *enlightened* compared to my animal-eating family and friends. I was educated, in-the-know about this essential moral matter, part of a still-small inner circle sworn to a life of non-harm to other sentient beings. True, I rarely discussed my conversion unless asked, certainly never boasted or preached. Simply enough, I proudly demonstrated by example each and every time I sat down to dine. Nonetheless, I harbored a bloated attitude about myself compared to the meat-eating "others." Oh, it was subtle for sure, nearly out of reach of my own awareness. Just enough out of reach that I failed to tell myself to *cut it out!*

> Flesh-eating friends and untold billions, I am now a devout vegetarian, embarking on humankind's new evolutionary path: lighter, healthier, more moral beings who save animals from suffering and death. And you who persist in devouring the putrefying flesh of our kindred creatures? You are definitely not on this path. But you can still make this choice! You really *must* make this choice!

I didn't actually tell anyone this malarkey. Nonetheless, in the enduring dwelling place of the ego, the comparing, judging ego that's absolutely certain it knows best, I most assuredly felt this way. How could my young self know that years later I would reject vegetarianism as the correct diet not only for everyone on the planet but for myself? It took me that long to renounce my sincere beliefs, born of the mind and emotions, and reconnect with my biological body. That long to realize that there is no "best, healthiest, most ethical diet" for all humans. Yes, it took decades for a hell of a lot of us rebellious, cock-sure, early plant-eaters to finally admit we are natural omnivores, that no matter how faithfully we worked our no-dead animals diet, it wasn't delivering for us as the years stretched out. Never in our worst or wildest dreams could we have foreseen this.

It's this same way of thinking that I still encounter among the hordes of new vegans. Rigidly, unbendingly, they cling to their unproven beliefs. An endless drone of online claims and condemnations reveals that nothing much has changed in all these years. Their ongoing themes? Immorality, ignorance, and sloth.

> Only your lazy habits and brainwashing by the animal exploitation industries permit this cruel abomination to continue unrestrained.

> *Allowing animals to suffer and be killed to satisfy your licentious appetite is heartless and immoral. Murderer!*

> Meat eaters, you are stealing straight from the mouths of starving kids. If everybody went vegan, we could free the land of all those miserable cows and sheep and grow enough food to feed everyone on earth.

Today I find this attitude more exasperating than infuriating. Why? Because it is genuine, based in not-knowing, and often comes from the mouths of babes. And although irksome, I can flick off these do-gooders like a high-pitched mosquito. But the persistent, disapproving, droning skeeters keep coming back to teach us a thing or two about animal ethics and environmental awareness, making omnivores "uncomfortable" in the words of activist Rod Preece, especially when these pro-veg opinions are "arrogantly, aggressively, pompously, or self-assertively expressed." (You said it Rod, not I.) Preece is a prime example of a seriously judgmental veg'n. In *Sins of the Flesh, A History of Ethical Vegetarian Thought,* he essentially calls meat abstainers higher moral beings. Omnivores who are not inclined toward vegetarianism, according to Preece, experience a sense of guilt "that the vegetarian takes the high ground they themselves have relinquished."

Funny, in all these years I have yet to encounter a meat eater who felt even the slightest twinge of guilt as he or she dove into Aunt Fiona's Irish shepherd pie or nibbled in delight on Uncle Luke's fresh-caught rainbow trout. No, in my experience it's the temporarily lapsed, obsessive-perfectionist vegans who feel pangs of guilt and regret, even abhorrence, at the tiniest morsel of animal food passing unbeknownst between their lips. *There was chicken stock in that broccoli soup? Gelatin in the chocolate mousse?!!*

Having been both veggie and omnie for separate, lengthy periods of time, I can assure you it's not omnivores who believe vegetarians live on a higher ethical plane. It is veggies who believe this about themselves, exercising a sense of moral exclusivity over the rest of us apparently fallen humans. In "Vegetarianism for Dummies," Lisa Turner defines a no-meat diet as "a requirement for the hip and enlightened," and Dan Morley concludes in *The Human Guide to North America* that vegans are "ethically superior, animal protecting liberals." Meanwhile, a large banner headline on *Above Top Secret* shouts: "If ending loveless orgasm is the fingerprint to enlightenment, then veganism is the full body resurrection!" On this same website, a pious plant-eater declares: "As a spiritual being who has already achieved enlightenment and as a vegan on his path to wisdom, I believe that any conscious and enlightened person would recognize the absolute horror in consuming animals...."

Other vegans are quick to point out that they don't consider *themselves* to be morally advanced but their diet most certainly is. "How do you define feeling superior?" plant eaters asked in response to NPR's *Culture* article, "Do Vegetarians and Vegans Think They Are Better Than Everyone Else?" If you interpret this as viewing meat-eaters as morally inferior, they explain, that's not the same as simply knowing we have more smarts and education on this issue.

132

Of course, to claim either type of superiority—either of self or knowledge—veg'ns must continue to wear blinders to blot out unsettling images of cropland wild animal deaths, stick fingers in their ears against the mounting testimony of suffering vegans, and pinch closed their noses lest they inhale the good earthy smell of conscious, compassionate farmers who take exceptional care of their animals and green fertile pastures.

It's the spanking new, totally lit-up vegan disciples who are most strident in their desire to convince and convert the "ignorant and uneducated" among us, their rhetoric the most grating. Although they have no clue what their own health outcome will be down the road, they know everything about what *your* lifetime diet should be—and apparently every person's on the planet.

One cocky new vegan, a male devotee, sent a letter to the editor of a yoga-spiritual journal—I swear this is true—demanding that commercial plant food be shipped to northern Canadian natives so they would stop hunting and eating local animals. Never mind the environmental absurdity of promoting recurrent 6,000-mile round-trip flights of highly processed, genetically-altered Iowa grains and California produce, versus local whole food. But do envision how the bodies of these high Arctic people have necessarily evolved over the centuries to consume, digest, and store high-fat, high-protein animal food. And do envision this urban veggie in cargo shorts and aviator sunglasses enjoying the sweltering Colorado summer while sipping an iced latte outside the millionth new Starbucks, believing he knows, oh yes he knows without a doubt, the appropriate diet for every human body of every age, constitution, and genetic stock in every corner of the world.

The blogworld is bursting with similar all-knowing vegans on a mission to convince and convert. Here's "Bailey" trying to persuade a feeling-paltry vegan who's contemplating an occasional therapeutic dose of pastured beef, that she's not only thinking illogically but tipping dangerously toward immorality:

> What are you saying, girl? Eating "animal-friendly meat" now and then isn't going to make you feel any better! Remember, you are VEGAN!! Is a grass-fed hamburger twice a month going to increase the protein you say you're missing? Don't you see the "humanely-raised" industry is a total load of crock? It doesn't stop the suffering of animals, it just brainwashes you to feel okay about eating them!

"Neva" dishes out her own Texas-style advice to another wavering veganite: "Listen it's quite simple really. It's not hard to be a vegan. I've been vegan for three years…I work at a bar and live in TEXAS…don't preach to me how hard it is. Our main food source in this state is the cattle in the backyard. I usually end an argument like this. Person: God put animals here for us to eat. Me: No, animals were Adam and Eve's companions….before sin. It wasn't until after sin, our punishment was to eat our companions. You're simply embracing life after sin!"

Rancor ensues when the comments get gritty and personal. Longtime rancher "Roger" is sick of hearing his profession smeared by vegans who want his cattle sterilized and denied existence, his pastures ripped up and planted with soy and grains for human consumption.

> Of course I am defensive of my livelihood and choice of diet. It is your intent to eliminate them by spreading false information and fear mongering. Using a moralistically superior attitude which does nothing but turn people off…You have also described people like me as being akin to "murderers, rapists, and child molesters." Yet [some of] you support the killing of human fetuses for population control….I have yet to see where you or anyone else has a right to preach your "superior evolved morality" to anyone. If anything you have changed my stance on the pro-life movement and how I feel about vegetarians in general….You're no better than Jerry Falwell or the man who shot Dr. Tiller.

Yes, maligned meat eaters are firing back, getting in their own cranky potshots. One group started their very own PETA: People Eating Tasty Animals. Poking fun seems to be the main objective, along with their own brand of disdain.

> In honor of true vegetarians, I'm going to have a bull roast in the backyard for all of my friends. I will post pictures of the carnage. I won't eat it but at least I will have satisfaction in knowing that liberal pansies….will be holding hands and crying together.

> *My theory is that all the douchebaggery comes from a similar high of being like a fundamentalist religious fucknut. I've seen many preach like it's a religion….it's fun to play with those types.*

Condescending and callous, this subset of omnivores is nonetheless not out to convert vegans to their own lifestyle. Actually, they're rather fond of splashing Nietzsche's classic quote on individuality across their website: "You have your way. I have my way. As for the correct way and the only way, it does not exist."

By and large, however, it's the pro-vegans who rule the righteous blogwaves. Sometimes they're simply defending their name against accusations of being too soft, too emotional, what one omnivore calls "a romantic swoony-emo teen club." At other times they come out howling, displaying a disquieting mastery of the zealot's language.

> If you chopped off your dog's tail and testicles, then whacked it over the head with a shovel and killed it, you'd be charged with animal cruelty and arrested. But you support this all the time for animals that you think are *tasty* and *juicy*, that you want for your *dinner*. Admit it, you vile, disgusting meat eaters! You are selfish animal exploiters.
>
> *Fascists!*

Perhaps I can uncover a more reasoned approach to diet and veganism. Oh here's one, offered by an online yogi:

> If you desire to live a life of higher consciousness, you cannot eat meat in any form. No fish, no fowl—not even eggs. The grosser, denser energy of animal food will coarsen your body, mind and spirit, leading to all the negative emotions of anger, envy, and anxiety. The karmic consequences of meat eating are severe! They manifest as ill health, disease, distress, and mental instability. A person who eats meat will never find peace and will be incapable of receiving spiritual truths and knowledge.

Now that's one bold and bizarre statement, rejecting almost every spiritual leader throughout time. It also doesn't speak the truth about my own daughter. Calm and serene by nature, after plunging into veganism on the advice of her yoga teacher and a profusion of popular books, Gabrielle slowly transformed into an agitated, distraught, nervous wreck. Yet some celebrated yogis continue to promote vegetarianism with missionary-like fervor, proffering dietary advice in their books and classes. "We agree that vegetarianism is not for everyone; it is only for those who desire happiness and peace," write Jivamukti yoga founders David Life and Sharon Gannon. "It is definitely a must for those who are interested in enlightenment." Really? Tell that to the Buddha, The Enlightened One.

In the birthplace of yoga, the subcontinent of India, vegetarians aren't even in the majority, comprising less than 40% of the population. Vegans barely exist.

And while almost all yoga teachers, like Life and Gannon, are soulful and even-tempered in their desire to inform and persuade, a certain class of militant vegans is on the rise, emerging more egoistic and vociferous over time. No doubt it's the ability to hide behind online anonymity that allows these types to come out slinging and screaming their holy doctrine.

> your [sic] a disgusting person....you choose to go with your shit family to hunt fish because you like it? or you think its yummy? over them feeling pain when you stab them with your rod and eat their carcasses. guess what, people that dont [sic] eat meat will always be better than people that eat meat, because they have one point that will shine over all your shitty qualities, they dont kill, but you keep continuing to hunt your fish and eat your steak and when the day comes i hope someone eats you and your shit aboriginal family :)

> *Corpse eaters, I hope you suffer and rot like the animals you eat.*

Extremism—especially arrogant loathing toward people different from yourself—is rooted in a paradox of opposites: insecurity and an inflated sense of self. Any psychologist worth her salt understands this, as does any conscious adult who has worked hard to overcome youthful delusions of all-knowingness. In her *FoodVibe* posting, "Confessions of an Ex-Vegetarian," Suzanne relates her evolving awareness of the high value of a flexible, generous mind—and diet. She now eats local poultry and fish for both health and cultural reasons.

> As a teenager I shunned meat and its unsustainability in reaction to what I considered to be my parents' bourgeois lifestyle. Like most reactionaries, I took great pride in my heightened consciousness. I took advantage of each opportunity, no matter how small, to point out the perceived social and ecological benefits of my lifestyle choice. I mocked how others lived. When invited to someone's house for a meal, I refused their unenlightened hospitality with the most enlightened of utterances: I'm a vegetarian.
>
> I was an asshole.

Occasionally, arrogant types get right in your face. One nippy autumn morning in southern Boulder County, I was scouting release sites for rehabilitated wild birds when a vegan-type greeted me at her door with a brash pamphlet intended to educate: "THINK YOU CAN BE AN ENVIRONMENTALIST AND EAT MEAT? THINK AGAIN!" A dedicated enviro since childhood, I felt mildly irritated until inwardly acknowledging that I once thought along these same lines, silently beating my drum against the ignorant masses. The masses have now been informed, I was forced to admit, however incompletely and with passionate bias.

What an enormous difference just a few decades of animal rights advocacy and slick magazine ads have made. In some social enclaves, it's now *de rigueur* to shun meat. While mockery continues in many rural areas of the country, among a certain class of urbanites *not* to be a vegan has become the ultimate seditious act. In an ironic reversal of veggie iconoclast George B. Shaw's famous *Man and Superman* quote—"the man whose consciousness does not correspond to that of the majority is a madman"—in many liberal-enviro circles it's now the meat-eater who has emerged as the madman.

When Heather Mamatey was attending college in Georgia, going vegan was "an honorable act that earned you a certain kind of clout and respect from your classmates and friends," she discloses in *Let Them Eat Meat,* "a declaration to your peers that you were *awake*, that you were not a brain dead suburban zombie, that you were not a mindless mainstream consumer of material goods, frequenter of Wal-Mart and McDonald's….a Future Corporate Drone." Those who didn't take the pledge were seen as selfish and environmentally ignorant and whenever she first met someone, ex-vegan Heather now admits, she immediately judged and classified them. "If I made a new friend and found out they still chose to eat meat, it'd be a definite mark against them in my mind, like a character flaw….I liked the *idea* of myself as a vegan, as someone who eschewed the dirty habits and addictions that enslaved others. I saw it as a huge, proud badge of anti-conformity. I wasn't a mindless automaton, following the masses like a sheep. Oh no! I was a VEGAN. "

It's a mistake to build arguments for veganism on a shaky foundation.

—Pro-vegan Virginia Messina, RD

MANY PROUD VEGANS are barely in their teens, prompted by their budding ethics and influential friends to commence a radical new diet. Yet I doubt most of them, nor their parents, realize this: no studies show that veganism is the healthiest of diets and some suggest that it definitely is not. "What a load of BS!" a lot of drop-jawed vegans are shouting right about now, energetically wagging their fingers and instructing us to read Dr. T. Colin Campbell's *The China Study.* "Rock-solid scientific verification of vegan health benefits!" they insist. May the truth, dear vegans, set you free.

Based on a 20-year body of research, Campbell's 2005 bestseller, *The China Study: Startling Implications for Diet, Weight-Loss, and Long-Term Health*, states what vegans everywhere want to hear: "People who ate the most animal-based foods got the most chronic disease....People who ate the most plant-based foods were the healthiest and tended to avoid chronic disease." This statement, Campbell's primary conclusion, is based on data gathered from 6,500 adults across 65 rural Chinese counties in an ecological study that *The New York Times* calls "the Grand Prix of epidemiology."

But hold on, not so fast. Critics have found deep fault lines in Campbell's published findings, including a handful of courageous pro-vegan dieticians and some of his own Cornell University colleagues. After exhaustively studying the original 894-page research monograph, crunching numbers and analyzing correlations for months, nutrition writer Denise Minger described Campbell's *The China Study* as "a foundation of unsupported conclusions upon which he has built his tower of vegan propaganda."

Professor Emeritus of Nutritional Biochemistry at Cornell and a vegan since 1990, Dr. Campbell has devoted his career to studying animal protein's effects on human health. In popular books and workshops, he advertises the many health advantages of a vegan lifestyle, declaring that a diet heavy in greens is as good as it gets. Sweet potatoes, beans, and brown rice are his other favorite foods, while meat, dairy, and eggs top his never-ever list.

First, let's allow a healthy skepticism for any dietary verdict offered by a committed vegan who's already concluded that an animal-free diet is the way to go. Second, less than 40 pages out of the 350 in Campbell's book actually pertain to the original study and its research data. Third and most important, the statistics collected from that study, *Diet, Lifestyle and Mortality in China,* do NOT support Campbell's personal conclusion that veganism is humanity's road to good health.

Even the authors of *Vegan for Life,* Jack Norris, RD, and Virginia Messina, RD, refuse to include anything from *The China Study* to augment their balanced, well-researched book. That's because they realize that any evidence to buttress veganism as a healthy choice isn't there. *The study participants were not vegans!* Most of them weren't even vegetarians. A few of the 6,500 came close but, no, the original study did not research plants-only eaters, nor prove one thing about vegan health outcomes. Yet the million-plus people who have read Campbell's book probably believe that it did. Or fervently, unconditionally believe this.

So let's bravely look at the facts. Statistics for *The China Study* came from an ecological study, one of the weakest types of research. These kinds of studies, which compare diet and disease rates among groups, can point to an association, at best, not cause and effect. They provide only rough estimates of what individuals are eating and *zero conclusive evidence* about health and disease. A hypothesis may arise from the data and *then* a proper study is designed to test it. Ecological research is "riddled with problems," admit Norris and Messina, citing too many factors that can't be controlled in the final analysis. They're called confounding biases and they always skew results, *making any conclusion impossible.*

Yet Campbell concludes: "The findings from the China Study indicate that the lower the percentage of animal-based foods that are consumed, the greater the health benefits. So it's not unreasonable to *assume* [my emphasis] that the optimum percentage of animal-based products is zero." Since when are dietary recommendations directed to millions of people based on an untested assumption? The original study indicated only a *possible association* between a *plant-based* diet and the health of this specific Asian population. To leap from this non-conclusive finding to a bestselling book which rigidly promotes *plants-only* for all humans of all ages is a very large, unsupported, and unscientific leap indeed. Plants, as every informed nutritionist knows, are deficient or wholly lacking in vital nutrients found in animal-sourced food.

Yet how many vegan promoters are advancing this same gratuitous conclusion? In an era where anti-oxidant research dominates the health headlines, few would argue against an abundance of vegetables, fruits, and greens. But what does any of this have to do with eating *only* plants and unflagging abstinence from animal food for the rest of your life?

It's at this point we really must ask everyone, including Dr. Campbell himself, to stop mixing the terms "plant-based" and "plants-only." *If you are endorsing a 100% plants-only vegan diet, please don't refer to it as plant-based or plant-strong.* This is deceptive, softening the reality of how severe this diet really is. Most omnivores follow a plant-based diet, with animal products added to the mix in varying degrees. Veganism is solely plants. Vast difference. So let's stop tossing around these two different concepts as if we are referring to the same thing. By being 100% clear with our language, we'll know who is recommending what. Those of you advocating veganism—it's time to use the correct term: plants-only!

IN HER CRITIQUE, "The Truth About The China Study," recovering raw vegan and statistical whiz Denise Minger primarily focused "on seeing whether animal foods were as closely linked to disease as Campbell insinuated.....they aren't. Not by a long shot."

What Minger found most disturbing was the contrast between the original research findings and Campbell's interpretation in his popular book. As just one example: "The bold statement on page 132 that 'eating foods that contain any cholesterol above 0 mg is unhealthy' is drawn from a broad—and highly selective—pool of research." In other words, Campbell appears to have cherry-picked his data to create a "plant foods are good/animal foods are bad" dichotomy even though a methodical analysis of the raw data doesn't show this.

But hey, it works great for me and my family! Indeed, Campbell is a kindly-looking gentleman and, no doubt, wonderful grandfather whose children and grandkids, he claims, are all either vegan or nearly so. However, it's clear to scholars who've spent voluminous hours poring over the original monograph that Campbell did indeed single out those correlations which supported his previously announced belief that animal foods are bad for us, while failing to point out those showing the opposite. "The only solid conclusion we can take away from *The China Study*," Tom Naughton declares in *Goodscience,* "is that rats who are fed a diet of nothing but casein (an isolated dairy protein) will become sick and die. From this, Campbell indicts all animal products."

Minger, author of *Death by Food Pyramid: How Shoddy Science, Sketchy Politics and Shady Special Interests Have Ruined Our Health,* dares to present the more complete picture that emerges from the data: "Sugar, soluble carbohydrates, and fiber all have correlations with cancer mortality about 7 times the magnitude of that with animal protein." Using Campbell's own numbers, she puts his leaps-in-logic through the shredder, showing us what the study truly reveals: total fat was negatively correlated with cancer mortality; those eating the most greens did not suffer less cardiovascular disease; and some of the healthiest Chinese live in counties with the highest meat intake.

Minger's smackdown of *The China Study* is so logical and compelling, it quickly went viral and vegans, ex-vegans, and math geeks are having nerd-gasms trying to punch through all the complex numbers. Her stinging critique eventually caught Campbell's attention who published a response, to which she countered with a second, more complete analysis. For those of us who did everything in our power to avoid Statistics 101, here's just a peek at her penetrating examination:

When citing the anti-disease effects of plant foods, Campbell points to inverse correlations with biomarkers for plant food consumption as well as plant food intake itself. One example is in Claim #5 when he notes that stomach cancer is inversely associated with plasma concentrations of beta-carotene and vitamin C (bio-markers) as well as with green vegetable intake….(Both of these claims are based on uncorrected correlations, by the way.) Yet when citing the purportedly harmful effects of animal foods, Campbell relies on blood markers (usually total cholesterol or apo-B) but fails to find direct relationships between disease and the animal foods themselves. He still indicts animal foods as harmful, but comes to this conclusion by enlisting the help of intermediary variables….to those who approach this discussion from a place of neutrality, the bias is unmistakable.

Minger is not after Campbell, whom she believes is sincere in his beliefs. She is after good science. "Science itself should be cool, neutral, and somewhat soulless," states Minger, who is disappointed that Campbell hasn't yet offered a more revealing look into his methods of analysis. Basing his pro-vegan claims on the raw and uncorrected data is misleading, she asserts. "Why didn't Campbell pay more attention to the role of confounders?" she asks. "Why did he accept the raw data….without conducting deeper analyses?"

The answer may be found in the author's original pro-vegan premise. But good science doesn't work hard to prove a favored supposition; it tries to disprove it. Good science doesn't narrowly look for specific trends; it sees with wide open eyes everything that's there. As Minger concludes: "The book, while not entirely without value, is not about the China Study….It would be more aptly titled, *A Comprehensive Case for the Vegan Diet*, and the reader should be cautioned that the evidence is selected, presented, and interpreted with the goal of making that case in mind….its bias against animal products and in favor of veganism permeates every chapter and every page."

As far back as 1990, Harvard researchers Frank Hu and Walter Willett also strongly disagreed with Campbell's conclusion, noting that the survey of Chinese counties "did not find a clear association between animal product consumption and risk of heart disease or major cancers." Of course, even association is nowhere near causality. In other words, not a thing has been proven. Yet Dr. Campbell and others keep sending out a black and white nutrition message: *Go Vegan! Everybody! Go!* But nutrition is not so simple. It is contradictory and complex, exactly like the diverse and confounding humans it studies.

When it comes to health, will we *ever* be able to reconcile what's slippery in our dietary choices with what is solid? We'd all prefer nutrition advice to be clear and absolute but quite often it just isn't. Thus, our collective angst and shaking of heads that researchers can't seem to make up their bloody minds about what's good for us and what's not! Yet it's far better to tell the whole story and present the often conflicting data than to oversimplify, exaggerate or fudge—especially if fudging elevates your own private beliefs to the false status of "nutritional truth."

Personally, I recommend that Dr. Campbell turn his attention to the hundreds of thousands of fans who followed his vegan lead and conduct an equally extensive western study, *The American Study*. This should not be ecological research but a respected cohort study designed to track a large number of vegans—how about 6,500—who are healthy when the study begins. Food intake patterns should be closely monitored over the years, with disease and mortality rates scrupulously recorded. It is not enough to draw vegan health conclusions based on studies of omnivores, as in the Campbell book, or diseased older people, as in the Ornish and Esselstyn studies. These are our children taking on this unverified diet, some as young as one year old. To determine their health outcomes, disease rates, and longevity status, today's young vegans should be studied for the rest of their lives.

MEANWHILE, PERSONAL TESTIMONY from suffering vegans and ex-vegans continues to pour in. Hollywood types get surplus press, like actress Angelina Jolie who claims her all-plants diet "nearly killed me," but lesser-known and similarly disillusioned vegans are wandering around like hungry orphans left out in the cold. Many did veganism "like a science," anticipating positive results but were rewarded instead with debilitating fatigue and faltering health. Here are just a few of their voices, distilled from veg blogs and my own interviews:

> At age 14 I made the tough choice to cut animals out of my diet. At first I felt fantastic about my decision, but a year later I was so exhausted I couldn't accomplish even the simplest task. I was so very tired and suffered from constant colds and stomach flu. My doctor put me on supplements, but they made me sick. I was desperate to be healthy again...I never realized what this kind of restrictive diet could do to my body. Eventually I made another hard decision: to add fish back into my life. I gradually increased the dosage....today I can happily report that I am healthy again and will not be cutting fish out of my diet.

I can completely relate to what you're going through. My severe fructose malabsorption and soy intolerance led me to stop being a vegan also. I was living off non-wheat grains and green veggies at one point and my health was greatly suffering....eggs were the first animal product I bought after I realized veganism was killing me.

Because of my love for animals and the environment, I long to be vegan again and wish I could embrace this lifestyle. For me personally, my body and health need more than a vegan diet can provide.

In my vegan phase I relied very heavily on soy and legumes and am now allergic to both.

I simply can't allow myself to slip back into the state I was in as a strict vegan. Though it seems long ago, I'm frightened it will happen again. I do feel disgusted to have to consume fish on a regular basis, this is the truth. People ask me, "well, if you feel disgusted, why are you eating it?" The answer is—for the good of my health.

Can you go online and find glowing testimony from non-suffering vegans who still believe in their diet? Of course, but we are here to discuss the growing army of largely unacknowledged plant-eaters whose health has taken a tragic nose-dive on this highly unnatural diet. And they don't need an epidemiological study of 6,500 non-vegan Chinese to tell them that.

VEGANISM IS A NOBLE aspiration but why would anyone assume this limited, little-studied diet is suitable for all? Exactly who are these activists who presume to prescribe the ideal diet for you, me, and everyone? Are they clairvoyants? Nutrigeneticists? Medical doctors? Forget that last one. The MDs we've been seeing since kindergarten know practically zilch about nutrition. Although the food we eat has a tremendous effect on our health, productivity and longevity, shamefully, only 1/3 of US medical schools require even a single nutrition course.

Here's the bigger question: Do vegan missionaries, with or without degrees, know your body better than you? Do they know what you experience when you pursue an all-plants diet, your short and long-term physical and mental health results? You'd think so by the way many of them lecture. But one-size-fits-all dietary thinking is not only absurdly simplistic, it is physiologically false and potentially harmful. And what a rip-off to your own intelligence to try to fit your-

143

self into someone else's dietary box! So vegan crusaders everywhere, listen up: *The only body you have authority over is your own.*

How revealing that the root word for zealotry, the obsessive pursuit of an ideal, is the Greek *zelos*, derived from *zeein*, to boil or simmer. But it also means to rage, fume or seethe, and there are plenty of angry vegan zealots out there telling the rest of us how to eat and live. And what's so problematic about the feverish conviction that your belief system is the right one? That because your specific diet/culture/worldview/religion works best for you, it is therefore best for everyone? Well, nothing, if you want to end up with the f'd up world we already have. By now we should all understand the dangers of this kind of misguided, absolutist thinking. It has been the mustard seed of many ill-begotten crusades throughout our species' history.

Where does this kind of fanaticism come from, this messianic zeal? Is it really a keen desire to help others? Or is it the ego that loves to be right, that's ashamed to be shown wrong? In the case of dietary priests and preachers, it's often an over-confident, do-gooder mix of both. Yes, there are plenty of humble vegans out there who simply believe they are following the right path for themselves. Unfortunately, it's the vocal and vociferous who grab all the attention.

Our food choices involve ethics, no doubt about that, but trying to impose a single moral code of eating on all people is profoundly unethical. In following a well-planned vegan diet, an unknown percentage of us will suffer, our health and quality of life. Surely the compassion that lies at the heart of ethical veganism extends to human animals.

A rigid insistence on plants-only is just as foolish as insisting that everyone eat meat. Attachment is attachment. Both directives are overboard. Both ultimately feed the ego as much as the body. As Michael pens in a vegetarian blog, "It's important to live conscious of your actions, eating and otherwise, but if you're doing harm to your own body in the process, it seems hypocritical to not eat meat out of cruelty to other animals. Vegetarianism might be a good philosophy, but it makes a dangerous religion."

Amen, brother.

23.

INTO THE WILDS

Swim through iced waters
My net will be your blanket
You will be my life

—Pamela Edwards

SURELY SEATTLE puts on the longest-running festival in the world, stretching October through May every single year. It's the slippery, socked-in wet season—endearingly christened the Seattle Rain Festival by its ever tolerant residents. And yet, to be fair, this radiantly green city receives far less annual precipitation than Mobile, Houston, or even Miami. It's the season's tenaciousness that provokes worries of leaving one's house without an umbrella. Downpours aren't the issue here. Seattle's is a slow rain, a leisurely, ongoing, blue-grey drizzle that's in no hurry to leave and quite happy to stick around for months.

But I was impatient, starting to feel more salamander than human and besides, something was decidedly *off* with my nourishment and my life, even if I refused to voice it. Back from the Midwest, hungry and restless as ever, I headed down to the waterfront to join the cast of quirky characters forever coming and going from deep, glacier-carved Puget Sound. From the eccentric to the romantic, they're always delighted to bend your ear with some strange, wondrous Far North tale. Overworked fishermen drowning in their Guinness; randy young cannery workers looking to get laid; big game hunters bragging shamelessly—even a wild one-eyed sailor in search of a compliant, good cook of a woman to stow below deck in the galley (I declined his salacious offer). Seattle was reveling in its anti-glam status long before grunge. Explorers, gold seekers, scoundrels and scalawags have used it as their jumping-off point for over 150 years, and the more I greedily inhaled their colorful and peculiar stories, the less I could come up with one good reason not to join them. What better way to ponder one's life and health than a crazy-wisdom journey into the wilds?

Then one night in the Tip Top Saloon I met a hearty, good-looking wilderness guide and it wasn't the golden hairs peeking out from his red plaid shirt that had my eyes nailed to his chest. It was the bear-tooth necklace strung casually around his neck. Turning animal parts into jewelry is a turn-off for any vegetarian, even when the death is natural, yet the idea that this tall, quiet, bearded young man lived and breathed among grizzlies excited me more than any naked male vegan in heat. Powerful emotions swept over my profusely sweating body right then and there on the barstool, and I knew it was a done deal. I was moving to Alaska.

By early April I was onboard, sleeping on the open deck of the *MV Columbia,* flagship of the Alaska ferry system, along with all the other cash-strapped twenty-somethings. Sharing lip-puckering cherries in the eerie foggy light, we meditated upon the endless, grey water/sky—it's all one piece up there—and read Gary Snyder's song-poems to our ancient continent, Turtle Island. As the soft persistent rain droned on and on, a rainbow-hued "tent town" blossomed in the ferry's wide stern and we huddled together with blankets and peppermint Schnapps, instant comrades on this grand adventure through the Inside Passage, 40,000 miles of intricate coastline, sheltered bays, and secret pirate coves. Early European sailors restlessly explored and then abandoned this same coast, questing in vain for the mythical Pacific-Atlantic route, but indigenous people continue to live in these lush forests as they have for millennia—nature and the supernatural shaping their lives and their art. Night descended, a darker grey, and we began to actually pity the other travelers ensconced in their stuffy little cabins, missing out—every one of them—on the dark, thrilling sweep of coastal mountains and the exhilarating freshness of the north wind.

Catching a ride from the Haines ferry terminal was a cinch. Dropped off in tiny Tok, junction of the Glenn and Alaska Highways, I grabbed some coffee at the White Bear Café, hitched up my leather boots, and started hiking my solitary way south and west through the sweeping alluvial plain drained by the immense Copper River Delta. In search of my gentle, dignified Grizzly Man. My heart was in my throat the entire way, enthralled by the silence and dearth of humans, the shimmering glaciers and massive, soaring Chugach Mountains pressing close. And then the empty road rose up and up to Thompson Pass where falls some of the deepest snow on earth—over 80 feet one freaky, white-out year. Onward and upward I rode in a beat-up Pontiac Trans Am with my latest kind stranger, a lean, animated young man with darting green eyes who fed me cheese sandwiches and confessed that, bar none, he'd rather dance than eat any night of the year. Down,

down we descended into the growing chill, through icy Keystone Canyon with its sparkling still-frozen waterfalls, following the path of generations of native Ahtna people and latter-day gold rushers. Then the road abruptly dead-ended and into the dreamy white-tunneled streets of Valdez my backpack and I tumbled.

There's really nothing to do at such a moment but lie back and gaze with open-mouthed wonder at the three-story-high piles of relentlessly plowed snow. Towering above the frosty, socked-in houses, they threatened to obscure street lights and utility poles and dwarfed the few hardy souls scurrying about in the glacial cold. This was pre-spill Valdez, little known in the lower 48 at the time. To me it was just another obscure, blizzard-doused village on Prince William Sound, southern terminus of the Alaska pipeline and home to a couple thousand freedom-loving souls, most notably my brown-eyed hero. Alas, he was hunkered down at a bush cabin with his horse when I showed up—what gypsy knows her arrival date? So instead of a squishy-warm, welcoming bed that night, I walked out onto the bleak tundra behind Buck's locked single-wide trailer, curled up on the hard white crust in my too-thin sleeping bag and started knocking my frozen feet together like flint and stone, hoping to spark some meager heat. And then I waited for the rapture.

WHAT EXACTLY WAS I hoping to find in this far-flung wilderness where emerald-gold lights danced across the cosmos like drunken angels that very first night? Certainly an experience of living beyond the confines of civilization in a raw, more natural state. Oh yes! I wanted to dwell among our wildlife brethren beneath a clarity of planets and stars guaranteed to take any rain-fogged, city-slicker's breath away. I'd be a rugged Saint Francis, conversing with eagles and lynx, a female Grizzly Guy communicating telepathically with primal bruins. And if my brawny wilderness male didn't work out (alas, he did not), I'd find myself another lusty backwoodsman who didn't even remotely like to hunt. Instead of rotting animal flesh we'd subsist on.....hmm, what precisely *would* we subsist on at five degrees latitude below the Arctic Circle? Why, humongous turnips, cauliflower, and kohlrabi, of course!

With 24-hour daylight at our disposal, surely this is a vegetarian gardener's paradise. No matter that summer is achingly brief, that winter can arrive in early September, because The Last Frontier's outrageously long growing days produce monster pumpkins weighing in at 1200 pounds and equally obese 67-inch gourds. I'd read all about it before leaving Seattle; veggie records are constantly being

147

shattered at the Alaska State Fair. Just recently 10-year-old Keevan Dinkel took highest honors at the Giant Cabbage Weigh-Off with his stunning 92.3 pounder named Bob, with not a single chomp from a marauding moose to mar its leafy beauty. Select the right frost-resistant variety and you can even grow potatoes above the Arctic Circle. Surely, I'd chosen the perfect place on earth to grow my own food. A veggie's determination knows no limits—we can thrive anywhere!

We'd split firewood all afternoon, my sweet strapping man and I. Then come long winter evenings, he would undress me ever so slowly and pour hot steaming water over my throbbing arms and shoulders, pour it languorously over my whole yearning body as I kneeled with curved back inside the sturdy tin tub (formerly a horse trough) smack in the middle of our one-room cabin. Tenderly, he would dry me off, inch by highly-receptive inch, and we'd glide as one into our overworked bed and I'd burrow my face in his warm scruffy beard and he'd slide his knowing fingers right where I loved them and those ecstatic gold and green lights would start flashing across the heavens all over again as the sinking 3 PM sun closed down yet another sub-zero day.

"Hold the fantasy!" I scolded myself, finally ready to acknowledge that two essential items were of more immediate concern than a hot-blooded wilderness mate in thigh-tight jeans and knee-high Sorrels. In reverse order of urgency they were 2) a strong desire to return to my former full health and vigor and 1) a dire need to put into my extremely emaciated wallet something green and substantial. So where did this tired yet still devout vegetarian end up finding work? Why, next to the shores of magnificent Prince William Sound, of course, surrounded by a blood-red sea of dead animal slime.

It's not why I traveled to Valdez, not even close. But slowly, grudgingly, I was forced to admit it was the only cash game in town. The only one within 300 miles actually, driving distance to Anchorage. There comes a time for many of us when we need to make money *pronto* in order to survive and I most certainly did, having never been paid as promised for my Skykomish farming stint. For refusing to bed down with the gangly young stud they'd picked out for me? (The thought did cross my mind.) Meanwhile, there was nothing else for hungry tenderfoots to do but head on over to the local fishing companies always hiring on the piers.

Frankly, the idea of adding fish to my diet had played on the edge of my consciousness for the past few years. As a young girl, I'd always felt content and well nourished after eating my uncle's fresh-caught bass or bluegill. And I kept reading about the amazing health benefits bestowed by our water-breathing kin, so I

148

dared to question (something bona fide vegetarians and vegans are not supposed to do) if just *perhaps* an infrequent to occasional repast of fish might revive my flagging energy and more fully meet my nutritional needs. If this were true, I wanted to see for myself the origin and destiny of the gleaming ruby, pink and silver salmon I had observed so elegantly arranged in iced rows every morning at Pike Market. Yes, absolutely, if I were to begin eating fish, I needed to know all the hidden-to-the-public, gory details of how they arrived clean and uncluttered on our dinner plates. No matter how appalling to my sensibilities, before making such a solemn dietary decision, I knew I had to participate in the killing of my own food. Murder vegans call it, nothing short of murder.

Early the next morning, I reluctantly headed to the crime scene: the Valdez City Dock. Besides some fresh-scrubbed college students in Reeboks looking to work a couple of days for a lark, I was joined on the quay by the strangest back-woods types imaginable: silent, scrawny, bearded, sometimes toothless white men who crawled out of the woodwork every spring to yank on their rubber boots, pull in their scant annual income, then head back to spend a long hard winter in hand-hewn shacks in Tonsina, Chitina, or even McCarthy at the foot of the Wrangell Mountains, population 28 and two hours to the nearest post office over a brutal gravel road.

Young, broke, vagabond-types from all over the lower 48 were showing up as well, thousands of miles from their places of birth. One scraggly-haired, modern-day Pythagoras arrived barefoot, skeletal thin, and eternally cheerful in the late spring snow, draped in a mice-nibbled, saffron-colored sarong and little else. The personnel office handed this genial vegan youth a pair of knee-high waterproofs, a slick black apron and a gutting knife, then put him on the slime line with the rest of us fools.

It is hideously hard labor, this fish processing business, an orderly mayhem, bloody guts and severed heads a-flying. It took me but one shock-filled moment to figure out how it all works: the header starts the line, a hulky guy wielding a colossal head-severing knife, followed by the gutters with their precision slitters, followed by the slimers using only their sensitive, aching fingers. Small women are often selected as slimers because they don't need to deploy a knife, just their rubber-gloved freezing hands to swoosh out the mass of wet complicated innards. Any flying fish-slime that doesn't make it to the take-away trough ends up on the floor next to your frozen feet or, more often, plastered like sodden worms all over your face, arms, legs, chest and burning throat. Luckily, I too was spared the knife and directed to the end of the line. Here I was instructed to catch all the cold, slippery, gutted and beheaded fish as they shot like polished baby torpedoes off the conveyer belt, ready to be sorted and packed in crushed ice.

Within minutes, my revulsion merged with utter astonishment at the sheer volume of glistening silver-finned fish. The herring runs were a done deal by now but the pink salmon were happening, and as fast as the boat crews could unload them into white plastic totes, they were speedily fork-lifted to the head of the line. Even this seemingly endless catch, I soon realized, was but a minuscule representation of the enormous bounty of the nearby sea. Tens of millions of these wild pinks—one of the most-eaten fish in America—valiantly, doggedly swim back to Valdez Sound during an average year, an outlandish 180 million to all of Alaska. They just keep coming and coming, shockwave after shockwave of wild pinks, a tsunami of returning salmon. As the hours passed my back and arms throbbed painfully, my heart ached unbearably and my eyes glazed over, inured to look at slender, intact, muscular fish by the thousands—whole gorgeous bodies one second, market meat the next. My mind floated out of my body and by late morning I had become so deeply cold and miserable, I wasn't sure if being a dead fish wasn't the better deal. Long before the mid-afternoon break, my numbed-out brain refused the deadening repetitiveness of the task. I quit.

Before my first day had even come to its shaky close, I slowly took off my guts-splattered apron and boots, wearily punched out, walked into the warm and merciful sun, and wept. Wept for all the beautiful dead and dying fish, for all the mind-demolishing jobs in this stupid industrialized world, and for the sustenance I could not seem to find in my life: not in my love relationships, not in my work, not even in my daily food.

I was ten years into my vegetarian way of life and although I was trying to be a good, honest, ethical veggie I knew something was not right. Wasn't this the recipe for excellent health? Wasn't this the prescription for a moral life? So why was my energy failing me? Why was my stamina a thing of the past? Shuffling past the town's quiet marina, emptied of fishing boats, I slumped cross-legged on the wood pier in the hazy afternoon light and gazed bleary-eyed and listless at the white-capped mountains rising out of blue-black Prince William Sound, twisting waterfalls rushing in. Broke and essentially homeless, I was steeped in my poor-me stupor when a brilliant sun suddenly erupted from behind dark clouds and the realization swiftly hit me: Here I am, this very moment, smack in the middle of one of the most spectacular, prolific, breeding, teeming ecosystems on earth and

I'm friggin' *whining?* Sucking in belly-deep, life-affirming breaths, I snapped to attention as the glorious scene unfolded before me. And then and there I vowed to stay and somehow make it work.

SO I JOINED ARCH-RIVAL Seahawk Seafood's packing and shipping crew on the other side of town. My feet and hands stayed warm and dry and I worked long and hard; but my back-to-the-land romanticism was bruised and battered. So I defended my new job with the knowledge that salmon are wild and sustainable in Alaska, that humans have eaten them for millennia and will continue to do so for millennia to come. Just as critical, I needed money for food. That, too, was a fact.

By August the coho salmon were arriving in full force. Upwards of 350,000 of these tough, resilient swimmers return to Port Valdez in a good season, averaging a hefty 10-12 pounds. My body loved the intense physicality of loading trucks but for some puzzling reason, the 24/7 breakroom caffeine had stopped performing its usual miracles. To stave off exhaustion and keep up the seven-day work week, I needed to greatly increase my calorie and protein intake. But how? How could I achieve this in a remote land of diminished food options? Plus a bloated gut which simply couldn't tolerate more legumes and fiber? As so often happens with our most confounding questions, the answer was staring me straight in the eye.

One night at shift's end, dog-tired, famished, 8 PM, I impulsively grabbed a wild coho from the thousands flowing through the plant with their hearts torn out. Wrapped and tucked it carefully under my arm, then wearily trudged around the harbor spit to my new abode after months of camping: a teeny two chair/one table apartment. There I stared, for long moments, at this resplendent, silvery creature's headless, gutted form. Its shiny, black, unblinking eyes were long-gone but still I saw them staring back at me, void of judgment, empty of sorrow, staring back from a taut muscular body ready to be consumed.

As I gently opened the animal's already-slit belly, its opulent scarlet flesh out-right shimmered in the 24-hour window light, beckoning me, summoning me. Consider—the salmon in my pale, uncertain hands seemed to be saying—my dense nutrition, my protein-saturated muscles, my wild riotous run to end up here before your hungry eyes, held in your open hungry arms. Consider my beauty, my stamina, the incalculable energy and passion it took for me to return home for my final few days, here to Valdez, your home now too. Consider all that I offer you. Will you deny allowing my body to become part of yours? Will you throw me back into the cold northern waters to disintegrate into food for other life forms when I am here in your kitchen, here in your warm hands, ready to sustain you? And I did at last consider, and I did at last stop denying. Without overthinking, I set the oven to 350 and purposefully, patiently waited for this handsome fish, bones intact, to bake to flakey tenderness. Taking out a 4-pronged silver fork, slowly flecking off piece after piece of dense red muscle, I sat on the floor and ate, and ate abundantly, right down to the soft spinal bone. And then I crushed the delicate vertebrae between my fingers and ate them too.

Sitting back on my haunches at the end of this ancient human-animal ritual, I looked out my living room window at the low-lying, all-giving sun and said a prayer of thankfulness to the shining waters that had delivered me this gift of utter and complete nourishment. My body was in absolute awe of the gift. Within the hour it surged with a raw energetic power it hadn't felt in over a decade. I danced around the empty room. I cried out my gratitude. The strength and spirit of the vigorous swimmer that had battled upstream for thousands of miles to complete its life cycle had somehow been bestowed, at least in part and temporarily, on me. That's exactly how it felt, no words held back. This was my body speaking its own unambiguous language and for once I refused to shut it off.

My mind, however, needed to rationalize my decision in order to live with it. *Veggie defector: Beware the slippery slope. Only because this is local fish from plentiful wild stock will I allow this. As soon as you leave Alaska, you must give it up. All of it.* I barely heard the authoritarian whines, the plaintive ideological whimpers. Freed from the indoctrinated mind's constraints! Freed to follow my own wise body's instincts! To self-preserve and flourish!

FROM THAT MOMENT ON, I consumed silver or sockeye salmon almost every day of the week: wild, fresh, succulent, nutritionally powerful, straight off the boat. My body had a lot of catching up to do and I could scarcely believe the physical and emotional changes sweeping over me. As the weeks and months passed, I found myself possessed of endless energy. *I never ran out of energy.* My brain became sharp and focused. My nerves calmed down. I tossed my morning coffee. I tossed my processed food. Compared to the previous spaced-out, draggy years, I felt like I was flying on jet fuel from early morning to late night.

For 12 hours a day, seven days a week, my crew and I packed and shipped protein-dense, omega-3-rich, fresh and frozen salmon to a hungry world. Barely

115 pounds in my work boots, I was hoisting 55-pound boxes into cold storage one after the other, loading them onto gigantic freezer vans bound for Anchorage and Seattle. By September I was directing a 10-person team, running around the plant like a frisky arctic fox, falling dangerously in love with my boss. I danced between forklifts with Mona, my fellow dancer-shaker, glided effortlessly between stacked totes, sashayed up and down steep metal ladders. When the late summer rain spit and drizzled into now-dreary Valdez harbor, my spirits only blazed brighter. People started asking where I had found the fountain of youth; what new drug was I on?

At the time I had no idea of the remarkable nutritional value of fish, wild salmon in particular. That is, my analytical mind had no idea. My body, of course, knew instinctively that I was onto something grand, that I was ingesting a truly superior food source—a food I had found no match for in the plant world, not even close. Is it any wonder Alaska natives, indeed all Pacific Northwest tribes, have long revered this audacious creature as a gift from the gods? When the first packed runs miraculously reappeared every spring, all the humans would shout out their joy and run to the river en masse. To watch in elation! Is it any wonder tribes still celebrate the cyclic energy input of these water masters in their totems and legends, calling them Salmon People, Life Givers? Any wonder why Pythagoras included locally abundant fish in his diet as needed? Why Jesus fed them to the hungry multitudes? Oh no, I will never, ever again wonder.

Many a long-lit summer night in southern Alaska, on the bountiful shores of Prince William Sound—where soars the eagle and roams the grizzly in quest of their own wild salmon—you would find this happy, healthy pescatarian sitting cross-legged on her kitchen floor, eating fresh-caught silver or sockeye, flaking off the tender morsels with joyous, greasy fingers. Chewing slowly and serenely. Sensing, with immense gratitude, the wild animal meat empowering her body and her mind. Feeling the old depleted self ebbing away and the new, vibrant energy invariably arise. The same vital energy she had known every single day as a child. A flesh-eating, fish-eating child.

24.

PROTEIN 101: DON'T GET WASTED

Is IT POSSIBLE for belief and objectivity to intersect? Walk up to any young vegan, inquire about his protein intake, and you're likely to get blasted: "Lose it! We're *really* tired of that question. Vegans get more than enough protein. I never even think about it." Then ask how many daily grams are recommended for his age, gender, and metabolic type and you may get a blank stare or, more likely, a prickly retort. "Americans are meat hogs and eat *way* too much protein—so cut the boring questions." I've also heard sadly misinformed responses like, "What's the deal? I only need 45 grams a day, right?"

Here's the deal: Individual protein needs vary widely, one might even say *wildly*, depending on an array of ever-changing factors, including your weight, physical activity and stress levels, even where in the world you live. A mere 45 grams might be adequate for Anna, a slender, not terribly active 15-year-old who writes poetry in Gulf Shores, Alabama. But Peter, 20, a muscular sea kayaker from Camden, Maine, may well need 100 grams of daily protein. Janet, a middle-aged, full-time keyboard-banger from Little Rock can get by with just 50 grams, while 30-year-old Erika, mother of three non-stop little tyrants in Toledo, needs in excess of 70.

Yet the current Recommended Daily Allowance (RDA) for protein is set in stone: 46-52 grams for teenagers and .8 grams per kilo of body weight (.36 per pound) for adults over 18, regardless of who you are or how you live. This easy one-for-all formula, advanced by the USDA and published just about everywhere, is employed in our children's school lunch programs, used to feed our elderly, endlessly repeated by professional dietitians, and waved in our faces by vegans and other low-protein advocates.

154

So the RDA has a huge influence on our society's nutrition practices. It's what you scrutinize to see if you are meeting the "correct" daily amounts of the macro-nutrients. And it's what vegan proponents use, in part, to justify the low protein intake of their restrictive diet. Just meet the RDA and you're good to go! Not true. What's little known is that the RDA for protein represents the *minimum* required to avoid progressive loss of lean body mass. In plain English: it's the minimum protein needed *to avoid wasting away.* Who knew that? Did *you* know that?

Is it any wonder the blogwaves are thick with ex-veggies grumbling about muscle loss and physical weakness? Here's one of many testifying for *Primal Living in the Modern World*: "I was a vegetarian for a little over three years with a short period of veganism. When I first went veg I felt great, but I now believe this was because I ditched the processed crap and started cooking all my own food. Three years later, my muscle mass and strength had wasted away."

Losing muscle mass means just that: your muscles become punier and your body grows weaker. There's a simple way to avoid this scary, unhealthy scenario: eat a balanced diet that includes sufficient protein and calories, accompanied by regular exercise. Eating high-quality protein at every meal works best, but exactly *how much protein* continuous to spark contentious debate—and the RDA isn't really helping us find individual answers to that all-important question.

Here's why misunderstanding abounds when it comes to the RDAs we believe in and dutifully try to follow. At various intervals the Institute of Medicine (IM) publishes recommended values for the macronutrients: proteins, carbohydrates, and fats. The goal of a recent IM report "was to extend, where possible, beyond the concept of a minimum requirement to the expression of a goal for consumption" according to the authors of "Dietary Allowance of Protein: A Misunderstood Concept" (Wolfe and Miller). In other words, the RDA of each macronutrient was going to be changed from a minimal to an *optimal* intake based on actual health outcomes, such as decreased risk of heart disease and osteoporosis.

While this optimal amount was published for some nutrients, it wasn't applied to protein and this uneven application has resulted in "considerable confusion," according to experts, regarding the most advantageous protein quantity for good health and disease avoidance. Some consumers even think the RDA designates the *maximum* recommended nutrient amount! In truth, the RDA numbers quoted by vegans and other minimal-protein activists are low-ball figures that might allow you to stay in the game, but just barely. They do not represent an optimal intake of daily protein for full health and disease prevention.

THIS HOT-BUTTON ISSUE has the low-protein crowd up in arms because a growing body of research reveals great benefits from higher protein intake: for bone health, muscle function, energy levels, weight management and wound healing. The current RDA for protein is, in fact, under fire from researchers who strongly assert that our daily needs have been significantly underestimated for years, due to the methodological limitations of the "nitrogen balance" technique. This just means finding out if your body excretes more nitrogen than you eat, putting you into negative/unhealthy balance—nitrogen being a component of protein, but not fats or carbs.) Using the newer "indicator amino acid oxidation" method, described as rapid, robust and reliable, researchers affirm that our optimal intake is nearly *double or more* the current RDA, or 1.5-2.2 g/kg daily (Elango; Pencharz).

Sorry plant eaters, but this is a whopper of an increase. Study authors conclude that there exists "an urgent need to reassess recommendations for protein intake in adult humans." What a far cry from the standard vegan line that our protein requirements are low, straightforward, and oh so easy to meet.

Moreover, the RDA assumes you are a sedentary human being! You know the drill: sitting on your keister all day, staring at those blinkity-blank pixels; driving four blocks to the nearest ATM instead of walking; texting your neighbor versus strolling over; or budging from your desk for potty breaks only—and more high-carb chow. Alas, this description applies to modern bum-sitting humans across the land, all of us dramatically increasing our risk for developing diabetes, heart disease, and death from all causes.

Studies reveal that those of us who sit four hours or more each day, without substantial bodily movement, are up to 80% more likely to die from heart disease and 50% more likely to die from just about everything else. This pattern has a chilling name, *sedentary death syndrome*: the slow decay process that ensues when you don't use your muscles for long periods of time, releasing a host of inflammatory factors.

Exercising after a long day at work won't prevent this; you need to be up and moving every hour of your day. So if an active lifestyle prevents sedentary death syndrome, why in the world is the RDA for protein designed for non-exercising or sedentary adults? Since every single one of us, except the bedridden, should be physically active, why pay attention to the RDA at all? Tossing it altogether, the International Society of Sports Nutrition (ISSN) is now advising us to increase our daily protein up to 150% of current recommendations, as part of a balanced, nutrient-dense diet.

As for athletic types, even the pro-vegan Academy of Nutrition and Dietetics is *finally* advising plant-eating sportsmen and women to increase their protein intake 50-100%, another enormous correction. These much larger numbers are quite easy for omnivores to meet; not so for vegans, many of whom struggle to meet even the current low-ball RDA. And you don't have to be an athlete to find yourself undergoing periods of stress-induced high-protein hunger. Think: exams, break-ups, divorce, job loss, money issues. During these events, common to all of us, protein needs likewise shoot up due to an increased loss of amino acids and a jump in demand for protein synthesis. Changing the moniker RDA (Recommended Daily Allowance) to MDA (Minimum Daily Allowance to prevent lean muscle loss) would be a good start to rectifying widespread misunderstanding about our optimal protein intake, especially among that segment of ultra-thin vegans who certainly do seem to be losing muscle mass, i.e., wasting away.

One concerned mother, whose entire family recently made the plants-only pledge, asked vegan guru John Robbins about this, remarking that all the vegans she knows "have in common a thin, frail look and a pallid complexion.....not exactly the picture of health." Robbins was quick to reassure her on his website, *The Food Revolution*, that there is absolutely nothing wrong with a frail, pasty-white appearance, especially as compared to oversized, flush-faced Americans. To understand this, he explained, just look at European autos!

Two-cylinder Citroëns look downright puny if you are accustomed to powerful 8-cylinder American autos, described by Robbins as gargantuan and grotesque. It's just a matter of what you're used to looking at on a daily basis, i.e., your idea of "normal." I seriously doubt Robbins' analogy is going to comfort concerned vegan mommas. When it comes to both the human body and automobiles, vigor and performance are everything. Asked about the everyday performance of the fragile Citroën—nicknamed the Little Freak in the former Yugoslavia—owners joke that it goes "from 0-60 in one day" and "you need to make an appointment to merge onto an interstate highway."

Yes, your level of vitality is a crucial marker when it comes to nutrition outcomes. And, o*f course*, an omnivore's diet is potentially lacking if food choices are poor. But once you pull out all animal-sourced food, a lot of nutrients have suddenly gone missing or exist in deficient amounts. "One of the biggest dangers of veganism is this restricted diet may cause malnutrition," admits Kate Pullen on a pro-vegan site. Protein, calcium, iron, vitamins B12 and D3 can all come up short, "deficiencies that can cause ailments such as anemia and osteomalacia, a condition that damages bones. In children these deficiencies can result in rickets and other potentially serious illnesses." A proposed law in Italy would, in fact, jail parents who impose a vegan diet on their kids if it leads to malnourishment.

"FAILURE TO THRIVE" IS REAL AMONG VEGANS

Despite the potential shortfall of so many essential elements, nutrition educator John Allen Mollenhauer once argued that by eating a wide variety of nutrient-dense plant foods, supplementing as needed, absolutely *everyone* can thrive as a vegan. Everyone, that is, except the many vegans he has witnessed suffering from the "Failure to Thrive" syndrome. Yes, this is how Mollenhauer describes the vegans he counsels who are doing everything right but remain unhealthy, beyond what he calls "a reasonable period of time." What a rare admission in the pro-veg world! "It's one thing to say that people experiencing Failure to Thrive are simply dealing with withdrawal symptoms from nutrient-poor and nutrient-barren foods," writes Mollenhauer, "but in reality it's more than that and this calls into question the nutritional adequacy of 100% plant-based diets for many."

To try to understand why some individuals are flourishing on a vegan diet (at least do date) while others clearly are not, Mollenhauer turned to Michael Klaper, practicing MD for 40+ years and a popular vegan enthusiast who has witnessed the benefits of an all-plants diet *as therapy for older folks who suffer from chronic degenerative diseases* (we've seen this theme before).

"I am aware that there is a significant population of long-term vegans who, despite their best efforts, and mine, to optimize their vegan diets, still remain pale, underweight, and unable to achieve the robust health they seek," writes Klaper in "The Failure to Thrive: Speculations on the Nutritional Adequacy of 100% Plant-Based Diets." *Thank you*, Mollenhauer and Klaper, for finally acknowledging this "significant" phenomenon in a pro-vegan public forum. This Failure to Thrive outcome, almost 100% denied, ignored or mocked in the vegan community, has become alarmingly obvious to those of us who know or live with one of those earnest, doing-it-right, can't-make-it-up-the-hill, Citroën-like vegans.

Klaper, whose background is not in nutritional biochemistry, nonetheless offers his personal speculations, i.e. guesswork, why so many people fail to stay healthy on the strict vegan diet he so covets and would like all of humanity to follow. Of course, the culprit couldn't possibly be the diet itself, with its inherent nutritional deficiencies, low-protein intake, decreased bioavailability, and high-fiber/phytate content which inhibits mineral absorption. Thus, instead of indicting a restrictive, nonhistorical diet, Klaper indicts the poor suffering vegans, possibly even their mothers. The roots of their ill health may go back to childhood, Klaper speculates on his *Nutrient Rich* site, based on zero data. They were probably fed a terribly SAD diet centered around meat and dairy, he guesses, which was "repeatedly slathered over the 26 feet of intestinal membranes," quite possibly becoming "a deciding factor in the structure and function of those organs." Totally out-there pro-vegan conjecture, as if human morphology and physiology evolve so quickly. Designed to put the onus on the suffering vegans, never the vegan diet.

Other, more reasoned doctors who work with recovering vegans believe it is insufficient protein, among other nutrient shortages, creating this clear Failure to Thrive outcome. That's sheer nonsense, advocates keep insisting: we get adequate protein while the average, steak-guzzling American grossly overindulges. "Twice the protein needed!" is their oft-shouted slogan. Really? Your sources? Statistics from the National Health and Nutrition Examination Survey (Fulgoni) reveal a far different story, debunking the myth that Americans are gorging on protein.

A startling 56% of all individuals studied failed to meet even the minimum recommended daily amount of protein, whether from animal or plant sources. The highest median intake was 16% of calories, found in men aged 51–70. Just 15% of daily calories for all Americans, on average, come from protein. These numbers are far from maxing out at the recommended upper limit of 35%. They are also right in line with historically healthy eating patterns, like the Mediterranean Diet. Researchers conclude *not* that Americans are greatly overeating protein (where do these people get their mock stats?) but that "higher protein intakes could be safely recommended."

Let's hope the next national nutrition survey includes a separate category for plants-only eaters, who tend to consume at the very low end of the range, 8-12%. Vegans are in great need of precise research on this subject. As of this writing, *zero* nitrogen balance or amino acid oxidation studies have been conducted on vegans to determine if they are getting adequate protein. What do we call belief without evidence? Blind faith.

I WAS PAST 4O BEFORE admitting, after years of denial, that I need a good 70-75 grams of daily protein to ensure sustained energy and full health, far more than I was intaking as a petite vegetarian. My veg books were very misleading in this regard, and even today's activists throw out arbitrary, one-for-all numbers, like "no more than 60 grams, tops, male or female!" Listen to this ardent vegan working his online food politics, trying to convince a rogue to get back on track where he belongs. It seems that Dylan has been feeling weak and despondent on his all-plants diet and wants to substantially increase his protein intake by adding wild fish to his regime:

> Dylan, you don't need to go that route. You just need to figure out what you're missing nutritionally that makes you want to eat fish. I assure you that a plant diet can offer anything you need. If it's protein you're worried about, just eat enough variety and calories every day; then you're for sure getting enough. Try a small scoop of sunflower seeds when you need a quick protein boost. Never abandon your animal ethics for health reasons!

A small scoop of sunflower seeds? That satiates me for about 30 minutes and I do a triple scoop. (Sunflower seeds are low in lysine, by the way, an essential amino acid.) Yet Vegan Man is convinced he knows not only the correct diet for Dylan but the specific foods and quantities that will energize his unique body. And here's the kicker in the above advice: *Never abandon your ethics for health reasons.* If stunted energy, crashing serotonin levels, and declining health aren't enough for advocates to cut with the ethical preaching, what is?

Yes yes, I know, V Man is saying that Dylan just needs to work *longer and harder* to find the right plant proteins, such as soy in its myriad forms, to support his full health. But you can say to a veg pundit after a decade of agonizing effort: my body hates soy, gets very tired after eating it, and he will respond, *There's no scientific proof of that outcome. Try tempeh instead of tofu.* I did; no go. *Then eat beans, lentils, and other legumes 2-3 times a day.* You don't get it, do you? My body truly loathes that many legumes; and he'll say, *Soak 'em, sprout 'em, cook 'em, then add kombucha, baking soda or Bean-o.* But dude, I tried all that and it's the same painful cramping and hellacious gas. I can't even function in that state.

So he'll insist, *Gas is good for you, fostering the growth of beneficial bacteria in your colon!* But, you inform him, humans lack the enzyme necessary to digest the complex sugar raffinose found in legumes, and I hate that this is happening but my body is telling me again and again: GET ALL THESE LEGUMES THE HELL OUT OF MY GUT! *Hey bro, just rise above all that fermentation and methane gas inside your spasming colon, knowing you are alleviating the suffering of animals.* Yeah right, and what about THIS suffering animal?

160

You see, it doesn't matter to a vegan proselytizer what your own truth is, your body's unique metabolic story and powerful messages. The problem is never the diet. The problem is always YOU. You're either lazy, lying, gluttonous or doing it wrong. (Or your momma did you wrong.) There are no exemptions to the Vegan Rule. *No matter how broken your health, never, ever give up your vegan ethics!* Here's "Miss Lisbeth" blog-counseling "Amber" against becoming a flexitarian who partakes of the occasional animal protein that her body is strongly signaling she needs for full health. Naturally, Miss Lisbeth knows the protein requirements of just about every human body out there.

> Amber, besides pregnant women, almost everyone needs no more than 45–55 grams of protein a day. Nobody should be losing sleep over how much protein they get! If you want to worry about some-thing, you can fret about the fluoride in your water.

The web is crawling with similar free vegan advice but here's another little discussed reality: plant eaters need an even *higher* protein intake than omnivores of similar weight and activity level, at least 10% higher, because of the decreased digestibility of plant protein—fibrous, tough, gassy—and thus its lower bioavail-ability compared to animal protein. (Another vegan myth busted: meat is *easier* to digest than plants.) This decreased bioavailability explains why true vegans, i.e., herbivores, spend up to 16 hours a day grazing, grazing, grazing. And ruminants like sheep and cows, with their multiple stomach compartments for all that heavy-duty digesting, still have to spend up to nine hours daily just eating.

Herbivores are anatomically and physiologically adapted to eat 100% plants; humans are not. (Shall we surgically insert more stomach chambers into omniv-orous humans? Is this the next vegan scheme?) What's more, low-calorie intake increases protein requirements as a percentage of total intake. These facts create a double whammy for plant eaters because they tend to take in far fewer calories *and* less protein than omnivores. So vegans: if you're consistently falling below your optimal weight, it's critical to start consuming a more protein-dense diet in order to maintain your strength and prevent muscle wasting.

After decades of denial that too-low protein is an issue, a courageous few are now ready to admit that vegans really *should* increase their protein intake. Some recommend bumping it up just 10% but Jack Norris, RD, acknowledging the growing research which indicates the RDA has been underestimated all these years, now counsels fellow vegans to err "on the side of more protein." Up your daily intake to 1.0–1.1 g/kg, he advises, a significant 25-37% gain. While we should all applaud this overdue recommendation, pity the millions of protein-marginal or outright deficient vegans who haven't yet heard the news. Especially those who desperately needed this advice years or even decades ago.

HOW VITAL IS adequate protein for your health? Consider this: other than water, it's the most abundant substance in your corporal being, responsible for building your muscles, nerves, blood, heart and brain. Among the human body's 50,000 specialized proteins are enzymes (catalysts for all your biochemical processes) and antibodies to fight off infections. Your body cannot create, heal, or repair a single tissue without protein. That's why dedicated athletes usually know more than their MDs about the quality and metabolic action of various protein foods. And that's why an attitude of indifference among vegans regarding daily intake is just plain foolish.

Big Mac guzzling Americans may indulge in excess protein (although the stats don't show this). Their task is to cut down and find healthy, humane products. But once you remove *all* animal protein from your diet, with its high biological value and diversity of sources, you do indeed need to be conscious of your daily protein intake and, just as important, how it increases as you age. You too will wake up one partly-cloudy morning and be forty.

Yet vegans remain confident of the protein-sufficiency of their diet, due in part to this commonly cited myth: *There's never been a single case of protein deficiency in the USA if enough calories are consumed; only Third World people are deficient.* Why then, do so many of us know committed vegans, even vegetarians, who took in adequate calories but still ended up exhausted and depleted? And why is at least one respected doctor in Boulder—arguably the veggie capitol of the world—treating veg'ns with protein deficiencies on a regular basis? What's more, he is treating clients who have access to a staggering variety of plant foods from local and global sources, such as I never dreamed possible in my youth. Doctors who work with recovering vegans can now be found in every big city across America.

Is it possible to get enough high-quality protein on a strict vegan diet? It *may* be possible for individuals with naturally lower-protein needs who can tolerate large amounts of legumes, lead low-stress lives (a low-stress life, what's that?) and keep a vigilant eye on daily quantity, quality, and amino acid completeness.

162

Easy? No, it is not. We live in a demanding, fast-paced society and emotional and physical stressors can greatly increase our protein and caloric needs. Add in anything out of the ordinary—illness, surgery, pregnancy, or even an injury trying to heal—and your body will start gobbling up protein stores, *requiring up to 50% more than normal.* Vegetarians and vegans are not exempt from the human need to eat regular and sustaining amounts of complete protein to keep their bodies from plunging into negative nitrogen balance, a polite way of saying starvation.

Diana Schwarzbein, MD, a leading authority on metabolic healing based in Santa Barbara, CA, has treated many unhealthy veg'ns who suffered from what she calls self-imposed but unintentional starvation. By and large, these were not people with eating disorders; they simply were not taking in enough protein to support the constant rebuilding going on in our bodies. And what happens if you keep doing this? Your lovely body will be forced to consume its own tissues to feed your brain and stay alive.

This means that too-thin vegans are eating animal flesh after all: their own. And not just muscle tissue but eventually—if inadequate protein continues for too long—vital organs like their heart, liver, and kidneys. It's called self-cannibalism and it might deliver an initial vegan high, but over time it's really not pretty to witness. Most of us have seen this in a stranger on the street or an elderly family member, that "wasting away" look of someone whose body is severely stressed from inadequate nourishment.

And you don't have to be deficient to the point of tissue starvation to suffer the effects of consistently marginal protein intake, including "poor bone health and compromised immunity," according to Virginia Messina, RD, and Jack Norris, RD, in *Vegan for Life.* Other telltale signs of inadequate protein include decreased energy and stamina, a lowered resistance to infection, and slow wound healing. It's simply not true, Messina and Norris concur, that vegans don't have to worry about sufficient protein. Yes, even here in beautiful, bounteous America, land of surplus crops and an almost embarrassing glut of food.

ARE YOU A CARB ADDICT?

When you suddenly feel hungry, do you reach for protein or carbs? Most vegans crave carbs. It's their stimulant of choice. Even veg guru Norris admits to seeking out cookies or juice when he's hungry and wants something quick. An almost sure sign of carb addiction, by the way, and possibly the worst choice any of us could make—especially if consumed alone. Simple carbs let loose a burst of energy and move through your stomach rapidly, creating that famous "empty and light" feeling. But they also spike insulin levels, resulting in a quick release of feel-good serotonin, *a temporary rush* that sends your mood soaring. Not long after, energy and serotonin levels plunge and your brain cries out for more carbs. A vicious cycle. An addiction.

When non-carb addicted people are hungry for a snack, they think of almonds or cheese, maybe a hard boiled egg, *not cookies*. Carb lovers who seek quick, get-happy energy have it all backwards because serotonin, as we've seen, depends on dietary protein, specifically the amino acid tryptophan, for sustained release in proper amounts. And if you're not eating enough tryptophan-rich foods, your brain will have difficulty synthesizing enough serotonin to keep your energy and moods stable. So when individuals on a low-protein diet give in to their cravings and binge on carbs, they are responding to a low-serotonin state and the brain's urgent message that they're not producing enough. This helps explain my friend Avery's strange, compulsive behavior last spring in canyon country.

It was an idyllic April morning in the Utah desert, warm and blue-sky bright, when nine of us met in downtown Moab for a hearty breakfast at Eklecticafé, an hour before our planned hike. This fun, funky outdoor bistro was mobbed as usual but once we finally got served, the omnivores among us enthusiastically chowed down on three-egg omelets or wild fish, accompanied by fresh vegetables or leafy greens. Avery, a steadfast vegan, chose homemade granola with blueberries and almond milk, along with whole-grain toast, no butter: a common, healthy-looking vegan breakfast that's quite high in carbs and low in protein. Because the group included a baby and an adorable but dithering 3-year-old, our easy hike through the lower end of Negro Bill Canyon ended up being just a few miles, with several streamside breaks. So in a little over two hours we arrived back at our vehicles: cheery, calm, and still satiated and energized from breakfast.

Calm and satiated, that is, except Avery, who straight away began rummaging through the food box, hauling out an entire loaf of her homemade gluten-free bread. Perched on the truck's open tailgate like a tall, graceful, very thin bird, she started pulling off hefty chunks of carbo currency and stuffing them with great urgency into her open beak, pounding half a loaf in ten minutes. Obviously, she was already hungry; obviously she was craving more carbs. Or thought she was. What her body was really craving was protein and a steady supply of serotonin, both of which she hadn't received in adequate amounts from her vegan breakfast.

It's a routine I have witnessed over and over again among my veggie friends: carb-heavy meals and snacks—and wholly inadequate protein. In fact, I am not convinced that protein consumption among veg'ns has improved all that much since 1970s Paris—or even 1870s London.

WHEN YOUR PROTEIN intake tends toward the 10% end of the spectrum, common among vegans, you end up consuming vast amounts of carbs in an unremitting effort to feel calm and nourished, versus agitated and running on empty. Some put away a shocking 70-80% of their daily calories in carbs, leaving little room for essential fat and protein. *Becoming Vegan* recommends 13-19 or more servings of carbohydrates *per day*, primarily grains, vegetables, fruits and beans.

This monolithic amount of carbs falls in line with the Ornish Diet, a way of eating praised as optimal by plants-only advocates. Yet legions of detractors and defectors—ex-veg'ns, paleo supporters, gluten-intolerants and researchers—have recently become more vocal in their opposition to high-carb, low-protein diets as an extended way of life.

Ex-vegan Jenna experienced ongoing symptoms of hunger, depression, fatigue and irritability before reluctantly giving her vegan diet the boot and incorporating free-range eggs and wild fish. She swiftly returned to full health.

> I was obsessed with the cleanliness of anything I put into my body....I vowed never to touch any animal products again. My diet consisted mostly of vegetables and fruit (usually blended into green smoothies), nuts, dried fruit, legumes and beans....I was not a junk food vegan .....but I was a sick one. For almost a year I held onto the belief that I was doing something wrong. Maybe I was missing a supplement? Was I not eating enough greens? Maybe I needed more grains to balance out the fiber I was getting from the veggies I was eating? Maybe I needed more fat....I constantly searched forums and blogs, desperate for an answer to my host of symptoms. I was completely exhausted—mentally, physically, and emotionally.

Jenna didn't need scientific studies to tell her that a low-protein/high-carb vegan diet wasn't working for her, no matter how scrupulously planned. Yet abundant research reveals exactly what Jenna discovered once fish and eggs were added to her nutritional arsenal: ample high-density, complete protein reduces appetite, boosts metabolic efficiency, and increases physical and mental energy.

Moreover, anyone contemplating a foray into plants-only will do themselves a favor by checking out all the research linking high-carb/low-protein diets and cognitive impairment; high-carb and several types of cancer (breast, endometrial; colorectal); high-carb and increased risk for metabolic disorder, stroke, and heart disease (Volk; Kerti; Klement; Romieu; Sieri; Nagle; Michaud; Feng; Yu; et al). A study comparing 40% vs. 60% carb diets found that the latter resulted in many more markers for cardiovascular risk. Indeed, these types of diets tend to lower heart-protective HDL cholesterol, and vegans consistently test lower in HDL than other dietary types. Other valuable research, such as the decades-long Nurses' Health Study, concludes that high glycemic loads from solo carbohydrate consumption—you know, like cookies and juice—are "directly associated" with higher risk for heart disease (Jeppesen; S. Liu).

To fend off potential dangers from a high-carb diet, always choose complex carbohydrates with high fiber content, in tandem with quality protein and fat. But let's be honest: what many of today's on-the-go veg'ns grab when hunger hits are heaps of tasty, stand-alone carbs: fruit, bagels, muffins and sugar-bloated energy bars. (God forbid they're still eating potato chips and soda for lunch like at my daughter's high school.) Sure, plenty of omnivores eat quick carbs, but at least they're usually accompanied by fat and protein foods which slow absorption and provide steady fuel and serotonin. Animal protein from nature comes pre-armed with healthy and sufficient fat—and few to zero carbs—but in the plant kingdom it is not so easy to find protein that isn't laden with carbohydrates.

Two high-protein veg choices not loaded with carbs are soy and spirulina, but the latter isn't even a plant. It's a cyanobacterium, deficient in lysine, methionine, and cysteine as compared to eggs, milk, and meat (while costing you 30 times more per gram). And what could be more robotically monotonous than a constant soy regime? Besides, it's just not that healthy to obtain your food from limited sources. Eating a wide variety, changing it up, is your best guarantee of getting all the micronutrients on a daily basis. Variety also keeps you much more interested in healthy choices, less likely to cave to the easy gratification of quick carbs.

Seitan, with its macrobiotic origins, is a processed, tasteless, high-protein, no-animal alternative, but its texture is so chicken-like some vegans report getting queasy ingesting it. Plus, it will work only if your body does well with large doses of wheat gluten. And that's an important "if." Recent research reveals that celiac disease, an autoimmune reaction to the protein gluten (naturally occurring in rye, wheat and barley), has *quadrupled* in all age groups in the US in just 50 years.

166

And this doesn't include those of us who are gluten sensitive or have the disease but are undiagnosed. Authors of this key study discovered a fourfold increased risk of death for individuals with undiagnosed celiac and are now labeling this autoimmune disease "a major public health concern" (Rubio-Tapia).

That's not really surprising given the fact that wheat and other domesticated grains are so new to the human body in evolutionary terms. For two million years our ancestors subsisted on wild plants and animals, moving with the seasons and the herds. Then came the rise of agriculture in the Mideast roughly 10,000 years ago, and if your family came from Europe that means just 5,000 years of ancestral grain eating. Clearly, the proliferation of celiac and gluten sensitivity followed the expansion of our first farmers across Europe (Mathieson).

Our modern high-grain diet is a mere blip in humanity's dietary evolution—we're talking just 0.4% of our long, enormously successful hunting and foraging existence. Furthermore, the estimated amount of genetic change (0.005%) in the human genome over this time period is almost negligible, "essentially unchanged from that of pre-agricultural man," contend the authors of "Origins and Evolutions of the Western Diet: Health Implications for the 21st Century." Thus, while evolution tends to be slow and conservative, humanity's jump to domesticated grains and legumes—let alone high-fructose corn syrup and grain-stuffed cattle—has been high-speed and radical. Scientists call this "evolutionary discordance" and evidence of its effect is highly visible in our dreadful disease statistics. This is why the paleo crowd may be justified in claiming that a pre-agricultural diet is more suitable from a genetic standpoint—specifically, lean muscle and organ meats from grass-eating animals, plus liberal amounts of nuts, veggies and fruit (while limiting grains, legumes and dairy). And if you think I'm pushing paleo, no way. I'm pushing smart, individualized nutrition choices.

I started investigating grains because of my own obvious energy-drag after eating wheat, plus a family member's recent diagnosis of celiac (100% photographed and confirmed—no villa in his small intestine: slick as a baby's bottom). When gluten proteins trigger a genetically-predisposed body to turn on itself and attack the intestine, complications can range from anemia to life-threatening mal-absorption of nutrients. Celiac aside, our guts' sensitivity to gluten is real and increasing in America, and theories range from a rise in wheat intake to higher gluten loads in modern wheat plants. Both these theories have flaws, however, as US per capita wheat intake has declined in recent years, following a rise from 1970-2000. It's now a substantial 100 pounds less than its 230-pound peak in the

1870s. And when USDA researcher Donald Kasarda reviewed data going back 100 years, he found zero evidence that gluten levels have increased in wheat plants. What *has* happened, though, is disturbing enough.

Average US consumption of gluten, not wheat, has indeed been escalating for several decades, in tandem with our shift to corporate food. Largely unnoticed by the public, "vital gluten" (fractionated from wheat flour and used for texturizing) is being increasingly injected into our food, up to 80% of it imported from places like China. (Scare alert: 13 million tons of crops harvested annually in China are contaminated with heavy metals.) Since 1977, our vital gluten intake has *tripled*, states Kasarda, the same time frame as our conspicuous rise in celiac disease.

Besides the newly touted, gluten-loaded seitan (pronounced "satan" by celiac sufferers), other fake meats contain extracted gluten as well. In fact, a continual intake of processed food, veg'n or non, all but guarantees elevated gluten levels— even more reason to be wary of consuming industrial food here in America. Yet for six weeks in France this past summer, having given up wheat back home, I ate bakery-fresh, all-wheat baguettes every morning and experienced zero intestinal complaints and never-ending energy as we hiked the Pyrénées and cycled through Gers and Languedoc. (Traditional baguettes are fashioned from non-GMO flour, fresh yeast, water, salt, and *that's it*.) I have heard similar stories from gluten-sensitive Americans who gleefully indulged in the forbidden wheat and rye while traveling across Europe. As for the presence of gluten in European *processed* food, that I don't know. My French friends would rather shovel horse manure all day than eat industrial pre-packaged food, let alone serve it to their guests.

ANTINUTRIENTS IN YOUR GRAINS & LEGUMES

ONE SURE-FIRE WAY to know our early ancestors ate minimal amounts of wild grains is their indigestible fiber. Like all primates, our gut doesn't possess the correct enzyme system to break down grain fibers for sufficient energy. Their tough cell walls have to be ruptured by milling and cooking, technologies that weren't available for most of our lengthy evolution. Additionally, the seeds of wild grasses are tiny: difficult to harvest and process. And then there's the issue of antinutrients in grains.

Antinutrients? If that sounds like another strong message from the plant world, yes it is. It's called "steer clear; we're toxic." To be blunt: cereal grains contain components that not only ward off plant enemies but can cause mayhem to human

168

health. One such antinutrient, phytic acid, is quite accomplished at blocking your body's absorption of calcium, iron, magnesium, copper and zinc, leading to impaired bone density, tooth decay, and zinc deficiency—all three have emerged as vegan health issues. Compared to omnies, for example, veggies must ingest up to 50% more zinc, a trace mineral critical for immune and neurological function. And spiritual elitists, take note: "The lightheaded feeling of detachment that enshrouds some vegetarians can be caused by hidden zinc hunger," according to Carl Pfeiffer, MD, "rather than by some mystical quality."

Other antinutrients in cereal grains that can inflict bodily damage include polyphenols, goitrogens, and enzyme inhibitors. And all those nuts and legumes favored by vegans? They too contain toxic substances. Nature designed it this way to discourage their consumption, allowing seeds to survive to germination. The best way to reduce antinutrients is to mimic spring rainfall and saturate these foods thoroughly. Overnight soaking or sprouting, followed by cooking, works best. However, it's not possible to remove all the phytic acid from plants, so nutritionists recommend deriving the bulk of your calories from nutrient-dense, low phytic-acid foods. That's tough to impossible for many vegans, who depend on grains, nuts, seeds and legumes for most of their daily calories. Our dietary needs vary but to keep antinutrient problems to a minimum, vegans should eat these foods in moderation, choose sprouted or fermented versions, and consume complementary foods high in vitamin C to increase mineral availability.

Love your five-grain bagels and heard enough? Sorry, there's more. Other antinutrients in cereal grains directly impair vitamin D metabolism, so critical for bone development, as it enhances absorption of calcium and phosphate. Vegans need to be aware that plant sources for this vitamin, D2, are inferior to the animal sourced D3, less than one-third as potent (Armas). So go for the sunshine, baby, to get the proper amount in modest daily doses. But wait! That's another reason veganism works best in warm climes, such as India. Above 37 degrees north latitude (San Francisco, Denver, St. Louis, Richmond, VA, etc. and further north), your skin makes little to zilch vitamin D from the sun other than in summer.

Furthermore, high levels of whole grains can impair biotin uptake, a B vitamin important for metabolizing amino acids and carbohydrates. Consider this grisly, high-grain tale from the anthropological annals: After digging up a 2,000-year-old mummy from a peat bog in Cheshire, England in 1984, scientists christened him Lindow Man (endearingly dubbed Mr. Pete Marsh by the locals). Although well preserved, Pete's body wasn't all that dear to look at, quite mangled actually

169

(murder is suspected), but it did reveal a last supper of unleavened whole-grain bread, indicative of the high-cereal diet of his time. His highly-ridged fingernails revealed yet more: acute biotin deficiency. Big grain consumers, you might want to take a close look at your own fingernails right now.

Legumes, too, belong in the non-evolutionary food class. "Hundreds if not thousands of citations document the antinutritional properties of legumes," warns Loren Cordain, PhD. Called the *unavailable carbohydrates* in legumes, raffinose and stachyose, among others, are not digestible and pass into your large intestine where they provide a perfect substrate for microflora to create bloating and the flutey-sounding *flatus*. (Would that our farts did sound like flutes instead of blasting trumpets.) So sure, go ahead and bathe your legumes for hours, then boil the antinutrient hell out of them, but that's no guarantee of disabling all the offenders. Moreover, these rather foul compounds "influence multiple tissues and systems," according to researchers (Liener; Cordain) "and normal cooking procedures do not always eliminate them." Plenty among us can testify to this distressing truth, having spent many a wicked night rolling around with painful distention and gas due to indigestible plant products fermenting in our gut.

You know that sudsy, grey, disgusting-looking froth that beans put out when you boil them? It's actually a type of poison, called a saponin, derived from the French *sapon*, or soap. Appetizing, eh? A natural protein digestion inhibitor, it's produced by various smart legumes to protect themselves from insect ingestion. No doubt it conveys a powerful message to humans as well: eat at your own risk. The sensitives among us get wretched results. Lentils and garbanzo beans, even double soaked and thoroughly cooked, plow through us like a rototiller. Trotting to the toilet at inconvenient hours is just part of the pact.

Yet some individuals apparently digest and metabolize legumes just fine and if you're a vegan reading this, I dearly hope this is you. Your plant protein options just expanded tremendously. As for the others, best wishes finding adequate daily plant protein without a shitload of legumes—especially at the new and higher recommended levels.

25.

SOY STORIES

To all creatures nature offers nourishment, whole and undisguised.

—Japanese Proverb

IF PLANT EATERS RARELY calculate their daily protein and amino acid intake, what about professional chefs who run the kitchens of all those holistic retreats serving "delicious gourmet vegetarian cuisine"? Surely they're doing a far better job of designing well-balanced meals. And yet, after visiting a well-known yoga center in the forested mountains high above Denver, I began to question even this assumption. Granted, I was there for just two days and four meals, but I figure every offering on any given day should include a healthy mix of high-quality proteins, healthy fats, and low-glycemic carbs, right?

Let me just say this: some vegan yogis sure do love their home-made muffins, pastries, cakes, and sweets sweets sweets! Lunch turned out to be the meal with the greatest amount of protein, consisting of ten sunflower seeds at the bottom of my tossed green salad, plus whatever small amounts were in the non-gluten bread and nutty rice. Maybe 10 grams, max? Personally, I need at least 25-30 grams of high-density protein for breakfast, around 25 for lunch, and 15-20 for dinner—no way possible on such protein-skimpy meals. Still hungry after every high-carb feast, just like everybody else attending the retreat, I bolted down a few more of those always available double-fudge-choco-chip cookies before we all took off — buzzed on sugar and serotonin—for our afternoon yoga in the woods.

To ascertain if these offerings were an aberration, I visited two other respected wellness centers to check out the carb-protein-fat balance in their guest meals. A personal growth institute near Big Sur offered *somewhat* more diverse protein, while further down the California coast, a yoga retreat north of LA was not as generous, although it did provide yogurt for breakfast the eight days I attended, along with granola, fruit and herbal teas. So a trifling amount of protein every morning, though hardly enough to kick-start our physically demanding days.

One Sunday holiday breakfast, the kitchen staff veered sinfully off-track and passed around an Easter basket full of pink and fuchsia-tinted hard-boiled eggs. *Just one per yogi, please!* We all cheered wildly, snatched our allotted egg and like the hungry animals we were, devoured it nearly whole, eyes darting around the room for more. Lunches and dinners were indeed organic and scrumptious but again largely carbs: pasta, rice, quinoa, beans, lentils and veggies. By the end of each strenuous day of ashtanga yoga, still restless and ravenous post-dinner, I'd sneak out to my truck camper and wolf down an entire tin of sardines: 32 grams of high-density complete protein, plus 2 grams of superior fat, including 885 mg of brain-nourishing DHA and 210 mg of heart-protecting EPA.

Add ample amounts of calcium, potassium, phosphorous, iron, selenium, co-enzyme Q10, and vitamins D3 and B12, and I had just inhaled a low-on-the-food-chain nutritional powerhouse packed into a teensy container not much bigger than your iPhone. (Eating sardines directly is sustainable; eating sardine-fed farmed fish is not.) Ah yes, on those salty piscine evenings, gazing at the dazzling Pacific sunset far below, I *finally* felt nutritionally balanced: fully energized yet calm. Then, feeling guilty for feeling so terrific, I washed out the oily little can and hid the evidence.

WHAT EVERY ONE of these yoga-veg retreats did serve for protein day after day was soy, always and forever soy, usually in the form of tofu—its blah taste and texture disguised by rich tomato or mushroom sauce. On planet vegan, soy is the protein god. Browse just about any veg cookbook and there it is: the essential component of snacks and soups, fake meats and faux dairy. Soy stocks the pantry of *The Vegan Divas, The Happy Herbivore,* and *Vegan with a Vengeance.*

Realizing that newbie veg'ns might be more concerned about a cow's well-being than their own, some advocacy groups now spell out specific meal plans. For example, PETA's Starter Kit (wrapped in silky images of female celebrities) offers tips for seemingly healthy all-plant lunches and dinners. Alas, like many vegan guides and recipes, it leaves plant-eaters in the dark about each meal's macronutrient profile. Moreover, with frustratingly few exceptions—I did spot a lone recipe for seitan "beef" casserole—its protein options are contained again and again in that same venerated word: *SOYA!*

172

Could the modern veg'n industry have survived, let alone flourished, without soy and its myriad processed products? Extremely doubtful. Too many craving-protein veggies would have jumped ship even sooner. Here's just the short list of processed soy foods flowing out of our industrial labs: concentrates and isolates, powders and sterols, soy cheese, soy butter, soy milk, soy cream, soy yogurt, yada yada, yada. You can also gulp down refined soy oil, soy flour and soy meal, plus the mainstay of many a plants-only dinner: texturized vegetable protein (TVP), cleverly sculpted to resemble pliant ground beef or supple pork bellies.

Do vegans even know how this TVP stuff is made? Invented by a corporate Goliath, Archer Daniels Midland, texturized soy protein is defatted thermoplastic proteins heated to 400 degrees F. and denatured into a fibrous, insoluble medium. Exiting the extruder, expanding like polymer gummy worms, this pressurized concoction is then molded into protein flakes, strips, and slivers for your eating "pleasure." Yikes, I almost forgot hexane, the highly-polluting petrochemical and neurotoxin used to bathe the original soybeans, separating the protein and oil. Independent testing by Cornucopia Institute reveals hexane residues as high as 50 ppm in soy products, including baby formula, burgers, and energy bars. However, the industry never bothered to figure out hexane risks (nor are they required to), so there's still insufficient data to know if you should or shouldn't be ingesting TVP every day. Chronic hexane exposure in factory workers (inhalation) is linked to neurological disorders; so play it safe, vegans, and buy organic soy foods only.

At 13 grams protein per patty, opting for a denatured soy burger does indeed make a nice dent in your daily protein needs but, hexane aside, is all this processed soy good for you? And is it smart to derive such a large portion of your diet from a single source? Like other legumes, soybeans contain a whole mess of antinutrients. That's why you can't chew them raw; they are toxic in that form. Soy is also a common food allergen, causing an overreaction of the immune system in sensitive individuals. American yoga pioneer Ana Forrest was forced to turn into a no-soy omnivore, joking to her students: "I'm allergic to everything vegan." Meanwhile, some plant devotees consume up to four soy products every 24 hours! Yet eating the same food over and over invites not only allergies, but micronutrient deficiencies and chronic fatigue.

NUTRIENT DEFICIENCIES WERE FAR from my mind when soy products began mega-multiplying in US supermarkets in the early 1990s. Western vegetarians were excited. *Finally* it would be radically easy to get adequate daily protein with this super-hyped miracle food. Wahoo!! No more smelly, beany concoctions that bloated our bellies like a gibbous moon; maybe we could even cut down on all that dairy many of us depended on to feel satiated and nourished, a protein source that was receiving, perhaps not coincidentally, increasingly bad press—including PETA's infamous, anti-dairy "Got Pus?" campaign. So veggies started downing soy milk instead of cow's milk, sautéing soy burgers and nibbling soy cheese—exactly as the shrewd industry giants had hoped. What better way to get rid of a waste product from the soy oil industry—foul-smelling sludge formerly fed to cattle—than to sell it at huge profits to a gullible public?

The industry's ambitious public relations scheme paid off, with the average shopper's perception of soy undergoing a dramatic shift: from indigestible livestock fodder to incredible human health food. To this day, vegan proponents recommend 2-4 daily servings of soy to meet protein needs, avowing that a surfeit of a single food is "not a problem." (*Becoming Vegan* recommends an astonishing 6-8 servings of fortified soymilk and alternates per day.) And it's not just vegans towing the company line; omnivores are likewise sucking down soy in record numbers. Following the FDA's approval of a heavily publicized health claim linking soy intake with reduced heart disease risk, sales in human soyfood soared, with a sensational five-fold growth to $5.2 billion in just 15 years (1996-2011). Other unproven health claims quickly followed: lower cholesterol, breast cancer protection, and hot flash cool-downs.

Today you can stroll just about any aisle of your local supermarket and find processed soy products hither and yon. Some are obvious—soy fake meats and beverages—but other forms are far less visible: tucked, folded, and injected into our frozen pizzas and packaged dinners, cookies and cereals. Restaurants cook with refined soy oil, and ice cream stores like Baskin Robbins blend soy into half their offerings. Cleverly camouflaged on labels, soy derivatives appear as mono-diglyceride, yuba, TSF (textured soy flour), TSP (textured soy protein), soja and lecithin. From 2000-2007 alone, food manufacturers introduced nearly 3,000 new soy-based foods to a trusting, soy-euphoric public.

Obviously, the United Soybean Board is quite pleased, announcing that "85 percent of consumers perceive soy products as healthful," and nearly as many "agree with the FDA's assertion that consuming 25 grams of soy protein daily reduces your risk of heart disease." Americans are decidedly, even giddily sold on soy. But don't grab your party hat just yet. A growing body of research indicates that soy is *not* deserving of all these health claims, and indeed may compromise

174

your health in significant ways. Vegans, of course, don't want to hear any of this, let alone believe it, because many of them are still ingesting large quantities of soy as their primary protein source, every day of their lives.

THE DARK SIDE OF SOY

"Studies showing the dark side of soy date back 100 years," Dr. Kaayla Daniel maintains, reminding us that the FDA-approved health claim arrived "despite massive evidence showing risks associated with soy and against the protest of the FDA's own top scientists." In *The Whole Soy Story*, called "the most important nutritional book of the decade," Daniel reveals hundreds of studies that link soy to digestive distress, immune-system disorders, infertility, thyroid dysfunction, cognitive decline, heart disease and cancer. This soy detractor is no slouch. Dr. Daniel holds a PhD in Nutritional Sciences and Anti-Aging Therapies, is board certified as a clinical nutritionist, appeared as an expert witness for the National Institute for Environmental Health Sciences, and specializes in women's health, infertility, and recovery from veg'n and soy-based diets.

At the very least, soy as health food is controversial, but you'd never know it from all the veggie books, blogs, and recipes extolling and amply employing soy in its myriad forms. Soy fans are fond of citing the industry's benign or positive research results, without even mentioning the mass of contradictory studies from independent scientists. Many don't acknowledge the controversy at all. This left Mary Terrain, a health-conscious vegetarian for over 12 years, terribly confused. Here's someone who actually took the time to plan meals with sufficient daily protein, fully embracing soy because the FDA had heartily endorsed it. She recalls studying food labels with strange new ingredients like protein isolate and hydrolyzed soy protein, but concluded they must be beneficial because the US government's stamp of approval is right there on the packaging.

Yet after several years of eating and drinking plentiful soy, Terrain started to experience stomach pain, bloating, and mood swings. Then her menstrual periods ceased, a sure sign of endocrine disruption. "It didn't occur to me at the time to question soy, heart protector and miracle food," Terrain admits in "The Dark Side of Soy," but after delving into the nutrition literature, she discovered the many risks associated with soy, including—what do you know—digestive problems and endocrine disruption. Jolted awake, Terrain began researching soy's deleterious effects on male and female hormones, sex drive, fertility, thyroid and digestion—

plus its potential contribution to cancer. Yet for every study that claimed a link between soy and increased disease risk, another study would suddenly appear to contest it. *What's going on here?* she asked, bewildered.

Here's what's going on. Soy has *not* been conclusively shown to benefit your health and many respected studies indicate the opposite. "On balance it doesn't seem that soy and its constituent isoflavones have met original expectations," writes Julia Barrett in "The Science of Soy: What Do We Really Know?" Despite industry claims, clinical results have been inconsistent regarding soy's ability to reduce cardiovascular disease risk, and a major review in *Circulation* reveals little to no positive effects (Sacks). Moreover, a key evidence report, *Effects of Soy on Health Outcomes*, concludes there exists "little evidence" to support a beneficial role of soy and soy isoflavones in bone health, reproductive health, cancer and neurocognitive function, plus other health parameters. And sorry, ladies, but the latest studies show "no advantages" for hot-flashing females (Balk; Levis).

THIS IS WHERE VEGANS start shouting me down with their own statistics about "the good health of Asians who have been eating soy products for more than five millennia!" Three factors appear to be at work here: genetics, the type of soy ingested, and daily amount.

Similar to their ancestors, whose diet they genetically favor, modern Asians consume much smaller quantities than soy-happy western veg'ns: just 8.7 grams of soy protein a day by the Japanese, on average, according to the UN's Food and Agriculture Organization. (Japanese kids are more likely to drink cow's milk, Tokyo residents claim, and soy drinks weren't common until Starbucks showed up with their soy lattes.) Average daily intake by the Chinese is smaller still: 3.4 grams of soy protein (Barrett). Even *The China Study* determined that not just soy but *total legume consumption* among participants averaged 12 grams of protein a day—just one valuable protein source alongside healthy whole foods like fish, poultry, and eggs: all staples in the Chinese diet. Compare that to the 25 grams of daily soy protein, in any form, promoted here in the USA.

But more is better, right? Apparently Americans believe this because we are scarfing down new-fangled soy products in record amounts. A single Crunchy Fudge energy bar offers 15 grams of processed soy protein. Multiple that by 2-4 daily servings of soy in its various guises, such as a typical vegan might dine on, and we are talking huge intakes that in no way mimic traditional Asian quantities. "Only in our country are we using [soy] in a free-for-all," laments Jatinder Bhatia,

MD, noting that soy "has a specific indication, and we tend to use and abuse in America."

The Chinese weren't even interested in eating soy until late in the Chou Dynasty, 300 BC, certainly not for the last 5,000 years as claimed by advocates. Before that, soy was simply "green manure," a legume crop plowed under to enrich the soil. It wasn't until entrepreneurs learned how to ferment it, creating a paste we now call by its Japanese name, *miso*, that soy transformed from indigestible cover crop into (for some of us anyway) digestible human food. By 1000 AD, fermented tempeh and natto were also being produced, still popular in Asia today.

Wisely, Asians almost always ferment their soy foods to disable most of the naturally-occurring toxins, antinutrients, and enzyme blockers. "These are not nutrients," soy researcher Dr. Lon White reminds us. "They are drugs." Leave out the fermentation process, as cheap, fast American soy production almost always does, and a whole bunch of us are pretty much guaranteed digestive and other health problems: nature's agonizing way of telling us we need to modify our food choices. Yet veg'ns who suffer from gut issues will usually look anywhere and everywhere but at the multiple processed soy products they endlessly consume.

This was definitely true for our good friend Jay from Chicago, a devout vegan who came to visit Larry and me at our mountain home in central Colorado, a rural location at 9,000 feet with limited food options. So Jay brought along his own nourishment, diligently packed into sturdy plastic tubs alongside his new Vasque hiking boots. Cramming our frig with soymilk, tofu, TVP, tempeh—and dozens of Chicago's best gluten-free bagels—Jay took in some form of soy as his primary protein two to four times a day, yet complained of ongoing digestive pain. When I dared to suggest an overabundance of soy as a likely culprit, he promptly denied it, looking incredulous at the mere suggestion.

Here was this really intelligent man, working as a business consultant by day, playing in a jazz band by night, completely blind to any possible connection between his vast, ongoing intake of soy and his body's growing complaints. His moral mind refused to make the connection, even though it was staring into his handsome 50-year-old face.

Since soy was his daily high-protein source, Jay couldn't imagine abandoning it, or even cutting down, because at 6'2" and 200 pounds, this strapping, outdoor-active man needs *a lot* of protein, 150 grams or more every day. I've seen similar blinders on other dedicated vegans, bright men and women who in other matters are perceptive and judicious. When it comes to diet, however, they are bound to their unbending belief system, and no amount of intestinal grief or malaise shall dissuade them.

To get a handle on his health issues, Jay would do well to increase his protein variety and drastically reduce soy intake. Andrea Nguyen, who explores Asian cuisine for *Viet World Kitchen*, argues for moderation in soy consumption. She calls these foods "an excellent alternative" to meat, but she also pays close attention to research and follows Harvard School of Public Health's recommendations on soy: "There's no reason to go overboard: 2-4 servings a week is a good target; eating more than that likely won't offer any health benefits and we can't be sure there is no harm." That's 2-4 soy servings *per week*, vegans, not per day.

Jay's health would similarly benefit from switching to the Asian way: whole and fermented soy, small amounts, very lightly processed. But we Americans like to do food our own way: super-sized, manipulated, and highly profitable. Take something whole from nature, then pulverize, isolate, and alter its parts—or concoct a new-to-humans recipe for our babies. Yes sir, that's the American way!

"Or we consume it in other forms that are highly processed and have a bunch of unpronounceable additives," states Ayurvedic doctor Claudia Welch. Then lo and behold: we're surprised when our health results don't mimic those of Asians! "We are even more surprised when, instead of delivering good effects," asserts Welch, "the soy is found to be harmful for our hormonal system, especially in infants."

Thus, both quantity *and* quality are more than likely skewing our soy health results as compared to Asians' favorable outcomes. Indeed, the chair of Harvard's Department of Nutrition, Walter Willett, MD, declared that soy supplements should be viewed as "totally new untested drugs." Such warnings make it all the more perplexing that many vegan activists don't seem at all concerned what kind of soy you munch on, nor how much. The overt message is to eat as much as you need in its various forms, including non-fermented and lab-isolated. *Whatever it takes to steer clear of all animal products!* They openly ridicule fellow vegans who've dropped out because they want to eat real, whole food.

Those who remain are often ingesting epic quantities of highly processed soy injected with protein isolates, including energy bars. High in sodium, sugar, fake colors and preservatives, these grab-and-go snacks have taken over soy beverages as the top money-getter in the industry—over a billion dollars raked in annually. Yet soy isolates result from a high-heat process that lowers their nutritional value, while increasing carcinogens like nitrates. Even a fermented soy food like tempeh presents a problem (as do spirulina, nori, miso, and other vegan foods) because of false B12 analogues that block this vitamin's metabolism. Eating these forms of soy can *escalate* the body's need for B12, already a major issue for vegans.

Soy foods also contain high amounts of isoflavones, bioactive compounds that mimic human estrogen. Isoflavones may be beneficial in modest amounts but harmful in the larger doses many vegans gobble up. They are known endocrine disrupters that interfere with thyroid function. Furthermore, an iodine deficiency greatly increases soy's anti-thyroid effects, and vegans are markedly deficient in iodine due to its low levels in plants. Up to 80% of all tested vegans suffer from iodine deficiency, a serious condition that can lead to lowered immunity, depression, slower brain function and thyroid cancer (Krajcovicova).

Soy isoflavones, sometimes called phytoestrogens, are also linked to elevated estrogen levels. They mimic estrogen so well that researchers have discovered alarming side effects in males consuming large amounts of daily soy, including low sperm count, decreased free and total testosterone, loss of libido and erectile dysfunction, even man boobs, i.e., gynecomastia (Doerge; Siepmann). *Should we even be surprised that researchers with paid connections to the soy industry have not found these same links?*

Here's the real kicker if you love your daily soy and demand additional evidence: monastic males who have taken vows of chastity report that abundant soy is exceedingly helpful in dampening their libidos. And it's well known in Japan that a woman will slip ever more soy into an oversexed husband's meals when she just can't take anymore.

Remember Mary Terrain, the soy-ingesting veggie whose periods vanished? Research confirms that soy-pounding females drinking just two glasses of daily soymilk receive enough endocrine-disrupting compounds to alter their menstrual cycle in as little as four weeks (Cassidy). In addition, a 28-year study of 8,000 Japanese-American men discovered a statistically significant relationship between tofu consumption during midlife and accelerated brain aging/loss of brain weight, plus an association with Alzheimer's. (Isoflavones that block an enzyme required by the memory-making hippocampus are suspected.) Unlike in *The China Study,* lead scientist Dr. Lon White controlled for possible confounders, yet "the effect of tofu remained apparent." The more tofu eaten, the greater the likelihood of mental decline.

At least 170 scientific studies reveal the dangers or potential dangers of human soy food. A leader in the explosion of research that began decades ago, Finnish scientist Herman Adlercreutz admits this about soy and its various components: "I am myself frightened a little bit by all this. There is so much we don't know."

WHAT ELSE IS LURKING IN YOUR SOY FOOD?

And that's before addressing the sneaky snake in the room: gene alteration. An astounding 94% of our nation's soy is now genetically messed with. Translation: an estimated 70% of our processed foods contain GMOs, mainly in the form of soy. They're in our breakfast cereal and pancake mixes, mayonnaise and bouillon cubes, herbal teas and vitamins. So unless all your food is 100% organic, you're likely consuming genetically modified organisms every day of your life.

And get ready for the next round of gene-tampered foodstuffs: bioengineered salmon, apples and russet potatoes, largely unregulated by our government and fast-tracked to market. Unlike in every other developed country, the USDA does not require external safety testing or even a label for our genetically altered food. Yet another brash human experiment in evolutionary discordance.

"So show us all the casualties!" proponents demand. Since GM foods are new to humankind, much like veganism, we won't comprehend all the health effects for several generations. And because money's corrupting influence on science is well documented, non-industry sponsored research on genetically modified foods is the only research worth your time. (Read the eye-popping *Heads They Win, Tails We Lose: How Corporations Corrupt Science at the Public's Expense*, by the Union of Concerned Scientists.) Independent studies are hugely underfunded, but the results thus far are extremely disquieting. In a detailed position paper, the American Academy Of Environmental Medicine warns that GM soy and all other gene-modified foods "pose a serious health risk" and should be avoided by not just vegans, but everyone on the planet.

> There is causation as defined by Hill's Criteria in the areas of strength of association, consistency, specificity, biological gradient, and biological plausibility....Multiple animal studies show significant immune dysregulation, including the upregulation of cytokines associated with asthma, allergy, and inflammation [plus] altered structure and function of the liver, including altered carbohydrate and lipid metabolism as well as cellular changes that could lead to accelerated aging....Studies also show intestinal damage in animals fed GM foods, including proliferative cell growth....

"But these are animal studies!" soy-happy vegans complain. "Show us all the human studies." Oh there's human research going on, all right. It's called *you and me.* It's called all of us manipulated-food-ingesting fools. The health results from DNA-altered, new-to-human victuals will take time to unfold, but independent studies from the US, UK, France and Argentina are giving us a grim preview.

Here's how it works: farming 21st-century style. Using a particle gun, industry lab-techs shoot foreign DNA under high pressure into our food crops, penetrating cell walls and tissues. The target is not precise and serious damage to the plant's cellular tissues can ensue. Moreover, the injected DNA can come from a variety of different species, including bacteria, viruses, insects and other animals, even humans. DNA shuffling it's called, and it allows geneticists "to create in a matter of minutes, millions of recombinant viruses that have never existed in billions of years of evolution," according to an independent panel of international scientists calling for a GM-free world. These instantaneous, new-to-earth life forms, called transgenic organisms, may bring unintended, destructive consequences to humans and the environment because the complexity of genetic networks is not yet fully understood. Playing God is a high-risk business.

Regardless, the high-profit plan proceeded with the synthesis of soy and other GM crops resistant to glyphosate, the active component in Roundup—the most widely used herbicide on earth and Monsanto's golden money egg. Cunningly, this behemoth corporation owns the patent to not just glyphosate-resilient crops like soybeans, but also their progeny. Farmers around the world can no longer save and plant their own seeds in the traditional and time-honored way, but must buy them instead from Monsanto, year after year. Jack in the Beanstalk is dead. The greedy Giant rules instead.

WHAT'S MORE, GLYPHOSATE is a systemic toxin that arbitrarily kills all plants in its path: grasses, perennials, woody shrubs, anything green and alive. Gaining entrance through the plant's leaves and soft tissues, the poison moves insidiously through its intricate interior, disrupting enzyme systems and metabolism. Most sprayed plants die an excruciatingly slow death that lasts for days or even weeks. Not one part survives.

Genetically modified soy and other GM crops don't die, of course. That's the whole idea. But they're likewise doused with glyphosate and residues of this toxic chemical are now present in nearly 80% of our processed food. Virtually any soy-containing food that is not labeled "Non-GMO-Verified" contains glyphosate. This includes soy flour in your non-gluten bread, "natural flavors" in your non-dairy milk, and soy oil or lecithin in just about everything, including your favorite gourmet chocolate bar.

So what? The levels of glyphosate are so low, soy advocates claim, there's no possible harm to humans. Independent scientists, with no industry money at stake, claim differently. "It's an endocrine buster," insists UK pathologist Stanley Ewen, a lead author of *The Independent Science Panel on GM Final Report*. Glyphosate "interferes with aromatase, which produces estrogen," disrupting the delicate hormonal balance of the female reproductive cycle. A growing, coherent body of research concurs, classifying glyphosate as a toxic endocrine disrupter which induces human breast cancer cell growth (Thongprakaisang).

Further studies confirm placental transfer of this toxin in pregnant women, with implications for birth defects. "Neurodevelopmental, reproductive, and transgenerational effects of glycogen-based herbicides must be revisited," Robin Mesnage, PhD, insists. Moreover, chronic toxic effects are being detected at recommended "safe" levels and lower, prompting researchers to challenge the industry's outdated science and assumptions of safety (Myers; Antoniou). Some have gone further, registering a plea to national governments to reconsider their policies regarding the safety of glyphosate residues in our food and water.

That plea has been answered, at least in Europe, due to a stunning 2015 report by the World Health Organization that has Big Ag foaming at the mouth, bleating for a retraction. "Probably carcinogenic to humans" is the honest conclusion of 17 experts from 11 nations, based on glyphosate-induced DNA and chromosomal damage in mammals and human in vitro cells (Guyton).

And that toxin is being sprayed in ever heavier amounts as more and more weeds become resistant and government agencies quietly raise allowable levels in our food, a whopping 200% increase for some. A recent Norwegian study found an average 9 mg of Roundup per kilo of food crops, nearly double what Monsanto deemed "extreme" in 1999. Residue levels in human bodies are also escalating, and a German study found substantially higher levels of this toxin in the urine of chronically-ill people compared to healthy ones (Kruger).

As mounting evidence links glyphosate to cancer and infertility, France and the Netherlands are the latest nations to ban its sale to their citizens. And humans aren't the only animals suffering. Glyphosate is genotoxic to other mammals, plus amphibians like fish and frogs.

Is this the industry you want to support with your food dollars, vegans? And don't think buying organic soy automatically exempts you. Many of our larger producers are bypassing American growers and importing from China, where lax oversight means that "organic" soybeans are being sprayed with toxic chemicals by exploited workers. Instead of purchasing from American organic farmers who labor with integrity to build our trust, corporations like the $11 billion behemoth Dean Foods/White Wave, makers of the top-selling soymilk Silk, opted for the cheap Chinese market, dealing a terrible blow to small farmers and the growth of organic acreage here at home. If this bothers you—and you'd like to know which soy products to buy and which to shun—read Cornucopia Institute's illuminating *Behind the Bean: The Heroes and Charlatan's of the Natural and Organic Soy Foods Industry.*

The innocent field laborers of the world also deserve our attention. Glyphosate has been detected in the air, water, food, blood and urine of agricultural workers, and after Argentinean farmers sprayed it on 50 million acres of GM soybeans, increased rates of human birth defects and cancers were reported. The director of the Laboratory of Molecular Embryology in Buenos Aires, Andres Carrasco, calls Roundup "a powerful poison," concluding that embryo malformations in the lab are "similar to human birth defects found in genetically-modified, soy-producing regions." Much of this crop goes to feed factory cattle, but vegans who blithely consume GM soy and lecithin in their protein powders and non-dairy milk are also contributing to this on-going tragedy.

So go ahead and eat a high-soy diet if you choose, but at least be conscious of the health and environmental risks based on research from independent scientists. And for anyone buying non-organic soy in the US or "organic" soy products from China, be conscious as well of the corporate worldview you are supporting with your food dollars: the manipulation of nature; the systemic killing of plants and animals; the disempowerment of the world's farmers; inadequate testing to secure the public's health and trust; and the corruption of science by money.

As for our nation's infants, an unprecedented 75% are now being bottle-fed industrial formula and one-quarter of that is soy-based, despite zero completed research on long-term cognitive, endocrine, and nervous system development. One has to wonder if all these loving mothers understand that their babies are drinking lab-created isolates and the hormonal equivalent of three to five birth control pills a day. The Swiss Federal Health Service compiled these statistics and Dr. Daniel Sheehan, soy researcher and retired USDA senior toxicologist, warns that soy-based formulas place these children at risk in a "large, uncontrolled and basically unmonitored human infant experiment."

And how morally disturbing is this: although the FDA mandates strict labeling for estrogen-containing prescription drugs, no such label is required for estrogen-containing infant formula. It is legal as well to keep silent about the genetically modified soy and corn in these lab concoctions. Nestle and Mead-Johnson flatly dismissed calls from concerned mothers to voluntarily remove all GM organisms from their infant products. Always, always remember: the corporate food industry is after your money, not your health, not even your newborn's health.

WHILE THE SOY DEBATE rages on among researchers, soy wars are also erupting across the blogsphere. Individuals are passionate about this issue because they're either consuming large daily doses of soy, notably vegans, or once did and gladly gave it up. Here's "Never Trust Doctors" with her shout-out:

> Doctors are all liars! You have to be completely insane if you don't think the medical profession is in cahoots with Big Business. SOY IS TOXIC. I don't care what the lying doctors say. There is tons of proof out there that shows the destruction soy does to the body, and so long as they can keep the people sick and in constant need of physicians, the physicians will support any evil thing....

"Louis" is delighted to respond:

> Bull Crap!! Soy is a super food and is better for all of us than some animal's milk; dairy is not natural for us humans to ingest, look it up, and soybeans are a natural food coming from this earth; my wife is Asian and yes, her grandparents and parents always had soy at mealtime and she eats tofu and seitan and drinks soy milk daily as did I for the last 22 yrs and me and my wife are healthier than most people our age, so don't believe the hype!!!

As conflicting research results continue to pour in, the truth about soy is much more complicated than many vegans want to believe. But surely we can all agree that real food from nature, whole and unrefined, is better for human health than food altered, isolated, and denatured in a for-profit laboratory. Notes Ayurvedic doctor Claudia Welch, "In Eastern medicine we tend to assume that Nature has a

184

wisdom that governs which active and non-active ingredients belong together and we are suspicious of teasing them apart." In the West we love to tease and tear, rupture and rip natural food apart in hopes of creating something better, i.e., more lucrative. Our industrial food complex now rakes in $1 trillion a year producing the most health-damaging, nutritionally-inferior food ever ingested by humans.

So, yes, vegans can meet their daily protein requirements by eating soy and more soy, but at what cost? Eastern medicine teaches that overuse of any one food will bring bad results. The idea of moderation is strong in both the diet and ancient philosophy of Asia. This is the homeland of the Buddha and Confucius, after all, and their enduring principle of the Middle Way: nothing to extreme.

Thus, moderate intake of a large variety of whole foods is the most beneficial eating pattern. The lesson for soy being this: limited amounts, fermented, whole or lightly processed, non-GMO, and not every day. But then, where would vegans get all their required daily protein—150 grams or more for the large-bodied and active—if they restrained themselves to 3-9 grams of soy protein like all those heart-healthy, fish-chewing Asians? What's a conscientious vegan to do? Here's "Isabelle's" honest appraisal:

> I've been following a vegan diet for a year now [and] eat a fairly balanced diet heavy on grains, beans, vegetables and fruits, nuts, seeds and soy products (soy milk, tofu, fake meat). I've always had low iron so I take plenty of iron supplements as well as B12 and calcium pills. So, theoretically, everything should be hunky-dory....

> But I have to say that after the first 9-10 months, I began to feel sickened by the thought of all the soy products. A typical vegan might consume the following in one day: two glasses of soymilk (straight or in cooking); one serving of tofu; one serving of fake meat. That's a whole lot of concentrated soy. Surely it can't be healthy to be consuming so much soy?

> Yet if I were to reduce my soy intake, I'd have even more trouble meeting my protein requirements than I do already. So now I am rethinking the vegan thing. I would like to follow a diet which is eco-friendly and allows animals to live healthy and happy lives....it seems unnatural to me to eat so much of one type of food. Maybe the occasional dose of organic meat from an animal-friendly farm makes sense?

185

Now there's a smart question from a thoughtful individual willing to think outside the rigid vegan box. Sadly, her sincere quest for truth was scorned and condemned in that same veg blog by all-or-nothing vegans firmly locked into their plants-only ideology, regardless of how processed, manipulated, or difficult to digest their food might be.

To decide which high-protein food might be healthier and more natural, this trusting but concerned young woman should consider undertaking a simple task, something that you, conscious reader, can do as well. And that is to compare the actual ingredients of two high-protein foods: a lab-concocted soy product, selling in America for about 20 years, and grass-nurtured bison, providing sustenance to humans on this continent for 20,000 years.

Here is the ingredient list for a popular fake-meat soy burger. And unless "USDA Organic" is clearly stamped on the front packaging, go ahead and add genetically manipulated, irradiated, herbicide-sprayed, and hexane-soaked to the inventory: *soy protein concentrate, soy protein isolate, textured wheat protein, wheat gluten, wheat flour, water, yeast, modified cellulose, spice, salt, onion powder, succinic acid, yellow corn flour, sugar, caramel coloring, natural flavor, and oleic safflower oil.*

Here is the ingredient list for bison: *bison.*

26.

THE NERVOUS VEGETARIAN

It's nature's way of telling you something's wrong.

—Spirit

Bison as food wasn't even remotely part of my consciousness when I moved from raw coastal Alaska to picturesque Missoula, Montana, on the banks of the Clark Fork River. Land-locked and liberal, Missoula sits near the entrance to Hell Gate Canyon, a high narrow pass where fierce Blackfeet warriors once hid in the dense brush, patiently waiting to ambush the Bitterroot Salish as they journeyed east to the vast bison hunting grounds.

Moving from Valdez to this northern Rockies college town meant I could once again proudly call myself a vegetarian. Fresh produce was everywhere and those physically demanding, protein pounding, 12-hour work days were long gone. I was here to raise my good-natured toddler, to be a graduate student and spend my days reading, teaching, and philosophizing—exactly like Pythagoras and those contemplative vegetarians of old.

The Human-Animal Connection, a required ethics class, confirmed my long-standing dietary values. Our environmental studies professors pounded us with graphic documentaries depicting the cruel realities of modern industrial farming and animal product testing, little-known truths at the time. It was 1987 and every person in the room was horrified. Brutality on this scale far surpassed anything I'd witnessed as a naïve teenager on the backstreets of Paris. We looked around the classroom with no-longer innocent eyes and inquired right out loud: *What do we do now?* We had just been exposed to the hideous truth of our mass-produced animal food. How could anyone in the room *not* convert to vegetarianism? Many did, on the spot.

With intense passion, we debated live animal research vs. computer modeling, read Jeremy Bethany and M.J. Fox, praised Peter Singer's *Animal Liberation* and condemned Descartes' clockwork universe that disconnected human minds from human bodies, influencing western civilization for centuries to come (including any vegans out there not listening to their bodies). Our final reading shoved the few students still harboring reservations over the edge. In harsh detail, Desmond Stewart's virtuoso story, *The Limits of Trooghaft,* describes a future earth where *Homo sapiens* serve as subservient animal stock for a highly advanced alien race. "Troogs took one century to master the planet," the twisted tale begins, "then another three to restock it with men, its once dominant but now conquered species."

Taking their cue from humanity's own hierarchal system, the Troogs segregate all humans into castes, raising some for pet-keeping and others for the delicacy of our flesh. Naturally, the youngest and most supple among us deliver the choicest, most tender cuts, with tart female tongues providing an especially treasured delicacy (and the sweet bonus of silence). Those of us who survive childhood exist in miserable small cages, defecating through rolling bars into a filthy sluice, never inhaling the freshness of morning, never glimpsing the open sky—the same living hell we've devised for our own industrial animals.

If that distressing image wasn't enough to make the most avid burger-chomper among us upchuck his lunch, our professors also hammered us with the environmental consequences of meat-eating: the wholesale destruction of rain forests to supply beefsteaks to gluttonous Americans; the enormous quantities of precious water consumed; and the pending worldwide disaster of global warming, toward which our factory-farm, non-local food habits contributed. The truths that I was exposed to very early in Montana only strengthened my original vegetarian creed. I was set for life!

My mind was on board, 100% committed. Once again, though, my corporal self had ideas of its own. But in our culture the yakking, insistent brain rules and the body must go along for its sometimes tragic ride. How strange and sad that we don't know how to listen to our own bodies, even when they are speaking very loudly to us, eventually screaming their messages and essential truths. Like food choices that do not sustain us; relationships that deaden us into lassitude; and jobs that send stress hormones coursing through our bloodstream, setting us up for illness or chronic disease. Your body's clear, repetitive, and eventually clamorous messages will tell you know in no uncertain terms when there's something you should NOT be doing with your life. But how many of us are listening?

BY NOW I WAS 15 YEARS into my vegetarian experience—"experiment" as I now call it—and other bodily signals besides hunger were pouring in that I failed to link to my diet. My beautiful ethical diet as the source of strange new maladies? The idea never entered my mind—or if it did, I unconsciously repressed it.

That's when the insomnia began. Dreadful, existence-altering insomnia for the first time in my life, along with a strange new nervousness, a floating anxiety that manifested whenever it felt like it, especially in the weird, mumbo-jumbo, middle of the night when our rational brain is on pause and a deeper self holds the space. When that grey Missoula dawn finally arrived, I would remind myself there was no good reason to be anxious—so snap out of it, woman! I was following my desired path through grad school, delighting in a new love relationship, eating mega-healthy plant foods, and teaching yoga four nights a week to students I adored, delivering me to a state of knock-out bliss every single class.

Yet over the next few years, my on-edge nerves escalated. I became not just anxious but hair-trigger jumpy, leaping out of my chair at the slightest unexpected noise: a drawer banging shut, a vehicle starting up. My family was beginning to look at me strangely. Not one of them (animal eaters all) was the least startled by these everyday sounds. What the bajeezus was going on? My parents had called me "Serena" as a pre-veg teen, guided by a palpable inner calm by day, sleeping long and deep by night.

Even more worrying, my brain power was diminishing, losing its ratchet-edged sharpness. My formerly awesome memory was likewise taking a beating. Trying to come up with the right turn of phrase was becoming out-and-out embarrassing; my brain waves were in slow-mo. Staring idiot-like at my professors, I could actually observe the more complex words leisurely forming themselves out of the ether—instead of my mind's formerly effortless snap! snap! snap! I was in my mid-30s, for God's sake, not some menopausal, neuron-challenged grandma. Ongoing poor sleep is a factor in reaction time, this I realized, but what was the underlying source of all this fatigue, rotten sleep and dreadful trepidation? Totally mystified, befuddled. Was it time to nix my caffeine addiction? Add new yoga poses? Join an ashram? Or maybe I just needed more fabulous middle-of-the-night sex.

That's when the image of exquisitely formed, iridescent ovals came dancing through my fog-wrapped brain. Eggs. Hundreds and hundreds of waltzing, spinning, fox-trotting, luminescent eggs. Out of nowhere they appeared like glorious cinema on the back lids of my closed and weary eyes: creamy beige, pure white, or tinged in subtle tones of bluish-green, like those I had seen hand-gathered by a local farmer—whose gift of fresh eggs I had adamantly refused. *Held out to me as a gift and I had refused.* This particular hazy, low-energy day, however, I didn't reject those oval-shaped whirring images spontaneously arising from my subconscious, nor the lucid message that finally pierced my thick, impenetrable beliefs. I got it.

Form follows function, as artists and architects love to affirm, and surely eggs possess the most perfect, most elegant form in nature. Besides providing the ideal structure for embryonic growth, these elliptical beauties serve as a nutritional power cache for protein-famished omnivores. That's why black bears swim out to the middle of our pond each spring to pilfer goose eggs right out of the island nest, parents madly honking from a distance. It's why coyotes will snatch 20 eggs at a time from a cluster of duck nests, burying half of them for future protein in lean times. And it's why farm-raiding foxes will risk—and replenish—their very lives for a messy, yolky meal.

The deeper I looked into the simple egg, the more it grew in nutritional and mystical power. Humans have long revered it, singing our praises through art and religion. As far back as the Rig Veda, 3500 years ago, the primeval egg motif started showing up in creation myths, and across the cultures these stories are remarkably similar: the universe comes into being after hatching, rising, or even radically erupting from one very fertile egg. For the Dogon people of Mali this primal egg represents the earth's placenta; it nourished our world's first animate beings. And in Chinese mythology, the dual energies of the universe, yin and yang, struggled mightily within one colossal egg until it shattered and the deity Pangu bounded out, his body forming the earth, his blood the rivers and seas. (And how fascinating that the fleas and parasites inhabiting his body turned into the first humans!) Modern cosmology centers its primary creation theory around the gracefully functional egg as well, declaring that 13.7 billion years ago the entire universe was fiercely compressed into a gravitational singularity—the so-called cosmic egg—followed by the violent Big Bang (or was it strangely silent?) and expansion of the universe into its current state.

If the universe could explode and expand for 14 billion years after emerging from a compact celestial egg, surely I could use this vital source for such a simple task as restoring my health. After all, humans have been utilizing real eggs for millennia to impart virility and fertility to their bodies, even creating elaborate rituals to invoke the mighty egg's condensed, life-giving power. Some of these ancient rituals are still in use today. Check out this modernized fertility rite between a man and woman trying to conceive:

> After gentle kissing and deep eye gazing, the couple makes a small hole in each end of an egg and then holds it between them....in their open mouths. As the man blows gently into the egg, its viscous fluid moves into the woman's open, highly receptive orifice. To aid the fluid's flow, she rhythmically sucks and sucks as he blows and blows and then she swallows it, all of it, whole. *Crazy erotic, yes, get those juices flowing!* Following a sharing of dreams and sensual massage, each unhurriedly removes the other's clothes and they engage in slow, sensual lovemaking beneath a waxing moon, white candles lit, peach incense burning. Following the sex act and dual climax, the couple continues to demonstrate care and love for one another for a good hour. *Quick, show this to every man you know!* And then they take the empty eggshells and bury them reverently in the soil.

I wasn't even looking for fertility, already had plenty of that—just ask my love child and sweet, raven-haired Alaskan boss. No, I just wanted my fair shake of the cosmic energy, enough to feel calm and energized throughout the course of a day. Enough to stop jerking at the slightest unexpected sound. Enough to get my sleep back. Enough to get my *brain* back. Was that asking too much? Of course not, and any vegan promoter who begs to differ can remain on his restrictive diet for a decade and a half—letting not one real egg or other loathed animal food so much as touch his impartial gullet—and then write with complete honesty his own body's story. This one is mine.

A healthy life, I finally realized, is not about perfection, deprivation and denial. It's not about being half-assed present to yourself and your loved ones, virtuous but fogged-out, draped over your desk by 3 PM, trounced by unrelenting fatigue. So out with the tofu scramble and in with the three-egg omelets crammed with red pepper, Tuscan kale, and pungent garlic. Sure enough: my energy *absolutely soared* on the days I downed plentiful eggs. Just like a smart, hungry animal, I inhaled them practically whole and deliciously guilt-free. And no, it wasn't the dark greens and garlic lending me this radiant new energy. I have always eaten my vegetables, the much-maligned bitter broccoli being particularly well loved. Clearly, it was high-powered poultry fuel that was sending me skyrocketing around my quiet Missoula neighborhood.

Seeking out locally pastured eggs with brilliant orange yolks, I felt just fine about my new protein source, not only because of rising energy levels and a growing inner tranquility but because it was suddenly clear that lab-extracted plant proteins, including pea protein and all the others, felt like foreign invaders that my body reviled. Along with intestinal complaints, a distinct drop in vigor followed their consumption, a feeling of lethargy, of blues and blah. By contrast, my wise body welcomed eggs like a long-lost friend, with joy and aliveness. As for those fake vegan eggs now being concocted in Silicon Valley, expect a rough ride ahead as humans once again try to replicate, in just a few years, food that has taken nature millions of years to perfect. Synergy, people! Complex synergy of incalculable numbers of non-replicable parts!

It's really rather obvious: denatured foods originate in sterile, for-profit labs, but eggs are dropped straight out of nature's vagina. (Or cloaca, in the case of birds.) Nutrition science, remember, is still in its infancy and new micronutrients continue to be discovered in natural whole foods. Yet the nutritional profile of a pastured chicken egg is already remarkable, providing high nutrient density in relation to calories. This compact oval package, nature's gift to omnivores, may be the healthiest food on the planet, earning a perfect score of 100 for biological value. It's oozing with quality protein and a perfect amino acid profile; good amounts of calcium and iron; vitamins A, D3, E and B-complex; trace minerals like selenium; plus high amounts of zeaxanthin and lutein for eye health. Egg yolks are a good source of vitamin K2 as well, dubbed "the forgotten vitamin" and critical for bone mineralization and heart and brain health.

Research on this group of fat-soluble vitamins has exploded in the past several years, and one science writer calls the incoming data and its implications "truly frightening." That's because K2 deficiency is now widespread in the American population. But why?? Because it is missing—once again—in our modern, lab-concocted, industrial foods.

Even our daily supplements don't usually contain any vitamin K2 and that's a major problem because when nutrients are deficient, according Dr. Bruce Ames and his respected triage theory, our bodies utilize what little is there for short-term metabolic functions only, at great expense to our long-term health. "If you are deficient for years, your body weakens, DNA becomes damaged, and you get sick and eventually die," Dr. Ames makes clear. "If you want maximum life span, your micronutrient needs must be met throughout life."

Actually, there are two naturally-occurring forms of this vitamin: K1 and K2. The former abounds in green leafy vegetables and is thus no problem for vegans who eat their kale and spinach, but its primary role is in blood clotting. That's a crucial function for sure, but it's K2 that's emerging as the champion in lowering our risk for heart disease, osteoporosis and cancer. The original 2004 study results stunned researchers: cardiovascular mortality risk was over 50% lower for participants consuming K2, with a 26% reduced risk for all-cause mortality (Geleijnse; Gast).

The scientific community expressed disbelief, but separate teams of German, Spanish, Dutch and American scientists have since confirmed that vitamin K2 significantly reduces risk of heart disease, severe aortic calcification, and death by all causes, while no comparable benefits were found for K1. Additional studies have found nerve protection benefits and a possible slowing of dementia. Vitamin K2 occurs primarily in animal products, with one of its most effective forms, MK4, found in animals only.

We now realize that K2 is the mysterious Activator X that Dr. Weston Price discovered in 1945 while researching traditional diets around the globe. "A vitamin-like activator," Dr. Price called it, a powerful catalyst for mineral absorption; essential for proper bone development, tooth decay prevention, and protection against inflammation and cancer. Yet for more than 60 years, the medical and nutritional establishments ignored Price's work, considering vitamin K2 of little value. Not until 2006 did the USDA finally determine the amounts of K2 in our food and recognize its vital importance.

Americans eat sufficient amounts of meat, eggs and dairy, so what happened to all the vitamin K2? Turns out our grandparents got plenty of it: butter and fat from grass-fed ruminants, rich egg yolks from backyard hens, and nutrient-dense livers from geese and ducks. As Price realized seven decades ago via chemical testing, K2 is produced by animal tissues from K1 and is found in the organs and fat of animals that consume fast-growing green plants.

Removing our farm animals from fertile fields and stuffing them with grains in sterile feedlots set off a cascade of serious health consequences that we're only beginning to comprehend. Moreover, as our nutritional knowledge expands, the French "paradox" further unravels. *Foie gras* just happens to be one of the richest known sources of K2 and Périgord, France, is the world's capital of foie gras: goose liver that's loaded with fat and protein. Périgord also enjoys the lowest rate of cardiovascular mortality in all of France, a nation already known for its low heart disease rates.

Getting your nutrients from a wide variety of whole foods is always preferred by your body, and pastured beef, chicken, eggs, milk, yogurt and butter offer K2 in beneficial amounts. To easily reach the recommended 45 mcg/day for disease prevention, some omnivores are also opting for Australian emu oil, worshipped as a sacred food by Aboriginals and part of their ancestral Dreamtime mythology. Science confirms its potent magic: 100% of emu K2 is the rapidly absorbed MK4 type found in France's revered, heart saving, goose liver pâté.

Along with reducing cardiovascular disease risk, vitamin K2 moves calcium out of places it shouldn't be, like your arteries and soft tissues, and shuttles it to places it belongs, like your bones and teeth. That's *huge*. It means that without adequate K2 our arteries and muscles calcify and our teeth decay more quickly. (Even more reason to believe all those vegan "dental horror stories.") But K2 needs to work in synchronicity with vitamin D and calcium. So if you're taking D supplements—as northerners should be—you also need to take K2. Ingesting a lot of vitamin D alone "could absolutely be causing harm if you are lacking the K2 to complete the job to get the calcium where it's supposed to be," warns Dr. Kate Rheaume-Bleue. If you're a mature female, it's critical to find the proper balance between calcium, magnesium, and vitamins K2 and D—preferably from your diet—to lower your risk for osteoporosis. *Taking calcium supplements alone can be very harmful, building up calcium where it doesn't belong, decreasing bone density and increasing your risk for heart attack and stroke.*

So if you're not eating good amounts of the following foods, your likelihood of being vitamin K2 deficient is high: pastured meat, organs, eggs and dairy (with aged cheeses like Brie and Gouda offering especially high amounts). I can already hear the rush of vegans as they descend on their local vitamin shop for yet another bottled-up nutrient that's missing in nearly all plants. Be choosy, my friends. Some K2 supplements are not biologically active and you must avoid synthetic K3, which has shown toxicity. Avoid the non-food, synthetic form of MK4 as well. The preferred variety from a bottle is MK7 and since vitamin K is fat-soluble, be sure to take it alongside some good dietary fat.

Vegans *can* obtain a very high amount of MK7 from natto, a fermented soy product common in Japan but still difficult to find elsewhere. Once you secure it, perhaps from an Asian market, be forewarned that natto is slimy and unbelievably stinky, described by one online foodie as possessing "the complex yet playful

28.

PRAISE THE LARD AND PASS THE BUTTER

The truth will set you free, but first it will piss you off.

—Gloria Steinem

"IT'S THE SUGAR, my dear."

Thus spoke the kindhearted voice of my long-gone, dear grandma Maggie as I lay in a tangled, anxious heap in the dead middle of the night, contemplating more magnesium. "Remember what a lively, healthy child you were? Remember how much you loved my stewed chicken and dumplings?"

A swelling body of research implicates not naughty fat in our soaring national rates of insomnia, obesity and metabolic syndrome, but mischievous sugar and high-glycemic carbs: sprinkled into our lattes, secreted into our salad dressings, and omnipresent in our dinners and snacks. Moreover, we're finally being told the truth our grandparents knew all along: satisfying, lip-smacking fat from grass-fed animals and other healthy sources is not only okay, it's good for you. So eat up! *Is your head spinning yet?*

Abundant, respected research now confirms that a reduced-carb diet is the best for lowering heart disease risk. But it's not so simple as extra carbs creating problems for vegans and others. Minimal fat intake is just as serious an issue. Now wait a minute—isn't low or even zero fat a good thing in the USA where a mind-boggling 70% of adults are overweight or obese? No, it is not a good thing. A diet too low in fat does terrible things to your body and brain. In fact, given enough time, this highly unnatural diet will likely make you, yes, fat—or at least poochy. It will also make you nervous and stupid, increase your risk for stroke and heart disease, and speed up the aging process. So let's set aside all the myths and distortions created by the food industry, media mongers, vegan gurus and bought-off researchers and look at the physiological facts.

Dietary fat does not create body fat. An excess of carbs creates body fat. And that's what vegans tend to eat, lots and lots of carbs, up to 70-80% of their total calories. This in spite of the fact that the World Health Organization recommends 60% tops. "I discovered I'm consuming 76% carbs in a single day!" exclaims a curious vegan who finally did his nutrition homework and posted it on a popular veg site. It wasn't clear, however, if he was proud or distraught.

Meanwhile, here's the short version of an important biochemical lesson, i.e., real science versus the scare tactics employed by those who profit from fat fear. Food fat, from both plant and animal sources, is not the same as the structural and insulating fat inside your body. When you eat fat, your body uses most of it to build essential materials—cell membranes, hormones, brain components—rather valuable stuff, wouldn't you say? Dutifully, meal after meal, day in and day out, good dietary fat from nature (versus refined vegetable oils and trans-fat trash) is constantly rebuilding your body. That's why eating good fat is imperative and why it's not the culprit in our national obesity epidemic. Need real-life confirmation? Just look at statistics following the *eat less fat!* advice that swept across our country starting in 1977. For three decades fat consumption fell dramatically—in absolute terms and as a share of calories—but Americans just kept getting fatter (B. Lin). Obesity rates for adults are now breaking records—more than one in three of us are having trouble reaching over our gut to tie our own shoes.

It's all those easy carbs that are transforming us into a nation of tubbos, brain-foggers, and cardiac patients. That's because any surfeit of carbs you eat is stored as energy, either in ready-energy form as glycogen or long-term as body fat. And that's why simply reducing calories, versus reducing carbs, often isn't enough to lose weight. An analysis of 23 peer-reviewed, randomized-controlled studies reveals that low-carb groups lost 2-3 times as much weight as the low-fat groups in 22 of the studies, and even the oddball one wasn't statistically meaningful (Gunnars). What's more, in most cases the low-carbers inhaled as much food as they desired, while calories were limited for the low-fat people. Yet the higher-fat groups still lost more weight and experienced less hunger.

Let's say you're out breaking vegan bread with your significant other. That Mushroom Lemon Risotto looks mighty tasty so you order it up, alongside a crisp green salad, sautéed veggies and non-gluten roll, no butter thank you. Because you've already put away an egregious amount of soy this same day, you prudently decide to skip the add-on tofu. So even if you brought along some chia seeds to sprinkle on your salad, your total protein and fat intake is going to be quite low.

Instead of a healthy dinner containing balanced proportions of the three macronutrients, you now have a meal composed chiefly of carbs, maybe even 76% carbs!

Unless you get moving and burn those carbohydrates soon after consumption, your body will convert them to triglycerides (glycerol plus fatty acids) that are then converted to body fat and stored for future energy needs, most often in your abdominal region. Elevated levels of triglycerides are linked to increased stroke and heart disease risk and they largely derive, experts agree, from carbohydrates. Of the 23 studies discussed above, 19 showed significantly *lower* blood triglyceride levels in the high-fat dieters versus the high-carb, low-fat ones.

The most flagrant offenders, besides alcohol? Fructose, sucrose, and an overload of carbs. Tragically, high-fructose corn syrup is pervasive in our processed food; read labels and get it out of your life. But even 100% juice, dried fruit, and other natural carbs spike triglyceride levels. A thorough review of the nutrition literature bluntly concludes: "The greater the increase in dietary carbohydrate and the greater the reduction in fat—the greater the increase in triglycerides" (Parks). Moreover, a higher saturated fat percentage is protective. One of the largest global studies ever conducted—over 145,000 participants from 19 countries—concludes that *your lipid profile suffers when saturated fat is replaced with carbohydrates* (Dehghan). Recommendations echo the Mediterranean Diet: just 45-55% of energy from carbs and inclusion of nuts, olive oil, and fish.

Despite mounting evidence, high-carb activists—especially vegans—continue to insist that the majority of triglycerides derives from the fat in our food, not the carbs, to which Dr. Andrew Weil responds: Recommendations for a low-fat/high-carb diet to lower triglycerides and cholesterol are "dead wrong in my opinion." An intentional choice of words: heart disease is America's number one killer.*

Now if you run 100 miles a day while eating loads of carbs, like Scott Jurek, a dedicated vegan, you don't store carbs because you're using them up right away. Most of us don't live in such a radical fashion, however; nor do we want to. That's good because many extreme athletes don't end up all that healthy. "Autopsies on top endurance athletes reveal signs of malnourishment," six-time Ironman World Champion Mark Allen informed me following a sports nutrition workshop. He wisely reminds us that fitness and health aren't always bed partners. In fact, studies on super-fit distance runners confirm a high level of inflammation, excess

*In response to vegans' concerns that their triglyceride levels have shot up, the T. Colin Campbell Center for Nutrition Studies admits: "Randomized control trials show that triglycerides may either increase or decrease when switching to a plant-based diet." Carb quality and exercise are cited as factors.

arterial plaque, and a *seven-fold boost in cardiac risk* (R. Schwartz). An omnivore during and after his racing years, Allen has since dialed back his physical output, way back, and makes certain to include healthy protein and fat in every meal.

Clearly, our bodies reject extremes. So after digesting that delicious veggie risotto, you might want to engage in some moderate physical activity, *not* a crushing marathon. And that doesn't mean diving into your favorite cushy-chair for a three-hour movie, allowing your high-carb dinner to be stockpiled for future fuel in the form of triglycerides and fat. In honor of this metabolic process—and in defiance of misinformed doctors everywhere—you might also want to repeat this dietary mantra: *An excess of carbs creates body fat. An excess of carbs....* And it heads, like a heat-seeking missile, straight to the middle of the compound.

"YOU'RE GETTING A GUT!" my trim, handsome, beef-loving boyfriend, Granen, announced one morning as we dressed for work. He had seen me naked many a time but I happened to be walking past a sunlit window so his view, regrettably, was a full-on profile that granted no mercy. "You're not pregnant, are you?!" That might have been a more agreeable explanation, actually, for a proud, svelte, active young woman in total denial about her expanding abdomen. That my lean, mean, vegetarian diet was the culprit never occurred to me, to anybody at the time. Fat made you fat. Fat gave you a big scary gut. Not brown rice and beans, not smoothies and raw juices, certainly not whole-grain bread! (Did you know the average glycemic index of whole wheat vs. white bread is negligible? 71 vs. 72.) So I trimmed off even more fat from my low-fat, high-plants diet and started to do crunches by the hundreds. *No Deal* was my body's unfathomable response.

Our mid-section is our "insulin index" and whenever you see someone with a not-so-glamorous wad of fat around the middle, you are looking at an insulin-imbalanced body. Insulin is the pancreas-produced hormone responsible for tightly regulating the amount of sugar in your bloodstream, moving it into body cells in an attempt to keep excess glucose out of your blood and brain, where it can do considerable damage. Fortunately, your muscles are filled with cells that provide insulin receptors for unloading that sugar. But remember, carbohydrates don't build muscle; those critically important proteins you consume do that. And since average vegan protein intake is on the low end, this means decreased lean muscle mass, which translates to fewer insulin receptors available to unload sugar.

So eventually, more and more of those carbs will be stored as extra fat around the middle, their preferred landing site. This can take years to manifest but go ahead, take a close look at the older vegan/vegetarian crowd and you'll often see a thin body propping up a spreading pooch. This is what happens on a high-carb diet if fat intake is adequate and hormone levels stay stable over the years. But if hormone levels drop significantly from inadequate dietary fat, the opposite will happen: *a thin person will start to waste away.*

But I don't eat sugar, the conscientious vegan insists, I eat legumes and grains —complex carbohydrates—big difference! Not such a difference in terms of how much glucose ultimately ends up in your bloodstream. Whether super-fast or not-so-fast, all carbs create a surge of glucose. If your veg diet tends to be high-carb *and* low-protein—as is common—it's a double whammy: more sugar/insulin and fewer insulin receptors. And watch out for a triple threat against your body if you aren't eating sufficient fat and cholesterol to keep hormone levels stable.

Yes, carbohydrates found in nature—especially veggies, fruits, and greens — are terrific sources of vitamins, minerals, phytochemicals, antioxidants and fiber. The problem arises with carb overconsumption, whether from raw apples or apple muffins, and the resulting insufficient intake of protein and fat. A chronic high-carb diet can cause repeated blood sugar spikes that may eventually lead to insulin resistance. And if you're not eating enough good fat, the consequences can be dire. Just ask ex-vegan Lierre Keith, who suffered from hypoglycemia and severe depression as a result of her two decades long, high-carb regime. A low-fat vegan diet, Keith concludes, "is not sufficient nutrition for long-term maintenance and repair of the human body….it will damage you."

Similar low-fat diets were once prescribed for diabetics. But doctors started recording spikes in blood sugar of 100-200 points after patients ate the "ideal" American Diabetes Association breakfast of whole-grain cereal with fruit, low-fat dairy or plant milk, plus juice—a meal remarkably like the one many veg'ns start their day with, including my carb-inhaling friend Avery and my young naïve self. When blood sugar spikes kept happening to Dr. Diane Schwarzbein's type 2 diabetes patients, including vegetarians, she put them on a temporary "zero" carb diet that eliminated all primarily carb foods and then asked them to eat more fat and protein. LOTS more, like full-fat cheese, butter, cream, poultry, fish and conservative amounts of red meat: *the forbidden foods*. Both doctor and clients were astonished by the positive, almost immediate results: blood sugars normalized and cholesterol levels improved. Patients gained muscle mass, experienced increased energy, and were no longer famished between meals. The most notable improvements were seen in the clients who ate the most "bad" foods every day.

217

The proverbial light bulb snapped on for the doctor. As Schwarzbein attests: "Both medicine and the media had promoted the belief that eating a low-fat diet while increasing complex carbohydrates caused people to lose body fat and stay healthy. But I had yet to meet anyone who was healthy or thriving on a low-fat diet." So she embarked on a rigorous search of the literature and was startled to find not a single long-term study showing that low-fat diets are good for you. What she did discover was an abundance of research showing that ample dietary fat is essential for good health.

THERE'S A REASON that nature, in all its wisdom, combines plenty of protein and fat within the same food item and in proper proportions: foods like fish, fowl, red meat and eggs. You need to eat these macronutrients together—in their natural form, in nourishing quantities—because protein *requires* dietary fat to be properly utilized. Look one more time at the mighty midget egg: in a mere 70 calories you receive an excellent balance of protein to fat that energizes you and then *bang*: immediately triggers satiety hormones. Furthermore, the protein causes your body to release glucagon, a hormone which encourages the utilization of stored fats. Eat high-quality foods like this in adequate amounts, and you'll not only obtain sufficient protein and fat but maintain a desirable weight.

Few plants offer this two-in-one advantage, so vegans have to work harder to find good protein/fat ratios in their food. Both avocados and olives are marvelous healthy fat sources but contain zero to negligible protein. You'll fare better with fat-rich seeds or nuts; pumpkin and sunflower seeds dole out a decent 7-10 grams protein per serving. A high-protein source like seitan, however, provides scarcely any fat. Only soy offers a good protein/fat balance from a plant, but loading up on the same foods day after day just isn't smart. And all those new protein powders? Some dish out a respectable 15 grams protein per serving, but many don't bother to list "Fat" as a category because there is none. Hemp powder does deliver a scant 3 grams per serving but also a common side effect: gastrointestinal distress.

Vegans can sure try to replace the two-in-one, high-protein/good fat sources found in animal-derived food, but even the conscientious don't always succeed. And that gets even tougher as intake recommendations rise. Spooked by all the recent fat-is-good news, a few vegan leaders are (finally!) advising higher fat intake, after vilifying such diets for decades. Yet many proponents still want to believe that 10-20% of total calories is sufficient.

218

Too-low calorie input continues to be an issue as well, judging by the plethora of pencil-thin vegans wandering around Whole Foods, looking as if they could slide through the cracks between all those massive, vibrating freezers packed with low-fat chow. Some vegans even boast how minimal their calorie and fat intakes are, but they really shouldn't. Anyone who rejects a more balanced approach may experience the preliminary symptoms of malnutrition, including depression, dizziness, mind-warping fatigue, itchy skin, and missing periods.

We're not talking third-world malnutrition, rapidly evident. We're talking slow-moving and insidious. A chronic low-grade fat deficiency can take years to manifest as a health issue. By then, the damage may be difficult to undo. "Every one of the vegetarians I have worked with has been metabolically damaged in one way or another," Dr. Schwarzbein revealed to me. Even the brainiest veg'n can be estranged from her own body, blinded by an obsessive devotion to a strict ethical diet, until she can no longer hide from the corporal truth. Ex-veg Keith testifies:

> Six weeks into veganism I had my first experience of hypoglycemia, though I wouldn't know that's what it was called until 18 years had gone by and it had become my life. Three months into it, I stopped menstruating…the exhaustion began around then too and it only got worse…My skin was so dry it flaked, and in the winter it itched so badly it kept me up at night. At 24, I developed gastroparesis, which, again, wasn't diagnosed or treated until I was 38 and found a doctor who worked with recovering vegans. Then there was the depression and anxiety…all those years of emotional collapse weren't a personal failing; they were bio-chemical, if self-inflicted.

Unfortunately, young vegans may not notice anything amiss those first years because the harm can be happening on a cellular level. Yes, everything looks and feels fantastic when you embark on your trendy new diet. Your body will use existing fat stores for energy, reducing your weight and lowering blood pressure à la Bill Clinton, Al Gore, and other celebrities—whose high-exposure testimonials convinced many that veganism is the way to go. *But any diet that skimps on good fat and stresses carbs may pose even more danger to your health than a calorie-scant one* because it often reduces not just valuable fat but critical protein, which you'll eventually be forced to take from lean body mass.

"I don't believe it," a lot of plant eaters are arguing right about now. "I know vegans in perfect health, including super athletes!" At what point in time an individual's long-term outcome begins to manifest is dependent on several factors:

age, metabolism, hormone levels at the start, and percentage carbs consumed. Whatever the starting point, however, the ultimate health outcome of a long-term, low-fat diet is detrimental.

"Since the destruction from eating a low-fat diet occurs over many years, the correlation is not an easy one to make," affirms Dr. Schwarzbein. Thus, while vegans and others may experience fabulous *initial* results from a high-carb/low-fat diet, many will eventually experience abnormal metabolism, imbalanced hormones, and a significant decline in health. Over time, the body will start making triglycerides at high levels because bad habits like too many carbs, too few good fats, and ongoing stress elevate blood sugar levels, while stimulants like caffeine decrease insulin sensitivity.

"Abnormal cholesterol panels are a *late* indicator of abnormal cholesterol metabolism," the doctor warns. "The damage being done on a cellular level from overconsumption of carbohydrates or use of stimulants has to occur for years before an abnormality will show up on a blood panel. That is true even if the damage is substantial."

That's why anyone pushing a vegan diet—whether in person, blogs, or best-sellers—has *an ethical obligation* to tell us exactly how long he or she has been on the diet and how faithfully it's been followed. And that's why newly minted or even 10-year vegans are not to be trusted with all their upbeat health declarations. Making long-term health claims based on a vegan diet of less than a decade—as many exuberant activists do—is jumping the gun, potentially misleading all those trusting newbies. We are only interested in the honest stories and *measurable health outcomes* of those who have been a strict vegan for 20 years, minimum. There may be disquieting signs before then, but that's usually when any long-term damage starts to manifest.

It took John Nicholson 26 years to admit that his low-fat vegan diet was killing him. Up to that point he was eating the healthiest diet on the planet, or so he'd been told: zero cholesterol, very low saturated fat, plants, grains and legumes. About eight years into his diet, Nicholson started experiencing serious digestive issues but ignored them despite the growing intensity of his pain. For 18 years he endured painful irritable bowel syndrome because it couldn't possibly be his pure vegan diet causing it. That's who he was. A disciple, a devotee, a lifer.

Nicholson was also an active man at the start of his vegan adventure but year after year, he put on the pounds until he finally weighed in at "clinically obese." In *The Meat Fix: How a Lifetime of Healthy Living Nearly Killed Me,* Nicholson admits he was waddling around his house by that time, drenched in sweat and short of breath. By the time he reached 40, his cholesterol levels were far out of range and he suffered from headaches, acid reflux, and constant fatigue.

The hard lesson for Nicholson is the same for millions like him who believed in the 20th century fat scare. Here it is: good health depends on a diet of sufficient high-quality fat, including saturated. Meanwhile, vegans continue to bash animal-derived fat, fanning outdated fears that sat fat and cholesterol are the twin boogie men of poor health and heart attacks. These vegans are either in complete denial or blissfully unaware that this harmful myth has been discredited. "This fear of cholesterol and fat is not grounded in scientific fact," asserts Dr. Schwarzbein. "I have found that the more good fats people eat, the healthier they become."

The French have known this for centuries, consuming liberal amounts of both cholesterol and saturated fat, as butter, cheese, cream, meat, organs and good old-fashioned lard, while boasting lower rates of cardiovascular disease than most western countries—where refined vegetable oils have replaced animal fat. In the Gascony region of France, fatty goose and duck livers are regularly savored, along with plentiful natural meat, yet the heart attack rate per 100,000 men is a remarkable 80 compared to 315 in the US. And females in France enjoy one of the highest life expectancies in the world. Living an astonishing 122 years, Jeanne Calment once remarked that "the only wrinkle I have is the one I'm sitting on!" The French present no paradox at all, once the truth about health's relation to good dietary fat (*and the ability to laugh at oneself*) is finally understood.

Obstinately ignoring this and other powerful evidence from fat-rich traditional diets that have stood the test of time, veg advocates focus on America's modern industrial diet with its altered, deleterious fat. They then arrive at the bogus con-clusion that an animal-based regime is inherently harmful. Listen to this typical statement endlessly repeated in popular veg books: "Diets high in animal products and processed foods—rich in saturated fat, trans fat, and cholesterol—increase chronic disease risk and lower life expectancy."

These kinds of statements are useless. Again, as with bad research, there are too many variables lumped together to support this spurious claim. Notice how "saturated fat and trans fat" are hitched together by these vegan authors, yet they have completely different chemical structures and metabolic effects. Saturated fat is natural, was consumed for millennia by our ancestors, and is easily metabolized by the human body. Trans fat, injected into our industrial food, is a chemically altered freak that clogs up our cells. Gosh, I wonder which one is killing us?

Notice that "animal products and processed foods" are also glued together in this coy vegan statement about disease risk, as if real turkey is the same as processed lunch meat; real fat the same as Olestra; and butter equal to margarine. Made from fresh or fermented cream, real butter has been enjoyed by humanity as a valuable source of high-energy fat since 6500 BC. Yet even hungry rats won't eat margarine, a lab-concoction from vegetable oils whose molecules have been rearranged. Common sense tells us which of these products is likely to escalate discomfort and disease in human bodies. (Side effects from Olestra, a fake fat with no nutritive value, include anal leakage—what fun.) Evidently, our easily manipulated, media-addled minds aren't as smart as rat brains when it comes to certain food choices. But surely our intelligent, impartial bodies know what's good for them and what's *not*—and they are churning out the evidence in the form of soaring rates of obesity and chronic degenerative disease.

There's actually a simple and reliable way to isolate the variables and study omnivorous diets that include natural animal products but *exclude* inferior foods like refined carbs, processed meats, and rat-repelling margarine. Indeed, an extensive body of research on traditional cultures already exists and the conclusions are firm: diets based upon grass-fed animals—high in natural fat and protein—confer excellent, long-lasting health to humans of all ages. It's our modern trans fat, high-carb, media-promoted fake food that's destroying us.

MAKING PERFECT BABIES

The anthropological data on traditional cultures consuming real food—animals and plants, wild and cultivated—reveals an absence of the modern diseases that are ravaging our families: cancer, diabetes, heart disease, autoimmune disorders, Alzheimer's, on and on. Among the population groups that have enjoyed robust health while favoring high-fat, animal-abundant diets are the Cretes, the Swiss, the Himalayans, Inuit, Maasai, Australian aboriginals and, of course, the offal-loving French. Total fat content in these diets varies from 30% to 80%, with the vast majority of calories derived from monounsaturated and saturated fatty acids.

In the northern regions of India, inhabitants put away 17 times more animal fat than their southern kin but live eight years longer. They're also seven times *less* likely to die from heart disease (Malhotra). And on three small atolls in the South Pacific, the Tokelauans thrived for centuries on a diet extraordinarily high in saturated fat. A good half of their calories came from coconuts—87% saturated—and

222

the rest largely from seafood. When 18th century British explorers landed on these tropical coral islands, they described the people as healthy, handsome, peaceful and happy, their graceful bodies "tattooed with geometric designs and figures of turtles and fish." Later research confirmed their remarkably low levels of obesity, diabetes, and coronary heart disease (Wessen).

Traveling the world during the 1930s to study isolated indigenous people and their traditional diets, Dr. Weston Price found none of our modern degenerative diseases, only superior health, strong bones, perfect teeth and superb immunity. All these people ate lavish amounts of animal fat and cholesterol—with hunters, herders, and fishers emerging as the strongest, most disease-resistant of all. Asked why they ate so many fish eggs, the women would just smile and tell the doctor, "So that we can make perfect babies."

And plants-only eaters? Purposely seeking out these tiny groups, Price noted the following: "I have as yet found no group that was building and maintaining good bodies exclusively on plant foods." Among those people trying to do so, he discovered a "marked evidence of failure." Why is that vegan supporters never bring up this rich cache of evidence? They cannot. Their anti-meat, anti-saturated fat, anti-cholesterol argument would die a fast death. So instead, they present studies based on grain-fed, factory-farmed animal products, lab-altered fats, highly processed foodstuffs, and other denatured and manipulated non-nourishment in order to make their claim that an omnivorous diet is *bad, very bad for you!*

Natural fats from animals and plants are not only good for you, they sustain your very life. They provide the building blocks for all your cell membranes, play a critical role in immune health, and help produce and regulate your hormones. Want to live a long life? Then eat healthy fat with every meal because those of us with the most balanced hormonal system will outlive everybody else.

Let's be clear: without sufficient dietary fat you will die much sooner. "Like cholesterol deprivation, fat deprivation disrupts all the biochemical processes of your metabolism," affirms Dr. Schwarzbein, "putting you on the accelerated metabolic aging track." Claiming it would be impossible to name every health issue that can result from a fat deficiency, the doctor offers symptoms to watch for. Any of these sound familiar? Carbo craving, caffeine craving, mood disorders, loss of lean body mass, expanding gut, infertility, disrupted sleep, poor memory, and the dreaded....what was that again? Oh yeah, *brain fog.*

Recall the importance of vitamins A, D, E, and K. Dietary fat is needed for the absorption of every one of them. The authors of *Becoming Vegan* admit that a low-fat vegan diet may compromise the absorption of fat-soluble vitamins, phyto-chemicals, and crucial minerals like zinc and iron, already less bioavailable from plant sources. Dietary fat also plays an important role in calcium absorption and bone health. So sure, you can get essential vitamins and minerals from plants, but they are not going to do you a lick of good if they're not absorbed by your body.

It's been drilled into our brains since childhood, but forget all the negative hype about dietary fat, especially saturated. Your body needs it. Now that better designed research is *finally* distinguishing between real fat and fake fat, natural meat and processed meat, the results are clear. "No evidence" exists for linking saturated fat from animals with an increased risk for coronary heart disease or stroke. Scientists analyzed over 100 research projects involving close to a million people, reviewed the results of 27 randomized controlled trials, and concluded that the evidence just isn't there (Siri-Tarino; Chowdhury).

Furthermore, a number of the studies show animal fat to be *beneficial* to heart health, including an association between the saturated fat in dairy and lower cardiovascular risk. As one example: in postmenopausal women, "a greater saturated fat intake is associated with less progression of coronary atherosclerosis, whereas carbohydrate intake is associated with a greater progression" (Mozaffarian). The omega-3 fatty acids in fish flesh were likewise found to be heart protective, and please note that *supplements did not have the same effect.*

It's a high-carb diet that should be getting greater scrutiny, claims Dr. Rajiv Chowdhury, who stands by the conclusions of his meta-analysis, despite a wholly predictable wave of condemnation from low-fat promoters. The smaller, artery-clogging cholesterol particles are increased by excess carbohydrates, the research shows, *not* saturated fat. Vegans aren't ready to acknowledge this truth because "sat fat leads to heart attack" is a vital part of their irrational, outmoded, anti-meat mythology. Yet it's a surfeit of carbs that lowers the "good" HDL cholesterol, the vegan profile that consistently shows up in research (along with their additional cardiovascular risk factors: elevated homocysteine; higher platelet aggregation; inadequate vitamin D). Adequate saturated fat, on the other hand, helps increase beneficial HDL cholesterol, studies now confirm, and replaces small, dense "bad" LDL particles with the large, light, fluffy ones that are generally benign.

That's not to say you should now stuff your pretty face with as much yummy high-fat chow as you please. (The average American downs 48 pints of ice cream per year—yazoots!—loaded with sugar, fat, and calories.) "Love moderately," as Shakespeare wisely instructed. Eat sensible amounts of saturated fat from healthy sources, along with polyunsaturates from nuts and olive oil, while reducing carbs, and you have a prescription for heart health.

Want to keep your brain healthy as well? Then feed yourself at the natural fat trough. Fully 60% of your brain's solid matter is composed of fat and cholesterol, with saturated fat one of its primary components. Our brains LOVE sat fat, with research showing that individuals who consume more saturated fat substantially reduce their risk for dementia (Roberts). It may even help *reverse* dementia.

Some caregivers are now giving Alzheimer's patients spoonfuls of sat fat on a daily basis. That's because Dr. Mary Newport made a dramatic discovery after prescription medicine failed to help her husband who suffered from early onset Alzheimer's. Steve Newport used to be computer savvy, but at age 53 he couldn't even turn one on. Yet when his wife began feeding him natural saturated fat every day, it wasn't long before he was enthusiastically reading again, tying his shoes, walking normally and even running. Trials are now underway to determine if simple, inexpensive saturated fat can help renew damaged functions in the brain.

HERE'S MORE GOOD NEWS for lipid lovers. Dietary fat not only imparts energy, it slows down nutrient absorption so you feel calm, energized, and satiated for hours. This grounding effect is well documented in controlled clinical trials. High-fat diets decreased anger, hostility, anxiety and depression, while low-fat, vegan-type diets had the opposite effect, significantly *increasing* hostility and anger (Wells). And you thought all that raging against omnivores was mere self-righteousness. Ironically, it may be diet-induced. Ahoy, hostile vegans and other angry types! Fats in their natural state are very good for you, very calming. So eat it up! As the truth about dietary fat leaks out to a deceived and incredulous public, the foodie bloggers are celebrating:

> Anyone scared to eat their egg yolks, butter, full-fat milk and
> bloody red meat can send it to me. I'll pay the postage.

> *Bring on the bacon and ducky fat, please!!*

Here are some quick facts to guide you. All forms of natural fat are beneficial, including saturated and monosaturated, but you need to eliminate heat-processed polyunsaturated oils like soy, corn, canola, etc. because they are inflammatory, highly unstable, and likely to go rancid (which you can't even smell due to all the chemical bleaching and deodorizing). For salads and other cold dishes, use pure, cold-pressed monosaturated oils—olive, avocado, most nuts—and cook at low temps with the much more stable saturated fats: butter, coconut oil, lard or tallow. Our sagacious grandmothers kept a metal tin chock-full of chicken or pork lard on the kitchen counter at all times, skimmed out of skillets and set aside for the next nutritious meal. Here's Alexandra commenting in *Simple, Good and Tasty:*

> My Nan, 90 this year and still going strong, tells me about the sort of food they used to eat. She talks fondly of "drippings on toast" and there was of course none of this low fat or vegetarian nonsense. They used butter, suet, lard, goose fat. I think it very strange that animal fats are naturally occurring and require little or no refining, yet apparently are really bad for you.
>
> I don't buy it—we have been conned. I happily consume animal fat when I want to…..Fat is satiating; if I eat animal fats I eat less food overall and I am less hungry; my blood sugar feels regulated and I have lost a stone in weight. I have more energy than ever….

Always avoid damaged fats; your body cannot metabolize them. They can be damaged by oxidation, high-heat processing (creating free radicals), or chemical alteration in labs, like adding hydrogen to vegetable oils to make them more solid (partially hydrogenated trans fats). Shun all of these but, veggie or omnie, you must avoid all industrial trans fats like the plague. They are terrible for the human body because we lack the correct enzymes to metabolize them; yet they are everywhere in modern food, concealed in our muffins and ice cream, restaurant fries and frozen pot pies.

Industry ends up the winner, churning out high-profit products with a longer shelf-life. *You* end up with speeded-up aging and a shorter shelf life. Some of the trans fats and vegetable oils in your food began their commercial life as soap, candles, paints and glue. *Are you starting to get pissed off yet?*

IT ALL STARTED IN 1911 when Procter and Gamble, dreaming up totally superfluous, never-before-eaten concoctions to maximize earnings, introduced Crisco to an unsuspecting American public. *"Better than butter for cooking!"* At the time, all Americans happily and healthfully cooked with lard, tallow or butter, but P&G needed to demonize animal fat in order to sell its new vegetable-derived trans fat, formerly used to produce, yes, candles. It seems candle sales were down due to modern electrification starting up, so a heavy-handed marketing scheme assured naïve Americans that plant-sourced CRISCO (*CRYS*talized *C*ottonseed

Oil) was a healthy alternative to saturated fat. Steadily, trans fat overtook animal fat in our nation's kitchens and we've been watching millions of Americans bung up their arteries and drop dead from heart attacks ever since.

Can you believe it wasn't until 2006 that the FDA required trans fats to even be labeled on all our commercial food? With an industry-approved loophole, of course: up to .49 grams can be falsely cited as "zero." This means hidden sources of trans fats are everywhere and quickly add up. What we need is a new product label for all the companies who continue to sneak trans fats into our food supply: *Fat profits pre-empt fat health.*

After decades of scientific evidence and public outrage, the FDA has at last admitted that trans fats induce systemic inflammation and are unsafe for human consumption, meaning they will be phased out. Some companies have already started the process. This is very good news for our children but it sure won't help the 7,000 Americans who are still dying prematurely from heart disease every year *due to trans fats alone*, according to the Centers for Disease Control (CDC). Procter and Gamble should light a candle made of Crisco to honor each and every life that fake-fats-for-profit have snuffed out these past 100 years. That's 700,000 candles for our loved ones. And that's not counting the additional 20,000 annual heart attacks the CDC also attributes to trans fats, all told killing or afflicting several million of our beloved family members and friends.

Besides clogging up cells and arteries, bad vegetable fats create an overload of omega-6 in our bodies. We need both omega-6 and omega-3 essential fatty acids (EFAs), derived solely from food, but they must be in the correct proportion. Historically, this has never been a problem. Eating real food from the earth, rivers and seas—plants, animals, fish, bugs—our ancestors received ample EFAs in the right ratio (approximately 1:1), allowing humans to survive and flourish. As Dr. A.P. Simopoulos writes in *Experimental Biology and Medicine*, this is "the diet on which human beings evolved and their genetic patterns were established." It's clear, however, that this grand evolutionary plan backfires in a plants-only diet.

Due to the hefty amounts of omega-6 in plant foods, a vegan's omega 6/3 imbalance is already elevated to begin with—grains in particular are disturbingly high in omega-6s. Add the typical intake of nuts, polyunsaturated vegetable oils, and baked goods in a vegan diet and we are looking at an extreme imbalance. Honest pro-vegan authors now concede this is a very serious issue, putting plant eaters at a great disadvantage. Omnivores who eat a lot of processed crap aren't doing so well either, with a typical 16:1 omega 6/3 ratio; but studies of vegans reveal *dangerously high levels of omega-6*, with ratios soaring as high as 120:1. An excess of omega-6 fatty acids spells big trouble for your body. They are dreadfully potent, increasing inflammation and platelet aggregation. Omega-3s, conversely, are anti-inflammatory and protect against harmful responses.

Having an imbalance of omega-6 is implicated in depressed immunity, disrupted hormone regulation, cell proliferation and cancer. Did anyone in the vegan industry scout out the deleterious health effects of an omega-6 overload and warn us in advance? Of course not. Omega-3s are seriously lacking in a plant diet, and 2,000+ scientific studies implicate omega-3 deficiency in hyper-activity, learning disorders, violence, arthritis, diabetes, stroke and heart disease.

We're still sorting out the metabolic disaster created by so swiftly and severely altering the natural balance of fatty acids in our foods. We do know this for sure: ever since industry began manipulating our traditional ancestral foods in the early 20th century, promoting processed carbs and replacing saturated fat from animals with refined oils from plants, our health as a nation has been in serious decline.

Other nations have been smarter. After adopting western-style diets high in omega-6 loaded vegetable oils, the Israeli and Japanese scientific communities outright condemned them, citing spiraling rates of depression, heart disease, and cancer. Authorities at the Japanese Society for Lipid Nutrition have called them "inappropriate for human use as foods" (Okuyama). Yet all across America, our grocery stores continue to stock refined vegetable oils, and much of the public remains ignorant of the dangers.

LEADERS OF VEGAN MOVEMENT DEVELOP PARKINSON'S

A lot of vegans are doing their own Nutrition 101 catch-up: how to consume enough omega-3 fatty acids for normal metabolism and good health. It's easy for them to secure the short-chain ALA (alpha-linolenic acid) found in plant oils, but much more difficult to obtain the critically important long-chain fatty acids found primarily in marine oils: DHA (docosahexaenoic acid) for brain health, and EPA (eicosapentaenoic acid) for heart protection. The premier source is cold-water oily fish: chiefly salmon, sardines, mackerel, cod and halibut.

Certain plant foods like flaxseed, hempseed, and walnuts do provide omega-3s, as vegans are quick to point out, but there's a big difference. While humans can directly metabolize EPA and DHA from animal sources, our bodies have to convert the very different, short-chain omega-3s found in plants into usable EPA and DHA. And that conversion is inefficient and incomplete. "Vegan levels of long-chain omega-3s are low, indicating limited conversion," admit the authors of *Becoming Vegan*, citing studies that show adult vegan DHA and EPA levels to be just 22-55% those of omnivores. (And less than 30% in breastfed vegan infants.)

Unfortunately for plants-only eaters, DHA is the primary fatty acid in human brains and low serum levels are linked to many neurological disorders, including depression, cognitive decline, memory loss, Parkinson's disease and Alzheimer's. In "Leaders of the Vegan Movement Develop Parkinson's: Case Studies," pro-vegan Joel Fuhrman, MD, reports on the deaths of two older vegan males who were leaders in the natural food movement and ate healthy plant food every day. Dr. Fuhrman had one of them lab-tested when the tell-tale tremors began and was "shocked" by the results: DHA blood levels close to *zero,* despite daily intake of nuts and seeds. By contrast, omnivorous diets rich in DHA are neuro-protective.

The grace of being part of nature is that humans *are* provided with abundant sources of essential long-chain omega 3s: animal fats that our bodies immediately use to protect our hearts and brains. But this doesn't help vegans because they're always trying to do an end-run around nature. Seaweed, anyone? Some vegans are growing it themselves. Yet even ingesting seaweed in concentrated, powdered form, you'd have to eat the equivalent of 300 grams every day to gain just 300 mg of EPA (and little to no DHA). Moreover, seaweed readily absorbs the ocean's toxins. High arsenic levels have been found in kelp and other edible seaweeds, and iodine content can reach hazardous levels as well.

As for a dependable plant source of essential DHA, there's only microalgae, microscopic sea plants eaten by small fish which in turn are eaten by big and then bigger fish, the same natural cycle that vegetarian Ben Franklin observed when he decided to return to his omnivorous roots. DHA-containing algae supplements are now available for vegans and sustainability is a big plus, but it's too soon to know their long-term effectiveness. Moreover, most research to date has been funded by the industry that profits from it. Like other nutrition experts, Andrew Weil, MD, believes fish to be the superior source because it comes directly from nature, not a patented lab process, and "contains DHA in the form our bodies require."

You do have to give these fish-boycotting, algae-loving vegans credit. They're trying very hard to revise *Homo sapiens'* innate position on the food chain. From all appearances, they'd rather be a fish than to ever have to eat one.

29.

BUSTED: THE CHOLESTEROL MYTH

Where there's an agenda to defend, people will believe anything.

—Anonymous

An EVEN MORE RADICAL WAY vegans attempt to flout the natural order is by denying the human body's need for dietary cholesterol. They are *required* to believe this because all plants contain zero cholesterol. Yet many will suffer the consequences of their obstinate belief system because we do indeed need dietary cholesterol. Strangely enough, those who consume too little may end up with elevated blood cholesterol levels. Let's look closely at this seeming contradiction because the truth will set us free from all the "cholesterol is evil" propaganda perpetuated by the medical, pharmaceutical, and vegan establishments.

As we witnessed with long-term vegan John Nicholson, eating a diet lacking in cholesterol can eventually lead to its overproduction and accelerate metabolic aging. Diane Schwarzbein, MD, explains how this works: "When you do not eat cholesterol, your body sees this deprivation as a time of crisis or famine, and during this 'famine' insulin activates an enzyme in your liver called HMG Co-A Reductase that begins to overproduce cholesterol." This happens when high levels of carbohydrates are taken in for long periods, something our ancestors did only when meat was unavailable, not by choice.

However, when you start eating enough cholesterol, your body sends a signal that the "famine" is over, and the HMG-CR enzyme is switched off. In other words, the cholesterol you get from animal food is of enormous benefit, keeping your blood cholesterol levels normal. The well-known Framingham Heart Study confirms this fact.

Involving 6,000 citizens from the small city of Framingham, Massachusetts, this oft-cited study was one of the first to identify risk factors for heart disease, including smoking, high blood pressure, and lack of exercise. Researchers noted that subjects who weighed more and had high blood cholesterol levels were also at increased risk.

This last statement was publicized far and wide—and is still disseminated by lazy media sources and uninformed vegans. But it leaves out the most valuable information of all: what all these at-risk, overweight people ate! *They all had abnormally high blood cholesterol levels but consumed the least amount of fat and cholesterol.* William Castelli, MD, former director of the study, clearly spells this out for us: "In Framingham, the more saturated fat one ate, the more cholesterol one ate, the more calories one ate, the lower the person's serum cholesterol."

Tragically, the media distortions persist and vegans are still insisting: "My body makes all the cholesterol it needs, so I never have to eat any. I'm going with my zero-cholesterol diet for the rest of my life!" So day after day, they choose cereal or granola and fruit for breakfast, never eggs and buttered toast. Again, the metabolic expert, Dr. Schwarzbein:

> But this strategy will not work. Carbohydrates stimulate insulin, and all the processes leading to plaqueing of the arteries are caused by the overproduction of insulin. Equally important is that carbohydrates do not have the same ability as dietary cholesterol to signal the body when it has made enough cholesterol. So the body keeps producing more.

You've heard of statins, of course. How could you not? Pfizer alone spends $3 billion annually to persuade the public of this drug's dubious merits via an army of 38,000 sales reps dispatched to medical offices around the globe. Oh yes, the pharmaceutical giants are fully aware that HMG-CR produces cholesterol, so they formulated some very expensive drugs to inhibit this enzyme. And because these wildly profitable corporations market statins to the tune of $26 billion in annual revenue, they're not about to tell you, nor your doctor, that the very best way to balance your cholesterol levels is simple and free: *Cut down on carbs, especially fructose, and get adequate cholesterol from a balanced diet of whole foods.*

They're also not going to tell you that for decades, statin advocates have been using a statistical sleight of hand, called relative risk reduction, to greatly amplify the drugs' trivial benefits (Diamond). When actual population benefit—a tiny 1%—is compared to the very real risks that these drugs present for decreased immune function, increased muscle atrophy, diabetes and cancer, the conclusion is clear: no net benefit for the millions taking statins who have high cholesterol and no history of heart disease.

Consider this supreme irony: statins deplete your body of coenzyme Q10—vital for heart health and muscle function—leading to chest pain and possible heart failure! Cholesterol-lowering statins are also associated with mitochondrial dysfunction, depression, and cognitive impairment. As Orli Etingin, MD, of Weill Cornell Medical Center admits: "Anecdotes linking statins to memory problems have been rampant for years."

Studies should be comparing statin effectiveness with nutrition management, enlightened researchers now insist. "We should acknowledge the inconsistencies of the cholesterol theory and recognize the proven benefits of a healthy lifestyle incorporating a Mediterranean diet to prevent coronary heart disease" (DuBroff). Over and over, the cholesterol-friendly/high-plant Med Diet has shown prolonged life and reduced risk for cancer, diabetes, and heart disease. Statin drugs have not. (Nor has veganism.) Yet the pharmaceutical cartel continues to push them.

KICKED IN THE GUT

Cholesterol is not your enemy. It's your powerful ally. You and every living thing wouldn't exist without it. This soft, waxy substance, called a sterol, has been part of you since the embryonic stage. It's in every cell of your body. Your brain and nervous system hold the highest concentrations, making it critical for neurological function, including memory making. And who doesn't love great sex, one of the benefits of healthy amounts of testosterone and estrogen? *All your sex and other steroid hormones are derived from cholesterol*—which also assists with serotonin function, keeping your moods positive and uplifted. If your blood cholesterol levels are too high, reducing carbs and eating cholesterol is the safe, healthy way to reduce them. If your levels drop too low, you may die.

Eating a balanced, nutrient-dense diet is how you get too-low levels back up. A healthy body can usually produce the cholesterol it needs, but this isn't true for too-thin, nutrient-depleted individuals who aren't getting enough calories, skimp on fat for long periods, or have abused their liver. These people *must* get their cholesterol from animal-sourced food to bring their levels into a healthy range. Overly-low blood cholesterol levels (which can happen with statins—and vegan diets) are linked to higher risk for cerebral hemorrhage, stroke, cancer, major depression and suicide.

"Insufferable" is how one loyal vegan described her slow descent into hell on her zero-cholesterol diet: life-sapping fatigue, constant carb cravings, extreme

232

mood swings, loss of menses, depression followed by anxiety, hope followed by despair, zilch quality of life. And eventually, total self-disgust. When Doreen finally consented to see a doctor, she was devastated by the lab results: a protein deficit and dangerously low cholesterol levels—the very deficiencies that vegans deny and deny and deny.

Hearing the verdict, she felt angry and betrayed, like she'd been slapped in the face and kicked in the gut by a best friend. How many years of quality life did she lose to this "fun and easy" diet?

EATING CHOLESTEROL from healthy foods is one of the best things you can do for yourself. Yet vegans, drug makers, and others with a vested interest continue to vilify cholesterol as the nasty, gluey creator of arterial plaque. Encouraged by Big Pharma, some doctors are even pushing statins for overweight children ($$$). But cholesterol is the good guy in this story.

If an artery becomes irritated or inflamed—whether from high insulin, highly unstable polyunsaturates, or infection—a protective scar or "plaque" is formed which itself contains minimal cholesterol. This plaque, along with the constriction of your blood vessels that occurs during the inflammatory process, does indeed boost your risk for high blood pressure and heart disease. So at this point, your smart body produces extra cholesterol and speeds it through the bloodstream to the exact spot needed. (High and low-density lipoproteins, HDL and LDL, are actually the *carriers* of cholesterol.) Once there, it helps cleanse the arterial wall of plaque and transports this to the liver for safe disposal. Renowned researcher Mary G. Enig, PhD, calls cholesterol a healing agent, "a repair substance that helps heal arterial damage."

"The fixation on cholesterol as a major cause of heart disease defies the last 15 years of science," concludes Ron Rosedale, MD, leading anti-aging doctor. "It deflects from the real causes such as the damage (via glycation) that sugars like glucose and fructose inflict on tissues, including the lining of arteries, causing chronic inflammation and resultant plaque."

A meta-analysis of over 160 research studies reveals that an increase in dietary cholesterol had a negligible effect on blood cholesterol levels and *no link at all* to heart disease risk (Colpo). Furthermore, hospital admission stats reveal that 50% of patients admitted for a heart attack have normal cholesterol levels. Okay, the drug industry says, so let's lower the guidelines, but smart doctors say differently.

"Serum cholesterol is not a strong risk factor for coronary heart disease," agrees Dr. Castelli of the Framingham Heart Study. Meanwhile, as Dr. Rosedale notes, hundreds of respected scientific studies have linked insulin resistance to coronary heart disease.

So what about that claim splattered just about everywhere that a vegan diet is heart protective? Remember, we're not focusing here on aged, overweight women and men *who already have heart disease*, as in the Ornish and Esselstyn studies. We're talking about basically healthy individuals who have plunged into a strict vegan diet. The truth is, there's so little completed long-term research on vegans as a separate entity that no claims can be made for heart protection. The statistics that we do have consistently show more protection against heart disease for those population groups who eat moderate amounts of fish, dairy, and eggs. These results may stun vegans but they come as no surprise to the authors of *Nourishing Traditions*. "Prevention of heart disease will not be achieved with the current focus on lowering cholesterol—either by drugs or diet—but by consuming a diet that provides animal foods rich in protective fats and vitamins B6 and B12," affirm Dr. Mary Enig and Sally Fallon, who sing the praises of adequate dietary cholesterol.

Your need for dietary cholesterol and saturated fat began the moment you were born. That's why human breast milk contains bountiful amounts of both. As a baby, you required fat and cholesterol-rich foods to ensure proper development of your brain and nervous system, likewise as a child and teen. As an adult, you need cholesterol for cell maintenance and repair, especially of brain tissue (ensuring you stay alert and don't get conned into those risky statins). And in our elders, memory function stays sharpest in those with the highest levels of cholesterol. From your day of birth, cholesterol works hard to keep you healthy.

If a new mother eats a high-quality omnivore's diet, her milk may contain an amazing 60% fat, with cholesterol levels up to six times what a healthy adult gets from food. Being breastfed is linked to higher IQs, cognitive advantages later in life, and a reduced risk for diabetes—so be grateful if your momma nursed you!

Perversely, infant formulas contain zero cholesterol—despite warnings from experts against formulas with cholesterol content below that of human breast milk. Dare we admit that 225 million years of mammalian evolution might exhibit more nutritional intelligence than modern lab techies working for corporates?

AN UNWHOLESOME CONSPIRACY

How did this modern demonization of dietary fat and cholesterol get started in the first place? Many believe it began largely at the hands of one man, Ancel Keys, a brilliant if ultimately flawed nutrition researcher.

In the late 1950s Keys offered to the world his very own Lipid Hypothesis. It's a theory, yes, an unproven supposition, but the public latched on as if it were Golden Truth. We need a villain to despise when bad things happen and Keys lassoed saturated fat, insisting that it causes cholesterol levels to rise, creating the obstructive arterial plaques that cause heart attacks. Everybody knows this "fact." Everybody, that is, except those of us who read more than trendy vegan books and recycled medical myths supported by the pharmaceutical and processed food industries, the same sources that want you to believe that eating *fat* is what makes you *fat*. (Different nomenclature from the onset would have prevented so much misunderstanding.)

So let's delve deeper into the evolution of all these anti-fat lies that have so deceived us, while vastly profiting industry. In the 1960s and 70s, research was zeroing in on—well, what do you know—high-carb and sugar consumption as the likely culprit in our nation's rapidly escalating rates of obesity, diabetes, and heart disease. Yet Dr. Keys—whose University of Minnesota lab had been accepting financial backing from the sugar industry as far back as the 1940s—was able to grab the national spotlight by advancing his "animal fat kills you" theory. For three decades, through the 1980s, Keys actively promoted his hypothesis, often clashing with his nemesis, John Yudkin, a leading UK nutritionist who pointed out the many flaws in Keys' data and adamantly claimed that sugar, not fat, was the primary culprit.

It didn't seem to matter. The word about animal fat was out and being pushed on an unsuspecting public. We Americans now had a tangible demon to blame for our increasingly poor health and ever expanding guts, one that allowed us to keep eating all the quick, convenient, addictive carbs we had grown to crave. Any alternative views were largely ignored by the press, as the cereal, beverage, snack, refined oil, and other processed food industries spent millions on their own research/promotion of the "fat causes heart attacks" model. What's a few million when you're raking in billions?

"Research on the suspected links between sugar and chronic disease largely ground to a halt by the late 1980s, and scientists came to view such pursuits as a career dead end," confirm Cristin Couzens and Gary Taubes in *Sweet Little Lies*. Based on recently released papers of deceased industry researchers, this inspired piece of investigative journalism relied on 1,500+ pages of reports and internal memos found secreted away in the archives of now-defunct sugar companies. In what is surely one of the most tragic events in our public health history—because diabetics often end up with heart disease—industry-recruited scientists even convinced the American Diabetes Association to relax restrictions on the amount of carbs in a diabetic's diet, while lowering fat recommendations. All this despite abundant evidence from the USDA's Carbohydrate Nutrition Lab, and independent scientists, that revealed *exactly the opposite*: sugar in its various dietary forms is a primary factor in our high rates of diabetes and heart disease.

"This decades' long effort to stack the scientific deck" explains why, according to Couzens and Taubes, the FDA to this day insists that all forms of sugar, including high-fructose, are *"generally recognized as safe"* (GRAS), and why the USDA's Food Pyramid (now a Plate) promotes carbs as our main food source, with grains, fruits, and veggies taking up nearly 75% of that plate. It's why our government reduced its saturated fat intake recommendation from 10% to just 7% of total calories. And it's the reason that oft-unaware yet trusting shoppers can stroll through any supermarket, anytime, anywhere in America and find hundreds of shelves stuffed with low-fat or zero-fat processed foods pumped full of sugar, corn syrup, and over 5,000 unregulated additives.

How many millions of diabetics have died from misguided endorsement of the "sat fat kills/profuse carbs are fine" theory? How many of our fathers or mothers have suffered from heart disease by adhering to the low-fat advice of our public health authorities and the American Heart Association—advice encouraged by the sugar/carb industry for the past 50-60 years, despite compelling evidence to the contrary.

This wasn't mere chicanery on the part of industry but purposeful distortion, one might even say lethal distortion, now that we are beginning to understand the real culprits behind diabetes and heart disease—and the value of appropriate amounts of saturated fat and dietary cholesterol for good health.

"The low-fat, high carbohydrate movement promised long, healthy lives and trim, athletic bodies, but instead it caused prolonged high insulin levels, which in turn increased the number of people with heart disease, Type II diabetes, excessive weight gain, and many more chronic conditions and diseases," affirms Dr. Schwarzbein, who has worked with hundreds of diabetics. Meanwhile, Dr. Walter

Willett of Harvard's School of Public Health reminds us of *the dangers in turning a working hypothesis into a Dietary Truth.* (Vegan proselytizers, take note.)

Dr. George Mann, a biochemist who studied traditional tribes and their lack of cardiovascular disease despite ingesting copious amounts of animal fat—up to 300 grams per day—calls the Lipid Hypothesis "the greatest scientific deception of this century." The Heart Mafia is how Mann describes those who profit from the Lipid Hypothesis, including researchers who should speak up but do not, for fear of losing their soft, easy money. When science discovers the real cause and prevention of cardiovascular disease, Mann clairvoyantly claimed more than three decades ago, "it will seem to many that there was an unwholesome conspiracy."

FORTUNATELY THE TIDE is turning and respected studies conducted by non-industry researchers are zeroing in on the real culprits snuffing out the lives of millions worldwide. "Scientists have now established causation," affirms Robert Lustig, MD, leading obesity authority. "Sugar causes metabolic syndrome." This condition, characterized by elevated insulin levels and excessive triglycerides, is recognized as a primary risk factor for type 2 diabetes, stroke and heart disease, with links to Alzheimer's and cancer. Excess carb/sugar intake—not sat fat, not cholesterol—is where we need to make drastic changes in our food habits.

Sadly, irresponsibly, many vegan advocates are still promoting the myths: "Animal fat is bad for you, and dietary cholesterol is *very* bad for you; so to lower your risk for diabetes and heart disease, just eat a high-carb 100% plants diet that contains zero of the wicked stuff." As T. Colin Campbell erroneously declared: "Eating foods that contain any cholesterol above 0 mg is unhealthy."

Meanwhile, educated omnivores and ex-veg'ns are quick to call this what it is: dietary fiction, an urban legend, a vampire fable that should have died years ago but lives on and on through endless repetition. Don't you dare touch cheese, red meat, or full-fat yogurt. Naughty cholesterol! Evil saturated fat! Artery cloggers! Their reputable scientific evidence? Absent.

BUT WHO NEEDS expensive, tedious research projects when any smart 7th grader, presented with some basic facts, could easily point out the inconsistencies in the sat fat + cholesterol = heart disease theory? Try it yourself.

FACT: Before 1920 just 1% of Americans were obese and heart disease was rare.

And what, you justifiably ask, was our traditional diet before 1920?

Plentiful whole plant and animal products, including grassfed beef, organs, eggs, poultry, dairy, butter and lard, with their attendant cholesterol and saturated fats.

FACT: Coronary heart disease did not emerge as the leading cause of death in the US until the mid-1950s. Today 40% of us will die from heart disease.

What then, you rightly inquire, changed in the American diet during that period? *From 1910-1970, our use of animal fat declined substantially. Butter consumption, for example—hailed in antiquity by Pliny the Elder as medicinal food—dropped sharply, from 18 to 4 pounds per person, per year.*

FACT: During this same period, Americans used 400% more vegetable oils in the form of margarine, shortening and refined oils, while our ingestion of sugar and processed foods climbed nearly 60%.

The beverage industry spends over $3 billion a year marketing high-sugar drinks to 2-19 year-olds, and one in three American kids is now overweight or obese. (How do these industry minions sleep at night?)

FACT: Following the recommendations of the original 1980 *Dietary Guidelines for Americans*, our intake of grains, cereals, vegetable oils and other omega-3-scarce plant foods shot up, while our consumption of whole foods like eggs and full-fat dairy declined for the next 3+ decades.

During this same period, America's rates of diabetes, stroke, and cardiovascular disease exploded.

FACT: In 1950 there were 500 cardiologists practicing in the US. Today there are 30,000—a staggering 60-fold growth for a population that merely doubled in the same time frame.

No doubt you've arrived at the same conclusion as that studious 7th grader: *we've been duped.* Fortunately, all the deceptions are finally coming into the light and the entire saturated fat + high cholesterol = heart disease hypothesis is falling apart at its poorly stitched seams.

Nathan Pritikin, who endorsed a low-fat, plant-based diet committed suicide while battling leukemia, and Dr. Dean Ornish, defender of low-fat, vegan-type diets, has been told to take a hike by a leading heart surgeon. Here's Dr. Donald Miller, Jr., of the University of Washington Medical Center:

Indoctrinated in low-fat dogma by health organizations, nutrition authorities and the government, I would instruct my heart surgery patients to eat a low fat diet, telling them to cut all the fat off their meat and not eat more than one egg a week. And following the USDA food pyramid, I did not express any concerns about how many carbohydrates they might consume.....I was wrong.

Closely scrutinizing the "incontrovertible evidence" linking fat and cholesterol to heart disease, Dr. Miller was appalled by what he discovered: poorly conceived industry-supported research and skewed data designed to validate pre-conceived theories. How about force-feeding enormous amounts of cholesterol to rabbits, herbivores in no way designed to metabolize animal food. These are the kinds of cruel, stupid studies conducted to "prove" that dietary cholesterol ends up stuck in our arteries. (They died of starvation, you idiots, not heart attacks.) Little publicized were studies dating back to 1950 that showed precisely the opposite but had no shock value. Feeding cholesterol to humans, even in large quantities, "consistently fail[s] to show a relationship between the cholesterol in the diet and that in the serum," wrote Ancel Keys (he got that one right). Most researchers went after dietary fat instead—because that's where the funding was.

Tweak the data here or there, put in this, take out that, and *voila!* You get what your sponsors want. In his Six Countries Study (which vegans love to cite), Keys cherry-picked the six nations that corroborated his fat-kills-us theory, deliberately excluding data from 16 other countries. Not exactly good or honorable science because if you stick those back in the graph, his perfect upward curve crumples into a much weaker one.

Keys' Seven Countries Study came three years later in 1956 and, once again, he selected those countries most likely to fit his fat-kills proposition, avoiding places like Switzerland, France, and Sweden that show the opposite. He also studied only middle-aged men, a sub-population known for increased cardiac risk. And get this: the dietary data for Keys' influential study relied on UN stats for food production, imports, and exports—not what subjects actually dined on, "a totally weird and unreliable way to measure what people eat," as nutrition writer Denise Minger so aptly described it.

Minger and Brendan Coburn, RD, who independently studied Keys' research in depth, both arrived at another startling conclusion. When you take a look at total mortality rates in these countries, the graph completely flips. "Fat now has the strongest *negative* association with mortality out of any variable," Minger notes, while subjects eating the highest percentage of calories from carbs had the highest mortality. Who lived the longest and experienced the lowest heart disease rates of all the population groups? Crete Islanders with their high-fat consumption (37% of calories) and large intake of fish and olive oil, along with wild plants, nuts, pastured meat, milk and eggs.

Unfortunately, Keys' lipid-heart hypothesis had a huge impact on the public's view of dietary fat as something to be shunned, especially after Keys appeared as a national hero on the cover of *Time* magazine. Even today, vegan blogs keep blitzing us with the same old propaganda. *Animal fat and cholesterol cause heart disease! Eat plants-only! Always and forever!* Likewise, the authors of *Vegan for Life* avidly encourage veganism for everyone as a life-long diet that "should" be healthy and risk-lowering for chronic diseases, while confessing 2/3 of the way through their book that, well, no studies exist that prove or disprove this outcome. It's just too early in this novel diet's history to know.

Is that an expression of regret? Or relief? Hard to tell, but either way it dismays me—and countless parents—to consider how many strict plant-eaters will take on the "don't worry, be happy" attitude that has overtaken the vegan media and never know how far off the mark they may be, year after year, from a balanced diet that supports not only adequate fat and cholesterol intake but a long, healthy, and productive life.

30.

RISING CASUALTIES / AYURVEDIC REMEDIES

I would give up milk if I could, but I cannot.

—Mahatma Gandhi

As VEGANISM continues to grow in popularity, Dr. John Douillard is seeing the casualties walk through his office door. His medicine? That is, if he can get his highly resistant patients to cooperate? Red meat. That's right. Raw, medium rare, or thoroughly cooked: your choice. Red meat is an ancient and potent Ayurvedic prescription for boosting health in undernourished clients.

A slender man with striking blue eyes and a calm presence, Dr. Douillard practices Ayurvedic medicine, humankind's oldest system of healing. Originating in the Vedic culture of India 5,000 years ago, Ayurveda translates as "the wisdom of life" and it's the alternative medicine of choice for yogis and vegans, whose worlds often blend. Yet the doctor's flocks of unhealthy yogi-veg clients are far from pleased with his cautiously considered advice. Incredulous or infuriated is more like it.

I remember those feelings well. Any suggestion from a concerned friend to toss in a bit of meat to restore my faltering health was met with a withering stare of contempt. However, it's now been over seven years since I reluctantly chewed that first ritual dinner of Colorado bison, alone in my daughter's kitchen, and felt the powerful rush of energy that initiated my return to a sustainable life. So as I sit down with Douillard at his LifeSpa Ayurvedic Center north of Denver, I feel compassion for all the suffering vegetarians and vegans he describes to me and hope they too are able to broaden their outlook and nourish their bodies in a way that works for them.

Why, I ask the doctor, do so many yogi types believe that Ayurveda espouses a veg'n diet for everybody when, in truth, it does not? *Yoga Journal* annoyed me for years by promoting the Ayurvedic lifestyle while refusing to include even the scantiest scrap of meat in its recipes, despite the fact that Ayurveda recommends animal protein for a specific constitutional type, Vata, and during certain life stages for others. The ancient Vedic scriptures describe not only for whom it's good to eat meat but which types to select. Hinduism, the historic Vedic religion, imposes rules on meat eating but certainly doesn't ban it.

Turns out I'm not the only exasperated yogi who questions this no-animal-food taboo in the Americanized version of yoga. Writing in "Meat and Yoga: Om….Yum," Meredith recalls reading "with a shudder" a *Yoga Journal* link to hundreds of recipes full of sweet and tangy fruits, nutty brown rice, and rainbows of vegetable kabobs.

> As a vegetarian for over 12 years, and a semi-vegetarian for 4 years after that, this menu sounded very familiar. It was the diet on which I developed insulin resistance, probably as a result of the high amount of carbs (whole grains) and sucrose (fruit). Don't get me wrong, eating a diet filled with fresh vegetables is great, but only when balanced with a good amount of fat and protein…..Curiously, although *Yoga Journal* takes a blanket editorial stand against recipes containing meat, milk, or butter, they have no such qualms about including recipes with sugar, flour, or soy. Because those ingredients are so pure and unadulterated, right?

So I ask the doctor to set the record straight. According to Ayurvedic medicine and his own experience with hundreds of patients, is vegetarianism recommended for everyone or not? Ayurveda singles out lean Vata types for a reason, the doctor believes: they generally don't do well on a no-meat diet and their health declines. ParaYoga teacher Barbra Brady concurs. "Vatas are drawn to veganism because it delivers what they are already familiar with: feeling light, pure, ungrounded and indecisive," she informs me. "However, their all-plants diet can exaggerate these tendencies to the point, sometimes, of non-functionality." Perhaps you know some of these individuals. I certainly do. They can't seem to make basic decisions and move their lives forward. Ayurvedic literature has a name for this condition: Deranged Vata.

As for those of us who remain functional, Douillard chooses his words very carefully: "In theory a vegetarian diet is probably the healthiest you can eat. Now, that being said, I've seen very few really healthy, vibrant vegetarians. Of course, I

242

see those who aren't well. I see the casualties." Every winter, in fact, Douillard treats "an inordinate number" of vegans, vegetarians, and near-vegetarians for, you guessed it, protein deficiency. "Most of them are health-aware and have made conscious decisions as to what they include and don't include in their diets. But somehow, despite their best intentions, they find themselves with this very significant deficiency."

In our culture it's difficult to be a healthy vegetarian, the doctor believes, let alone a vegan. He reminds us that in India, vegetarianism has been part of the traditional culture for more than 25 centuries. "Genetically, Indian people are able to metabolize and do reasonably well on a vegetarian diet. But when you look at Americans, you have to add in a couple of vital factors: westerners who are not genetically able to do as well on a vegetarian diet; plus high levels of stress in our workaholic culture which is simply not the same in much of India. If we were able to sit under a fig tree and meditate in warm weather throughout the year, I'm sure you'd agree that many of us would fare much better" on a low-calorie, low-protein diet.

The majority of Americans don't live in a year-round warm climate, nor do we spend a lot of time meditating under shade trees. So here's a good question for all would-be veg'ns to ask themselves: A hundred years ago would I have been able to live as a vegan, or even a vegetarian, in the geography and climate of the place I call home? For most of us in temperate zones and colder, the answer is a resounding no. "A hundred years ago if you lived here in Colorado, you either ate meat or you died," maintains Douillard, author of *The Three Season Diet: Eat the Way Nature Intended*. "It wasn't like our ancestors had a choice. Even today the Brahmins in Kashmir eat meat to survive the colder areas of northern India."

"But in America we now have a choice!" vegans will forcefully respond. Yes, we do, *if* we persist in our dependence on a global food industry that floats on oil and destroys entire ecosystems (animals included), in order to have our veggies, fruits, legumes and coffee delivered via long-haul, carbon-spewing transporters. Now let's get back to the original question: What would a true Colorado diet look like if we were to eat only regional, seasonal, organic whole foods, living off the land as honestly and efficiently as our ancestors? You certainly would not be a vegan, not here, not anywhere close to here—not unless you want to try surviving chiefly on grains. Barley, wheat, oats, millet and sorghum grow well in Colorado; and our summer gardens and orchards abound in greens, beans, cabbage, squash, sunflower seeds, apples, cantaloupe and peaches—but that covers only half the year and these are largely carb foods. Where are your regional high-protein, high-fat foods to survive the grueling winters and live a hormonally-balanced long life? Actually, you can find them here in variety and abundance: wild birds, game and fish, grazing bison and cattle, grass-raised pigs, turkeys, sheep and chickens, plus eggs, butter, milk, cheese and other good-fat pastured dairy.

Historically, humans have always stored up protein and fat when most needed, after the autumnal equinox, in order to rebuild and insulate their bodies. And the source was animals. That's why the majority of Douillard's ailing veg'ns show up in the winter months. "When our ancestors were living off the land, they had a strongly meat-based, high-fat diet in the late fall and winter, followed by a mostly vegetarian, low-fat diet in the spring and summer. This is how nature organizes it," the wise doctor tells me. "The harvest is the medicine of the season."

The harvest is the medicine of the season. These words jump out at me as something we should all recognize as simple truth. But how many of us do? Good food is our medicine, keeping us hale and healthy, and the genius of nature provides the right medicine at the right time. During the winter—or times of intense physical labor, life changes, or extra stress—it's a high-protein/high-fat diet that's absolutely needed. As Douillard elaborates on his theory, my fish-heavy meals in Alaska make more sense than ever. Harvested in late summer/fall—when natives worked long and hard to shore up protein and fat for the bitter winter ahead—salmon's rich flesh provided critical nourishment for their labor, while also being dried and stored for the coming season of cold and ice.

But what does any of this have to do with skinny, carrot-munching yogis in the Lower 48? Well, the majority of us here in the States do live in a four-season or at least three-season climate, and nature does provide precise foods for every season in every region. Regrettably, we have become so dependent on continent-hopping industrial food that most of us don't even know what our own bioregion shrewdly delivers, month after varied month, to energize and strengthen our bodies.

TO BE CLEAR, Douillard is not talking about a pathological protein deficiency in his veg'n clients. He's addressing what he describes as "a chronic subclinical lack of protein that forces the body to adapt and compensate for this nutritional imbalance." To correct this harmful state, traditional medicine prescribes the strongest and most acidic protein, red meat, to replenish a weakened body. That's because Ayurveda recognizes that alkaline foods like fruits and vegetables are terrific cleansers, helping the body to detoxify and flush out wastes; however, following that process, your body needs to rebuild: muscles, tissues, and joints. And to accomplish this, you need plenty of high-quality complete protein. And the more acidic a protein source is, according to Douillard, the deeper it penetrates your tissues for rebuilding and the better it is stored.

"This is nature's way of balancing," affirms this Ayurvedic advocate. By eating naturally-occurring alkaline foods in the spring and summer, like greens and veggies, we cleanse our body, and by eating naturally-occurring acidic foods in the fall and winter, like wild game and grains, we rebuild our body.

"Many acidic foods are actually very healthy and essential," asserts Douillard, deflating the anti-acidic craze. There is a reason nature doesn't offer us very many alkaline foods in the colder months: our bodies need something else. That's why the harvest before a frosty, long winter is traditionally loaded with animal organs and meat—primarily acidic and rich in protein for rebuilding. "And that's why people who are yoga teachers, or simply do yoga and eat vegetarian or vegan for 15 or 20 years, oftentimes, just like yourself, find that they need meat because they are fading," the doctor explains. "And their bodies are looking for acidic protein to be stored, to build the body's reserves. Once you build those reserves back up by eating meat, you can really get back to having that resiliency and hardy health again."

So how do his yoga-veg patients react when he tells them this? "I see a lot of vegetarians and vegans in my practice who are having trouble, and in Ayurveda there's a health-building protocol that's basically a protein replenishing program where you put someone on 4-ounces of red meat every single day for two weeks. Naturally, vegans are like, *Oh my God, are you crazy? I can't believe you're even suggesting that!*"

And then the conscientious doctor patiently recounts to the vegans all their expressed symptoms of a protein deficit: the debilitating fatigue and drooping energy; the moodiness and jangled nerves; the mid-afternoon crash and desperate craving for carbs or caffeine to quickly re-energize; the emergency chocolate bar stashed in the Subaru glovebox. Other common symptoms include unstable blood sugar, sore muscles, and ongoing failure to get a restful night's sleep. So the good doctor says to the genuinely shocked vegans, "*You may be protein deficient. And the best proteins for this problem are the acidic proteins in red meat. You need to pay back the original protein debt. If you eat red meat for two weeks and feel phenomenally better, you have just proven that you are protein deficient.*"

245

If the patient is still squirming or horror-struck, Dr. Douillard will often say, "Let's just do it. This may be your best bet." The doctor, himself a long-time vegetarian who suffered from deficiencies, does not shy away from the truth: "I have yet to have a patient to whom I suggested this red meat remedy who didn't have an amazing outcome." He always tries to hear the side of not having to go down that road but when he sees the problem clearly, Douillard doesn't hesitate. "I say to them, 'You know, I really think this would be the best thing for you.' Some of them just won't go there and I back off, but the ones who are willing to take a look at the possibility have had literally *miraculous* results."

There's no shame in wanting your health back, but most ethical vegans would consider the doctor's protein-replenishing protocol to be heresy. Yet even veggie iconoclast George Bernard Shaw reverted to meat-eating during his recuperation from smallpox. And vegetarian devotee Mahatma Gandhi, who famously wrote that "man was born to live on the fruits and herbs that the earth grows," was nonetheless forced to admit: "I would give up milk if I could but I cannot. I have made that experiment times without number. I could not after a serious illness, regain my strength unless I went back to milk." He went on to say that his need for animal-sourced food "has been the tragedy of my life. But the basis of my vegetarianism is not physical but moral. If anybody said that I should die if I did not take beef-tea or mutton, even under medical advice, I would prefer death." Of course, Mr. Gandhi was not confronting death when he uttered those idealistic words, and he did indeed choose to consume an animal product when it came right down to the wire of self-preservation.

Siddhartha Gautama *was* confronting death at the end of his ascetic period in the forest, the traditional biography tells us. Attempting to discover enlightenment through austerities, including food restrictions, had utterly failed him. Near death from starvation, he collapsed by a river and almost drowned before being found by Sujata, a village girl. And what saved the future Buddha and revived his will to live? A pudding made from milk, offered by Sujata. The vitality received from that animal-based nourishment delivered Siddhartha to a focused, blissful state and in that pivotal moment, he rejected asceticism and began to reassess his path.

And in the 21st century, staunch vegan-promoter Michael Klaper, MD, now publicly admits that a sizeable number of long-term vegans need to put animal products back into their diets in order to amend their failing health. "A significant population of long-term vegans....despite their best efforts, and mine, to optimize their vegan diets, still remain pale, underweight, and unable to achieve the robust health they seek," Dr. Klaper concedes. "When, out of frustration with years of trying to overcome their nutritional challenges by using various supplements and vegan food regimens," Klaper continues, "a number of them reluctantly, but finally, reverted to adding some meat or eggs back into their diets, they often achieved significant benefits—sometimes with dramatic results. Increased energy levels and muscle mass became evident in many of them."

All these devout, doctor-seeking vegans didn't fail the diet, as plants-only proselytizers love to insist. The diet failed them.

31.

YOUNG AND VEGAN: GET WORRIED

nobody peaceful and civilized murders helpless, defenseless,
pseudo conscious beings for any reason. nobody needs
to eat dead animals to live a long, healthy life.
these are the rules of our existence.

—"Vegan Thug"

"I HAVE THESE VEGAN NAZIS who come see me," Annie is telling me, her fork poised mid-air, her soft feminine voice rising in dismay. On this delightfully warm September day, we're sharing an outdoor lunch on my front deck, including ripe cherry tomatoes and fresh basil from the garden. "I want to help them with their health problems but they won't let me!"

Annie, a compassionate woman, is venting her frustration. For more than 30 years she's been practicing Traditional Chinese Medicine, and much of her work involves helping young women who have hormonal imbalances, have lost their menstrual periods, or desperately want to get pregnant. Unlike western medicine, this ancient medical tradition teaches close scrutiny of each individual's diet and that's exactly what Annie practices, especially when a woman is experiencing infertility issues. At the moment, she's recounting the story of an unidentified vegan who recently visited her office, a slender athletic type, about 35, who longs to have a child after years of trying. Noting the woman's weight and very low BMI, Annie carefully studied her food diary, which listed only spirulina, nuts, and legumes as her protein sources. She then gingerly asked the young woman, "Would you consider adding eggs to your diet?"

You'd think Annie had asked her to wrestle down a screaming chicken and extract a still-hot egg with her bare hands. She immediately turned to stone and cried out, *No! Never!* Annie didn't even get the chance to tell her that eggs are rich in choline, and deficiencies are linked to infertility in women and failure to

248

thrive in newborns. Egg-craving stories during pregnancy are legendary—*I've been a passionate omelet eater all three pregnancies!*—a telltale sign that these women's bodies are ordering up more choline and fat. But Annie wasn't able to share her stories with this client, who also tested deficient in sex hormones but refused to take progesterone to correct the deficit because there was something in the filler that *might* have a teensy bit of animal product in it.

"I wanted to reach out and gently shake her. Tell her: I'm trying to help you get pregnant but you're not letting me!" Annie's sincere consternation shows in her face as she continues, "Here I am trying to strengthen and nourish her to support a pregnancy, but she's just sitting there frozen-faced, clinging very hard to her beliefs." Soon after the woman heard the tainted word "egg," she got up and left, never to return.

Another vegan who badly wanted a child became defensive and started to cry when Annie discussed her limited food selections and kindly questioned whether they contained adequate protein, fat, and cholesterol to produce all the essential hormones in the right balance to support a pregnancy. (Low serum cholesterol levels are strongly associated with adverse birth outcomes.) Annie also wasn't given the opportunity to talk to this young woman about B12, zinc, and calcium supplementation as well as other possible nutrient shortages: vitamins D3 and K2, plus long-chain fatty acids. Nor was she able to advise that vegans are more likely to be deficient in both taurine and methionine, the former essential for fetal and neonatal brain development, the latter's lack associated with neural tube defects and premature delivery. This young woman cut Annie out of her life before they could explore concerns about infant soy formula (should she become pregnant), and the very real dangers of feeding soy milk to a baby. "She stood up and said she wouldn't take any more questions about her diet," Annie tells me with a sigh. "I never saw her again."

And then there are the even younger female vegans, many of them still in their teens, whose periods have disappeared due to insufficient calories and fat. Girls so thin and undernourished their bodies are incapable of supporting normal hormone production. Vegan athletes so driven they're down to 12% body fat and end up with amenorrhea, the loss of menses for three months or more. This loss is no blessing: amenorrhea has serious implications for reproductive, heart, and bone health. *With each missed period your risk for osteoporosis significantly increases.* Practitioners like Annie have seen them all. Vegans as young as 15 with bodies so bony you have to keep from gasping, with periods gone missing for a year, even more. The blogwaves are rampant with female vegans who've lost their menstrual cycles and urgently seek advice. Yet very few of these young women would consider giving up their limited diet; some won't even look at it as a probable cause. To even suggest this can elicit anger or panic. "I've concluded veganism is a type of eating disorder," Annie states succinctly. "There's so much control around food. It's extreme eating."

Annie knows all about eating disorders and how they function; as a young woman she took up the macrobiotic diet to cure herself of bulimia. Introduced to Americans in the 1960s by Japanese philosopher George Ohsawa, macrobiotics emphasizes simplicity. Meals consist largely of organic whole grains and cooked vegetables, with added seaweed and Asian condiments. Short-term, it did bring results for Annie and established some good eating habits but when she became pregnant at 27, she knew instinctively that this restrictive diet didn't offer enough. "My body told me exactly what I needed to know. I was craving dairy every day, especially yogurt." And it worked for Annie, increasing her intake of protein, fat, calcium, B12, potassium and probiotics, contributing to a successful birth and healthy baby boy.

Not all of Annie's vegan clients have run away. One who was suffering from years of infertility decided to add eggs and yogurt to her diet and went on to have a full-term pregnancy. Nor is Annie saying that a vegan can't get pregnant and deliver a healthy baby, but in her considerable experience "it's very hard for these women to balance all the needed nutrients and achieve the optimal hormone levels" that encourage fertility. A tendency toward sub-par calorie consumption is also an issue among vegans, as this greatly affects protein totals. "I'm *always* talking protein to these women because their daily intake is usually low," she continues.

"There's an old traditional saying in Chinese Medicine: if you want to deliver a baby, have a chicken a day. Of course, those Asian women were rural and poor, laboring in the rice fields all day long. They needed lots of nourishment to build their energy and their blood." Yet she sees a correlation between these hardworking female laborers of old and the modern young women who come to her office: overloaded, multi-tasking, not knowing how to relax. "So different from my laid-back, mother-earth clients from the '80s!" Annie laughs. "Young women today are driven by *unyielding perfectionism*: to be strict vegetarians, career women, super moms and first-rate athletes. You can see it in the way they move! Intense, purposeful, always in a hurry."

She believes this kind of stressful, non-stop lifestyle demands extra calories, extra protein, and ample natural fat, not all that different from those Chinese women in the fields. Annie's idea of a perfect meal is a half-plate of fresh veggies and greens, quarter-plate of slow-digesting grains, and another quarter-plate of lean protein with good fat sources like chicken or fish. "I hate to break the news to plant eaters," she says, "but beans are correctly categorized as a carbohydrate. They are *loaded* with carbs."

Why does she think so many young people are embracing a vegan diet? "Not knowing," she says without hesitation. "Immaturity. Powerful advocacy groups." She believes most of our youth will figure it out as they progress in years and self-knowledge. To stay blindly fixated on one diet over the decades rarely if ever works. Eventually our ever-changing bodies will demand an alteration in course, signaled by diminishing energy and worsening health. The Taoists who created Chinese Medicine saw the human body as a microcosm of the universe, its well-being dependent on finding equilibrium amidst constant change. Annie concurs: "Over the years my own diet changed so much because my needs changed."

"MY BODY WAS SUFFERING," admits Sylvie an ardent vegan for over a decade who finally cut loose—and with no regrets. "It was a good thing for me to do. I had to get my health back." Sylvie converted to vegetarianism at the tender age of 16 for one simple reason: she did not want to eat animals. Echoing a familiar theme among teen veg'ns, especially females, she states, "I didn't think animals should have to die just so I could eat."

A lacto-veggie for over a dozen years, Sylvie then adopted a macrobiotic diet, but for a very different reason than Annie. She wanted to clean out all the dairy she'd been eating to fill her vegetarian hunger pit. She then practiced full-fledged veganism for 11 years, six of them raw. But over time Sylvie began to notice tell-tale changes in her health: coldness, fatigue, poor sleep, and a worrisome lag in energy. Yet she was unsure of the cause and entertained zero thoughts of changing her diet or ideology. Her body, however, had different plans and Sylvie's sputtering, ultimately unsatisfying romance with veganism came to a roaring halt around the communal fire. She recounts her tale:

"I arrived at a friend's house for dinner one summer night and there was this big backyard pit with a fire going. Someone had caught and cooked fresh trout, and it was sitting right out on the table. My friend, who knew very well I was a vegan, asked: *Sylvie, do you want some fish?* My usual response to such a brazen question would be shock and irritation, but I looked at the fish on the table and for the first time in all those years, no emotions came up. My mind was empty, a blank slate, and I heard myself saying as if in a dream: *Yes, I want some fish."*

A tall, stately blond, Sylvie is speaking in measured tones, vividly remembering the transformative scene. It's the miraculous fish story all over again. *"So I had a taste and then I had some more and a little more, one serving in all. It tasted so very good."* When she arrived home a few hours later she had all kinds of new energy, too much energy to go to sleep, like she'd ingested some kind of magic potion. "I was up half the night doing all sorts of projects," she recalls. "It was a good energy. A very good energy. One I hadn't felt in a long time."

So Sylvie started eating fish once a week for breakfast or lunch; it was simply too energizing to eat in the evening. "I started feeling better, looking better," she tells me, sharing noontime tea at a crowded café this bright, blustery day in the Rockies. Eight months later she cautiously considered chicken. "I realized that I'm okay watching a fish die and then eating it, so I think I can watch a chicken die. I knew I couldn't watch a cow die; I couldn't do it. Strange as it sounds, that was my criteria at the time."

A decade later, ex-vegan Sylvie now starts each day with a "really substantial" breakfast featuring animal protein. To maintain her current good health she faithfully eats high-density protein and omega-3-rich fat several times a day: eggs, fish, chicken or bison, and occasionally wild elk or deer from hunter friends. She refuses to support factory farms and consumes 100% pastured livestock raised without hormones or antibiotics, local and organic whenever possible. "Actually," she admits unabashedly, "I prefer fresh in-season game meat." Is she familiar with John Douillard's *The Three Season Diet*? She nods her head approvingly. "It's what the earth is producing at the time. It's what our bodies are longing for."

Sylvie embodies the long-term veggie who's done it all since birth: omnivore, vegetarian, macrobiotic, vegan, and 100% raw vegan. But after 26 years devoted to vegetarianism in one form or another, she's now come full circle and returned to what she calls "the most sensible diet of all," the omnivorous ways of her childhood. "If I was ever to do anything with my life, I needed stronger protein sources, stronger energy sources," she says. "This whole idea of sacrifice, of giving life to another being—I decided my own life is worth supporting, too."

Today's new crop of vociferous vegans will insist she was weak, gave up too easily, did it wrong. Sylvie just laughs at such scornful judgments; these people

252

have no clue how hard she tried, how dedicated she was to veganism. Let them pay attention to their own body's needs, she says, as I am finally paying attention to mine. "It's not like I was some unconscious junk-food vegan. I was a very conscientious good eater, lots of different healthy foods." I started naming protein sources to make certain she'd tried all the new plant offerings, but she shot me an impatient "not this again" look and swiftly cut me off. She'd been drilled on this by righteous vegans too many times before. Read my lips, she says: "*It made no difference which plant foods I ate, how much, or what combination. It wasn't working for me anymore.*"

As far as protein intake, Sylvie remarks that "the veg literature has always emphasized low numbers, but now I have osteoporosis and veganism may well be the cause." In truth, the matrix of all bones is protein, hardened or "calcified" by calcium, and research reveals "significantly lower" bone densities in vegans versus omnivores, with nearly double the incidence of hip fractures. Far too late for Sylvie, the word is just now getting out: vegans, you need to increase not only your protein intake but your calcium and vitamins D and K2 as well.

Now they tell us. This is the problem with historically new diets: insufficient data and unknown lifetime outcomes. Vegans are plunging into the unknown. "A long-term protein deficit probably caused my low bone density," laments Sylvie, who required hip surgery. Asked if she regrets being a vegetarian for 26 years and a vegan for nearly a dozen of them, she says, *absolutely.*

SYLVIE IS NOT ALONE with her regrets. Now that many western vegetarians and even some vegans have hit the quarter century mark, similar testimony is spilling out online, frank and unfiltered. Today's new batch of plant eaters will do themselves a great favor to read them. "It's the rare person who wants to hear what he doesn't want to hear," author Dick Cavett noted. So be that rare and courageous person, vegan sister or brother, and allow yourself to sincerely consider opposing viewpoints without the usual denial or derision; to read the honest and unbiased stories of ex-veggies who did everything right but ended up wronged in body and broken in health. These people are not trying to market a diet philosophy—or sell you the latest vegan cookbook, making money off their beliefs. They are simply trying to insert caution and common sense into the dialogue.

Here's the tale of vegan Diogena who crashed and burned after two decades on her constrained diet:

For over 20 years of my adult life, I ate first according to a whole-some, organic, and complex-carb vegetarian diet and soon after elim-inated all dairy and eggs. Little did I know the reason I felt good for awhile was that I was running on adrenaline because I was starved for protein and animal fat....Once my adrenals were exhausted, I crashed and developed severe hypoglycemia. To remedy the problem, I was prescribed a hunter-gatherer diet and essential fatty acid supplementa-tion. It has taken me over 10 years to finally get over the reactive hy-poglycemia problem that according to my naturopath was directly caused by my long-term veg diet. After a year on the hunter-gatherer diet, I stopped catching respiratory infections. After 10 years....all of a sudden my cognitive abilities skyrocketed. Even though I was by then a middle-aged adult, I was able to teach myself computer lan-guages and learn to play button accordion. While I was [vegan], I never had the brain power to cogitate complex computer languages or play a musical instrument that required so much lateral independence.

Yes, there are healthy and happy plant eaters out there. Thus far anyway, the diet suits them and that's to be celebrated. Yet I rarely go a day without reading or hearing heartfelt tales of debilitating fatigue and brain drain as the vegan years unfold. I'm on the lookout, for sure, but disillusionment seems to be rearing its hungry head wherever I roam.

An international mountain climber based in Colorado, Andrew reluctantly re-nounced his vegan diet and started eating high-density animal protein to maintain his strength and endurance. A Utah MD advised a young friend to add grass-fed meat to her meals to get her carbohydrate intolerance under control, a precursor to insulin resistance. And of the hundred or so women I have had the privilege of performing with in Montana and Colorado, it was a vegan who couldn't make it through a two-hour performance without post-dinner food. A fellow soprano, she was often moody and high-strung. I can still see her willowy self, slumped on the backstage floor in her strapless, pink satin gown just before the curtain rose, pounding nuts and bananas in a frantic attempt to energize and focus.

Anecdotal evidence? Of course. Our young people have little solid research to rely on regarding this unverified, restrictive diet designed for celibate cleric and aging cardiac patients. As personal evidence continues to pour in, some of the most in-depth, intelligent testimony can be found on the blog that vegans love to hate, *Let Them Eat Meat*. Since 2010, writer Rhys Southan has been conducting extensive interviews with ex-vegans like himself, publishing detailed accounts of their failing health and broken beliefs. Here are three poignant examples from home and abroad: Saudi Arabian women's rights activist Tasha, Turkish college student Erim, and long-distance American runner Devon.

Many people mistakenly think my abandonment of veganism was an overnight decision, when in reality it was anything but. I'd been feeling very sick and weak for awhile, but when I went to the doctor they took blood and told me it was normal. I remember telling myself to ignore my deteriorating physical condition and celebrate the "hard proof" that I was healthy.....I found another doctor.....insisting upon a complete blood panel. When I got the results and saw the deficiencies, I was devastated. I felt like such a failure....It took me months of visiting doctor after doctor, feeling weak, depressed, and miserable before I finally made a change. I think many vegans underestimate just how life changing it can be to go through such a serious health crisis. I had been robustly healthy for my entire life up until then, so this complete physical deterioration was devastating. Once I finally decided that I deserved to be healthy and embraced an omnivorous diet, my health returned within two months.

Sickness happened and as a result, a whole lot of questioning. I really was a true believer in the low-fat raw vegan lifestyle [and] followed it perfectly for three years. About a year and a half into it, I started to get weak mentally....Talk about ups and downs. Cloudy sky meant bad mood. Cold weather meant bad mood....My teeth started getting incredibly sensitive, and there were clear signs of heavy acid erosion; my gums started to recede.....months later my dentist would find six cavities in my raw vegan mouth. I started to get more and more fatigued....I also had no sex drive. Now, believe me when I say there is a difference between LOW sex drive and NO sex drive. Because I had NONE. And it wasn't just because girls were evil, smelly, meat-eating murderers. I was even indifferent to Jenna Dewan Tatum's PETA ad, so that says something. But it didn't bother me much. After all, getting rid of those nasty animalistic desires was a bonus! All in all, this "healthiest lifestyle ever" gave me the shining gifts of....low energy, pale skin, anxiety, and a mouth that looked like battlefield ruins.

A vegan diet stopped supporting my health and when I stayed on it anyway, I ended up with a whole host of problems that I still have to deal with. I was rundown, anemic, had developed hypothyroid and had severe adrenal fatigue. And on top of that, being vegan made me neurotic about my food....Before I went vegan, I had a healthy balanced relationship with food. I was in tune with my body's signals and ate intuitively. When you take on a strict definition of yourself as an eater....you become hyper-aware of what is in everything. Knowing what is in your food is good (*In Defense of Food*-style) but being rigid and neurotic is not.

AND BEAUTIFUL LINDA? The super-cycling Renaissance woman from Sarasota, California, and original inspiration for my vegetarian leap of faith? She of the cornsilk hair and ripped body, who instructed me in the fine art of body piercing in a small Parisian flat so very long ago? After years of limited communication, I stumbled upon her inspiring Facebook account of traversing the Alps' classic and challenging Mont Blanc Circuit, joining her comrades every alpine evening for some tasty hut-cuisine, like *stewed chicken with roasted vegetables and panache.*

I was stunned. If anyone could make it as a life-long veg, surely it was Linda, anti-establishment superwoman. Immediately contacting her in England, I was further startled to learn she began eating animal flesh just five years after our wild hitchhiking spree through Spain and Portugal. "I felt tired, deprived of protein," she told me forthrightly, practical woman that she is, the kind who changes her own car tires and maintains an orderly garage full of sensible tools. "I just didn't feel I was getting substantial nutrition." A smart, realistic, no-nonsense move for Linda; she's in excellent health now.

Exactly like Sylvie, Linda remembers the precise moment she renounced her vegetarianism: "I was on the island of Phuket, off western Thailand, and the local men were hauling in fresh fish each morning, putting them in ice boxes on the beach. Then the women would arrive and set up yellow and pink umbrellas for impromptu restaurants. I remember the fish exactly: it was bonito, not even very large and it fed 13 people, including me. Just delicious and right off the boat— you couldn't get it any fresher. I don't think I've enjoyed a better meal since."

Linda now eats fish and eggs on a regular basis, yet her English friends still consider her a vegetarian and a bit on the outskirts of proper British life due to her ongoing abstention from red meat. "When I show up for a roast beef and Yorkshire pudding dinner," she admits "I feel apologetic after all these years, refusing my host's main dish." While in the States for Christmas recently, she made the conscious decision to start eating the long-boycotted holiday turkey. "I wanted to start participating in my family traditions," she tells me candidly. "Now I make free-range turkey enchiladas and freeze a dozen at a time, but I'm beginning to wonder if my once-a day, high-protein meal is enough."

Linda still bicycles and treks with zest, but her dietary needs have undeniably changed over time. "I can't digest lentils at all anymore and only a small amount of beans, forcing me to seek ample protein elsewhere. I finally kicked coffee; it was giving me unbelievably nasty migraines. And I can't miss meals now, not a single one. For years I didn't eat breakfast but now I just can't cope without it."

It's so true. In our teens and 20s, we can get away with *a lot* when it comes to diet, be it junk food, raw veganism, or skipped meals. Unfortunately, sub-optimal nutrition or simply the wrong diet for your metabolic type eventually catches up. Big time. And the catch-up usually arrives by age 35-45 as any deficiencies start to manifest and your body undergoes sometimes dramatic hormonal changes, asserting its nutritional needs in non-conditional terms. *You ignore your body's pleas for reconsideration at your own risk.*

Personally, I want to get the word out to our youth *now,* before the years roll by: investigate the facts versus the hype; and pay close attention to the unbiased messages of your own body. Yet I know all too well the tenacious power of a beautiful idea that has taken hold of a young person's mind, constantly corroborated by special interest groups and your own tribe.

Vegans have taken the valid model of a plant-based diet to its non-validated extreme, 100% plants only, carefully controlling what they will allow into their mouths, to the point of revulsion at the mere thought of biting into an egg or licking a drop of animal fat. Unfortunately, until the day arrives when they too might start looking and feeling poorly, our youth have no incentive to change and will continue to hold fast to their brilliant-in-theory, all-plants diet.

"The young ones still look good" is the dry observation of Sylvie, the former long-term vegan with osteoporosis and hip reconstruction. "Make sure you come back and interview them in 25 years."

32

SKINNY VEGAN BITCHES OVER 35: BEWARE

I can spot a Vata vegan in perimenopause from fifty feet away.
She seems to be aging before my very eyes.

—Anonymous yoga teacher

I WONDER IF young vegans even know what perimenopause is. There's no real knowing, of course, until it whacks your unsuspecting body like a heavy, cranky centrifugal juicer falling off the top of your refrigerator.

This usually happens in your early 40s, give or take about five years. By that time your poor head may already be spinning from an overload of responsibilities, coupled with financial insecurity. If you're a mother, you're likely to be raising teens while working full-time, trying to save for college educations *and* retirement. Women of this age are three times more likely to be single parents than men and twice as likely to be the primary caregiver for family members with disabilities or Alzheimer's. Make that the primary, unpaid caretaker. Let's just admit it—most females heading into their 40s lead hectic and stressful lives.

Add wildly fluctuating and then plunging hormone levels to the mix and you have a prescription for going bonkers. The natural transition that a woman's body undergoes before her ovaries close shop, perimenopause brings with it a dreaded list of possible symptoms: irritability, fuzzy thinking, insomnia and night sweats. And what, besides the natural aging process, radically affects hormone levels? Yep, your diet.

Advocates often flaunt low estrogen levels as one of the benefits of a vegan diet for females. Sure, that might work well when you're young and have an abundance of estrogen, maybe even an excess driving you crazy with PMS or unbridled horniness. Low estrogen levels may also be protective of breast cancer over a lifetime, although age, diet, genetics and a host of other factors are more significant. In fact, new research points to the role of carbohydrate intake and glycemic load in increased breast cancer incidence (Emond; Muti). Carbs—again! One study of 10,000 women found that "fasting glucose is a predictor of breast cancer." Moreover, the association was "strong" in perimenopausal women.

Authorities in alternative therapy have long known that cancer feeds on sugar. PET scans show cancer cells lighting up like a Christmas tree when radioactively-tagged sugar is injected in patients. And as new research pours in, confirming a cancer link, some experts believe that within a few years most of us will understand that sugar—especially in the form of fructose—is a leading cause of not only cancer, but diabetes and heart disease. Without being obsessive about every bite of birthday cake, we will purge it from our diets as much as possible.

Lewis Cantley, director of the Cancer Center at Beth Israel Deaconess Medical Center, already refuses to eat the stuff, flatly proclaiming: "Sugar scares me." Interesting, is it not, how the evidence regarding modern degenerative disease is swinging away from animal-based foods and toward plants? Highly processed and manipulated plants.

NOW BACK TO THOSE LOW estrogen benefits claimed by vegans. Excess estrogen over a lifetime isn't good; however, too-low estrogen in teens and young women can lead to serious health issues, the most common being cessation of menses or even its complete lack, causing delayed development. Normal female cycles are a prerequisite not only for fertility but somatic health, according to Zsuzsanna Suba of the National Institute of Oncology. "Anovulatory infertility," she warns, "is a very strong risk for breast cancer in young women." Vegans losing their periods from low estrogen is cause for alarm, not celebration.

Mid-life females should be concerned also. Decreases in circulating estrogen can bring "significant" undesirable changes in skeletal, cardiovascular and brain functions, leading to increased mortality (Spangenburg). Want to age gracefully? Then care about your estrogen levels. The protective effect of this sex hormone keeps your bones sturdy through the decades, promotes the synthesis of proteins, and maintains healthy vaginal skin, vessels, and flora. To be frank, low estrogen can cause your once plump vagina to atrophy—not something a 40-something wants to contemplate. Adequate estrogen is also critical for sustaining a woman's mental health through the years. No slouch, this oft-maligned hormone.

In many respects, estrogen is what makes you a female. It develops your hips and breasts, giving your body its curves and that unmistakable female shape that signals fertility to receptive males. Indeed, from antiquity until the 20th century, voluptuousness defined the ideal woman. As men gazed upon her, visions of twelve handsome heirs or, more likely, a dozen laboring children went dancing through their heads. (My late uncle was one of 13 hard-working farm kids.) It matters not the culture or social group; when males view females with hourglass figures, all their brains light up in the same area, an internal enticement system that signals rewards of sexual pleasure and healthy offspring. Is this why today's growing number of noncommittal, just-cruisin' young men prefer thin girl-bodies, against all historical and evolutionary precedent? Some dim, primitive awareness that these females are less likely to be fertile? It's low-risk assessment, albeit sub-liminal. Jennifer Lopez excepted, "I love your skinny ass" is what young women are most likely to hear nowadays. This presents a fascinating scenario because two symptoms of low estrogen in too-thin females are lack of sexual desire and painful intercourse.

Who dreamed up the anorexic model look anyway? No doubt some androgy-nous artistic type, lover of linear lines, whose idea of children was "somebody else's problem." Today's average runway model has a dangerously low BMI of 16.5, lower than poverty stricken women in food-insecure Zimbabwe. They may be raking in the money and the men, but these skinny-by-intention women are flirting with hormonal disaster.

Besides menstrual issues and infertility, symptoms of low estrogen include fatigue, forgetfulness, moodiness, depression and insomnia. Sounds like a real party, huh? Women with depleted estrogen may also experience panic attacks and low self-esteem. Decreased HDL ("good" cholesterol) and increased LDL ("bad" when the particle number is too high) are other possible outcomes of low levels of circulating estrogen. Osteoporosis risk likewise shoots up. And then there's the possibility of early menopause, a rough wake-up for a 40-year-old—menopause is tough enough after 50. Its premature arrival brings higher risk for heart disease, neurological problems, and overall mortality.

So why do female vegans have statistically lower estrogen levels than female omnivores? Two factors are at work here: low body weight and low-fat intake. More weight usually means more body fat, which means more stored estrogen. That's why thin women, including vegans and hardcore exercisers, often have insufficient amounts. (Eating disorders and thyroid dysfunction can also decrease levels.) Just as crucial as *how much* you eat, the amount of estrogen in your body is determined by *what* you eat, day in and day out.

Do you recall that most of your hormones are generated from protein and fat? That all your sex hormones are derived from cholesterol? Despite swigging green smoothies from high-speed blenders—instead of patiently hunting and foraging in verdant meadows—we moderns have the same basic physiology as our ancestors, a physiology dependent on sufficient cholesterol, fat, and protein to produce and regulate our hormones. So when females consume a low-fat, zero-cholesterol vegan-type diet, their estrogen levels can drop markedly in a very short time. If they choose to remain on that vegan diet, their circulating estrogen will be significantly less than omnivores of the same age group. "Significantly less" may spell big trouble, depending how low those estrogen levels go, for how long, and what other bodily systems are impacted.

LOTS OF TALK ABOUT hormones, antibiotics, and cattle out there in Veg World, but I've yet to hear an animal rightist talk about female hormones—that would be *human* females. Nor do they ever discuss how dependent all of us are on optimal dietary fat and cholesterol to ensure a healthy endocrine system that will support us through our peak years and into old age. Nor will you hear them admit that your body doesn't always produce all the cholesterol it needs. No need to talk ethics or philosophy here; our bodies don't follow those fuzzy systems. *It's time for vegans to start discussing human physiology with appreciation and precision.*

Not only do plants-only advocates fail to recognize the real risks of too-low estrogen in young vegans, they also conveniently omit any talk of these women as they age. But existing low estrogen can turn into a debacle when vegans hit their 40s and hormone levels start to take their infamous dive. Deficiencies can have enormous ramifications on a woman's health because estrogen affects just about every organ of the female body.

Starting anywhere from your mid-thirties to early fifties, perimenopause typically lasts several years. Some women apparently sail through it—although I've yet to meet one—but for others it's like a bad, sweaty dream they must endure for up to a decade. It's puberty in reverse, with your sex hormones defiantly acting up and then rapidly diminishing, especially if nutritional intakes are too low and stress loads too high. Perimenopause brings not only lower hormone levels overall but also "changes in the cycling and ratios between estrogen, progesterone, testosterone, luteinizing hormone, follicle-stimulating hormone, and DHEA," according to Marcy Holmes, Nurse Practitioner at the Women to Women Health Care Center in Yarmouth, Maine. Translation: emotional rollercoasting, possible hot-surge havoc, and increased bone loss risk.

Many Vata women have a particularly tough time with this transition. Vata, remember, is the Ayurvedic constitutional type that's energetic and enthusiastic, always on the move. (Each of us is a unique blend of the three types, *doshas*, but one usually predominates.) This woman naturally tends toward thinness, lighter bones, faster metabolism, and dry skin and hair—qualities that may become exaggerated during this volatile period, especially on a plant diet. It's true: you can often spot a Vata vegan in perimenopause, even from a distance. If I haven't seen a 50ish plant-eating Vata friend for a couple years, she can look to have aged ten years in just 24 months. And no, I do not offer these observations lightly. Being a Vata myself, I offer them out of concern for other slender mid-life females who are long-term vegans/vegetarians. I have seen these women in my dance and yoga classes, delicate-boned and slight, and watched them change quickly and dramatically as their already-low estrogen levels plunged.

Estrogen is stored in fat cells and these women just don't have that many. So when their mid-life ovaries start to naturally shut down, leaving the estrogen in fat-tissues as their major source, these skinny veg'n females have set themselves up for the classic symptoms of vanishing estrogen: thinning skin and wrinkles, decreased bone density, urinary tract infections, hot flashes, depression, vaginal dryness and declining interest in sex. We are not looking at a healthy, libido-filled scenario here. To counter low estrogen levels, experts recommend cutting down on carbs and loading up on a variety of high-quality proteins and fats. But even vegans who make a concerted effort to increase their fat/protein intake often unwittingly send their estrogen out the other end. That's correct: *female veggies are pooping out their estrogen.*

Why the heck? Because estrogen absolutely loves binding with fiber. So it's a sure bet—given the high-fiber content of a plant diet—that veg'ns have a higher fecal output than omnivores and more estrogen in their feces, 2-3 times more actually (Goldin). And that is *not* the place you want to send your estrogen as you get older. You want to store it inside your body, protecting you from osteoporosis and brain fog, keeping your libido strong and your skin supple and smooth.

Veganism over age 35 is much more suited to Pitta or Kapha women, if anyone. (Doubtless the reason these types keep annoyingly insisting that *everyone*

262

can be a healthy vegan.) These larger-bodied women have much more abundant fat stores, thus more stored estrogen and less likelihood of "crashing and drying" when they reach their middle years and beyond. For slender Vata types, however, the Ayurvedic literature prescribes a high-fat, high-protein, meat and dairy-based diet, along with specific lifestyle habits. In sum:

> The Vata constitution is characterized by dryness and lightness, speedy metabolism, and swift, sudden hunger; thus, these people greatly benefit from sticking to a daily routine with consistent meal times. Vatas should eat hearty, moist foods like homemade soups, meaty stews, whole cooked grains with vegetables, and hot cereals with ghee—plentiful, tissue-building foods that are heavy, oily, and warm in quality. Specifically, Vatas do well on a meat-based diet and can handle ample dairy. In addition, they should drink lots of warm fluids like herbal teas. Raw fruits, raw vegetables, legumes, and cold beverages aggravate this type and should comprise only a small part of a Vata-balancing diet.

Remember, these are evidence-based medical recommendations built on 5,000 years of methodical study of diverse diets and actual health outcomes. Compare that to veganism: a diet philosophy plucked out of the ethical ether not that many decades ago, with absolutely no data to back it up. Yet many vegans are exactly that: thin, fruit-eating Vatas. They believe, just as I once did, that they are eating the best diet on the planet. And they just might be if they were fleshier, less reactive to carbohydrates, and living a low-stress life in a year-round warm climate.

So instead of following the medicinal wisdom of the ages, we now have these millions of thin Vata vegans closing in on 40, living in cool or even frigid zones and eating heaps of cold, fibrous carbs, egged on by books and blogs with animal rights or raw food agendas. More likely, they should be pulling up their collective kitchen chairs to a generous, greasy meal of roast chicken, steamed root vegetables, and dark leafy greens. And to get the K2 needed for metabolizing the calcium in those greens, just smother them in some sweet pasture butter.

A single four-ounce serving of chicken in this well-rounded meal provides not only essential dietary fat but 30-35 grams of complete protein, going a good distance in meeting a mid-life woman's daily protein needs. You can *try* to meet this increased need with plant protein alone, but many former vegans, as they reached their middle years, found this to be impossible.

263

OH, YOU DIDN'T KNOW your protein needs increase with age? That's not really surprising, since even the Academy of Nutrition and Dietetics fails to recommend additional protein for older adults in its 2009 blanket endorsement of veganism for all comers. But as you age, your body becomes less efficient at processing dietary protein and less able to hold onto its stores (Chernoff; Bauer). As we jog past our middle years, specialists are now advising *25-30 grams of high-quality protein at every meal* in order to maximize synthesis and maintain muscle mass. That's a lot of protein for a plant eater to come up with.

Furthermore, in discussing veganism apropos to major life stages, Academy authors elaborated at length on pregnancy, lactation, infancy, childhood and adolescence but failed to even mention perimenopause. Yet this is the very stage in a woman's life when plentiful dietary protein, fat, and cholesterol are critical for balancing fast-diminishing hormones and creating stress-fighting neurotransmitters. Incredibly, the words "hormones," "menopause" and "perimenopause" don't even appear in the indexes of popular veg health books. The special dietary needs of older males during andropause aren't discussed either. These are serious omissions, a disservice to mid-lifers everywhere and reflective of just how young and experimental this diet really is.

Are we even surprised that the Academy's recommendation of an all-plant diet for every life stage was co-written by a vegan and a vegetarian? This is the very same position paper endlessly cited as "validation" that this restrictive diet is healthy for everyone. I'm sure interested readers initially assumed, as I certainly did, that it was written by an independent, impartial group of clinical nutritionists and dieticians. In fact, Ann Reed Mangels, PhD, RD, is a longtime veg promoter who advises the Vegetarian Resource Group, serves as nutrition editor for *Vegetarian Journal,* and has written a slew of pro-vegan books and papers. Her fellow author, Winston J. Craig, PhD, is a Seventh-day Adventist and Professor Emeritus in Andrews University's Department of Public Health, Nutrition and Wellness, whose stated mission, as God's stewards, is "to influence the community-at-large to affirm the Adventist lifestyle, including the vegetarian diet."

So here we have a devout vegetarian and an equally devoted vegan (committed to their diet for life, by way of religion or entrenched belief) charged to examine the research data and arrive at a science-based recommendation. *Why weren't these co-authors tagged for conflict of interest?* If one of them had been a paid adviser to the Beef Resource Group and the other a fervent hunter and best-selling publisher of paleo books (both possessing impeccable nutrition credentials, of course), you can bet your sautéed tofu that vegans would be howling to the moon about any recommendation against an all-plant diet, citing blatant bias.

The Academy's highly influential position paper also sidesteps confounding factors like genetic predisposition, ethnic ancestry, and metabolic individuality in advancing "a well-planned" vegan diet for you, me, and everyone. Unfortunately, this generic endorsement doesn't offer the specific dietary guidelines we all need, especially a mid-life female trying to maintain her hormones at healthy levels.

If this woman's life is free of emotional stress when perimenopause begins its assault (and whose life would that be?), then her body can sometimes adjust and cope without a great deal of intervention. However, as Marcy Holmes, NP, notes, "Women carrying extra burdens tend to have more extreme hormonal imbalance." When I asked Dr. John Douillard about this, he concurred: "What happens is that most mid-life women are already stressed and when the pre-menopausal years hit, the body needs more sex hormones but the progesterone usurps to make stress-fighting hormones instead. So it's no longer available to support the menopausal process and that can create a very rough transition. If you add a vegan or vegetarian diet into the equation, it's often not supplying the protein needed and all this combined makes a woman inclined to eat meat as a medicine. For years she's been mitigating and borrowing from her body to keep it all going and now, all of a sudden, perimenopause hits and she realizes there's no money in the bank."

I'm hanging onto his every word. Douillard is describing nearly every woman over 40 I know. "There are three places your adrenal glands will borrow from your body when they're exhausted from your lifestyle and possibly insufficient diet: your reproductive hormones, blood sugar, and thyroid—thyroid dysfunction being epidemic in our culture. Your adrenals borrow this energy in the form of cortisol to keep you going, and usually the body will burn out all three places before anyone stops to realize they are totally out of gas. And that's, of course, our minds driving our bodies into exhaustion in order to keep everything going."

My brain sparks wildly at these last words. The good doctor has just defined our entire manic culture. *Our minds driving our bodies into exhaustion to keep everything going.* But more to the point of this book: "If you add a veg'n diet that's not delivering the protein to maintain stable blood sugar, that blood sugar will go into fragility, into highs and lows, into a hypoglycemic state. And you're going to need energy to mitigate that, so your body will take progesterone from the reproductive hormones, making that system vulnerable. So when you actually go into menopause, you're in big trouble."

I explain to Douillard how I had to cut carbs, give up all sugar, caffeine and eventually, my sacrosanct veggie diet—plant protein was absolutely not working for me—and start eating large doses of animal protein in order to stop dragging myself through life. He heartily agrees: "Yes, what you had to do is exactly what I just described. Your body was under stress for a long time—from an inadequate diet or your lifestyle or both—and your blood sugar became unstable [so] you had to cut out a lot of carbs. As your cells age, they do not process sugar as well. The other issue is that your protein levels weren't there to stabilize your blood sugars, so you had to start pounding protein. When the blood sugar is crashing, that's an emergency state, and without adequate protein and fat, your adrenals will borrow from the reproductive hormones."

So is hormone supplementation the magic bullet? *Give them all progesterone; they'll be fine.* Douillard disagrees and believes women in this imbalanced state should add high-quality, grass-fed, complete animal protein to their meals, as well as healthy fats. Mary Vance, NC, who specializes in female health, fertility, and hormonal issues in San Francisco, recommends a healing protocol combined with a nutrient-dense diet.

"Organic, fatty-acid-rich foods like wild fish, grass fed beef, organ meats and eggs should be the base of every meal," she affirms, along with lots of "mineral-rich veggies and sea veggies because the adrenals require minerals to function." And stop chugging coffee, but do add healthy traditional foods like bone broth and fermented vegetables, plus good fats like olive oil, coconut oil, and butter to keep hormones balanced. All three—Vance, Douillard and Holmes—believe our stressful lifestyle is a primary culprit, exacerbated by an inadequate diet that pushes hormones severely out of synch. In today's rush-rush, eat-run world, Holmes contends that it's no surprise "younger and younger women are experiencing perimenopause-type symptoms."

At Women to Women, the first line of defense is a deliberate diet that phases out sugar and caffeine and incorporates, you got it, extra protein and quality fat. Brooke, a satisfied client, confirms this protocol has made a huge difference in her life. "I enjoy eggs most mornings for breakfast. Protein, protein, protein—gets me through the day with energy and really cuts those sugar cravings....I have learned to take care of myself, and when you *know* you can do that, life becomes pretty glorious."

266

BROOKE'S NEUROTRANSMITTERS are kicking into high gear as she heals and regains energy. Largely produced from amino acids in the protein you eat, these brain chemicals motivate us to take charge of our lives and....*get the hell moving!* So if your diet is too low in quality protein, over time you'll experience depleted levels of neurotransmitters. And how does that feel? Like a stranger has taken over your body.

Affecting not just the brain but your entire nervous system, these chemicals determine whether your life feels fantastic or flat. They act as mood mediators and, if unbalanced, the results can be life-altering, creating sudden mood swings, sadness, depression or compulsive thoughts. Depression is, in fact, a common complaint among long-time vegans before they reluctantly put animal protein back into their diet. Their frank, often gut-wrenching testimonials speak to the dull gray nothingness caused by waning neurotransmitters.

Twenty million-billion calculations per second. That's how fast your brain works when you're feeling good, on top of your life. But to accomplish this rapid-fire feat, your brain needs even more than plentiful protein. It needs ample dietary fat to speed those transmitters on their way. That's why low-fat diets have been implicated in decreased brain function and memory loss, while diets high in good fats lower your risk. Important new research reveals improved brain function in older adults who consume 35-40% fat compared to those on a low-fat diet (Valls-Pedret). Meanwhile, an alarming number of vegans continue to view just 10-20% fat as optimal.

Assuming your memory's still clicking, serotonin and dopamine are the key neurotransmitters to remember here. We know that low levels of serotonin lead to depression, while depleted amounts of dopamine can create difficulties in concentration and memory. These symptoms sound all too familiar to mid-life women walking around in a fog of melancholia. Fortunately, one of the most potent ways to bring your neurotransmitters into balance is through exacting food choices. Once again, *food is your power.*

Foods rich in protein can boost dopamine and its derivative, norepinephrine, within minutes, speeding up your thoughts and increasing feelings of joy and alertness. This explains the exhilarating swiftness with which Linda, Sylvie, myself, and so many others felt our well-beings lifted and our bodies empowered as we ate protein-dense animal food for the first time in years.

A mere 3-ounces of fish, red meat, chicken or eggs greatly increases dopamine and norepinephrine in just 20-30 minutes. Vibrant foods like beets, blueberries, and leafy greens also contribute to their production. You just need to figure out which foods work best for *you*, noticeably increasing your energy, stamina, and smart-brain output. As for those all-knowing vegans who insist you can't possibly feel any effects from your food (e.g., meat) until it's completely digested and absorbed....*whoa*....these people are seriously out of touch with their bodies.

And too-low serotonin? Again, you can prevent this abysmal depressive state by eating sufficient protein containing the amino acid tryptophan. Game meat and organs offer the highest quantity per calorie, while crustaceans, fish, eggs and poultry offer good amounts. Tofu, beans, oatmeal and quinoa offer fair amounts but keep in mind that you also need adequate magnesium, calcium, and all the B vitamins to achieve level moods. Sustaining your estrogen at optimal levels is likewise essential for satisfactory serotonin production. This might seem like a lot to keep track of, but depression is your body's powerful signal that you need to do exactly that.

When you enter your 40s, your body also increases its demand for choline, found primarily in cholesterol-rich animal foods and known to improve cognition and slow the brain's aging. Recall, however, that vegans have trouble meeting even the minimal RDA for choline. Bottom line: scientists at Life Extension Research warn that diets which restrict animal foods, cholesterol, and fat "may not contain sufficient amounts of the essential nutrients that support cognitive function and membrane structure." As for females over 35 trying to lose weight or get skinny, Debra Waterhouse, RD, author of *Outsmarting the Mid-Life Fat Cell*, cautions them to steer clear of a strict vegan diet.

Clearly, as we climb toward our middle years, a mindful diet becomes more critical than ever. Deficiencies that aren't taken care of when we're younger, will come back to bite us in our 40s and 50s. And that bite can be ferocious for any woman heading unprepared into perimenopause. So female vegans—especially slender Vata types—you would be wise to reevaluate your diet with complete objectivity as you move past your 30s. Depending on your lifestyle and nutrition choices, this vital passage can be an exhilarating period of transformation, or a downhill spiral into vanishing hormones, diminished brain function, and accelerated aging. It's in your power to make excellent choices that will support your health through mid-life and beyond. Do it, oh strong lovely woman. Do it!

33.

RAW AND EXPOSED

LIKE VEGANISM, eating all raw sounds quite beautiful in theory: naked and unadorned, so very pure. Indeed, beauty is a dominant force in David "Avocado" Wolfe's pursuit of the perfect diet for all.

A leader in the raw food movement, Wolfe espouses 100% raw for everyone, 80% if you're not quite there, and 51% minimum for those of us still enslaved to the gratuitous habit of cooking our food. A "frontier science" is what this health guru calls all-raw nutrition, yet he offers no science at all. That's because there is no scientific evidence to offer. He does, however, offer us poetic words, undocumented health claims, and alluring photos of buxom, plump-lipped California babes who've jumped aboard the raw food brigade.

Want to become ever more attractive? Wolfe's bestselling books explore how to eat consciously to achieve this enviable feat. Your face is a canvas and your body a sculpture, this art-loving raw foodie declares, painted and chiseled by your daily food choices. Clearly, Wolfe resonates with the classical ideal of beauty and openly praises the ancient Greeks. Describing them as "startling" in appearance, he quotes the Roman Admantius: "They had square faces, fine lips, straight noses, and powerful eyes with a glittering gaze. They were a people with the most beautiful eyes in the world."

With his curly dark hair and long classic nose, Wolfe strikes his own Greek hero pose on the back cover of *Eating for Beauty*. How intriguing, therefore, that the diet of these gorgeous, sparkly-eyed Greeks of the Hellenic Age was neither raw nor vegan but included copious amounts of cooked animals. Historian Colin Spencer informs us that upper-class Greeks were fond of serving their guests anything from pigs and pigeons to pheasants, ducks, and fried cicadas—even dogs and puppies. The common people cultivated crops but also hunted their fair share

269

of bears, boars, lions, deer and asses—stewing the bones and tongues separately. Raw ass, anyone?

And let's not overlook the water creatures, as Mr. Wolfe apparently has. Above all other provisions, the Greeks loved and continue to love their seafood—well cooked. Spencer notes that tunny, fished by the Greeks for millennia, "would have been sliced in steaks, fried on iron skillets in olive oil and while cooking be sprinkled with aromatic herbs and cumin. To be served only with a green salad." Sounds like a yummy meal straight out of an Alice Waters' cookbook, doesn't it? Barring a few exotic imports for the elite, ancient Greeks ate locally and seasonally, grounding their cuisine in the natural riches of their seabound home: fresh fish and olives, mustard greens and fennel, fava beans and grains. Very similar to the plants-and-fish diet touted by our more balanced 21st century nutritionists: some raw, some cooked; many plants, some animals.

But the Greeks didn't eat just for health and sustenance. They revered their food and considered the act of ingestion a truly aesthetic experience. In *Eating for Beauty* Wolfe describes his own enjoyment of raw food as a thrilling and creative event, each carefully selected item conveying its unique sound, tone and color, transforming the eater into a veritable work of art. Eat high-quality raw foods only, according to Wolfe, and every meal will turn into a climactic experience, "as if cells in various parts of the body are having orgasms!"

The literature doesn't reveal if these early Greeks experienced simultaneous orgasms throughout their comely, well-chiseled bodies whilst sitting down to wild boar and crisp bacon, but they did take great pleasure in consuming their food, both raw and cooked. They were also master bakers, according to Athenaeus, and would have scoffed at the idea of giving up bread, all 70+ varieties. Yes, from their rocky seascapes, fields and forests, the beauteous Greeks of the Hellenic Age pursued all things edible that their homeland provided, gathering plants during periods of warmth and plenty, storing away animal protein and fat for the leaner months. Even today, winter for Greeks means cold and wet.

Raw eater Wolfe has a home in Hawaii, the tropics, where winter temps can shoot up into the 80s. The sun shines 270 days of the year and plenteous fruit and vegetables grow year-round. It makes sense that a raw diet might work on the Hawaiian Islands. Many in the raw community do in fact live here—or in other pleasant, hot-weather locales like the southern reaches of California, Arizona and Florida—surrounded by fresh avocados or oranges, eaten on the beach in skimpy shorts beneath a blazing sun. And raw goddesses hold their cleansing retreats in sultry Costa Rica or Indonesia, dining on kelp, pineapple and papaya. Excellent tropical fare!

What we'd all love to witness is these same all-raw pushers living year-round in the truly raw, wind-scoured plains of Minnesota, Wyoming or Alberta, while continuing to eat cold, naked food at every meal. Yet in their promotional books and videos, raw foodies—exactly like vegans—make no distinction whatsoever as regards climate, ancestry or lifestyle, preaching their odd dietary principles to all individuals in all places. Do these rawdies really believe that wheat farmers in Saskatchewan, construction workers in Maine, and coal miners in Chile should come in from the bitter cold after a long day of hard physical labor and sit down to a meal of cold cauliflower, parsnips and cumin seeds? Hey, it works splendidly for me, lounging around the pool in San Diego. Follow me! Eat like me!

I dislike pointing out the obvious, but many of us here on planet earth don't live in places where fresh, varied plant food is available year round. And for those who care about their health—and the planet's—eating in-season and locally is fast becoming imperative. Actually, Wolfe and other 100% naked foodies would be wise to study the original native diet of their warm-weather locations. Ancient Hawaiians for example, well known for their fine health and knock-down strength (Kamehameha was crowned King after allegedly hoisting a bruiser of a boulder), subsisted on a diverse diet of wild birds, taro root, seaweeds and over a hundred species of fish and shellfish, fresh-plucked from the sea. And how refreshing that Hawaiian women did the hunting and gathering while the men were consigned to the kitchen!

Tragically, modern Hawaiians are not fit and healthy like their ancestors. Of all our ethnic groups, they have the shortest lifespan and claim some of America's highest rates of obesity, diabetes, and cardiovascular disease. An appalling 70% of deaths among native Hawaiians are diet-related. So researchers took a group of natives off their modern industrial-food agenda and put them on the traditional diet of their pre-western-contact ancestors: bounteous plants alongside fresh fish and chicken. After three weeks, the data revealed major weight loss, lower blood pressure, decreased triglycerides, and reversal of other heart disease markers.

Our distant ancestors weren't naïve boneheads. They were smart—far smarter than we are when it comes to diet. Harvesting fresh, varied nutrition from the sur-rounding land and water, they lived in synch with the natural world. That's how all indigenous cultures survive and endure. "The most profound influence is the harvest of nature. That's what really got us here," John Douillard reminds us.

"The nutritional cycle on this planet is an annual cycle. So that's a critical step: you need more of what's in season where you live." To even attempt to eat all-raw for 12 months of the year only makes sense with a year-long growing season. Even a cooked vegan diet works best for someone who lives in an equatorial zone like Hawaii, 100 miles south of the Tropic of Cancer. But for most of us humans scattered across the latitudes and longitudes of our curvaceous, light-angling earth, 100% vegan/raw diets are perilously inappropriate.

The inter-mountain West is definitely *not* a good bioregion for raw foodists to sprout. Same goes for New England, the Midwest, our northern states and most of Canada. Then again, if eating platefuls of cold plant food in the dead of winter, a foot of snow on the ground and arctic winds howling out of the north appeals to you, go for it. However, no culture on earth does this unless forced to, unless the alternative is not to eat at all. Yet raw advocates act as if this is the most natural of diets. They cling, like unapprised vegans, to a make-believe mythical age when we subsisted on raw plants only. The discovery of fire and thus cooking, rawdies mourn, marked the beginning of the end for humanity's earthly paradise.

Yes, there is a time and a season to eat naked food in abundance: in the spring and summer when cooling green salads and chilled cantaloupe abound. Most of us of us do this quite naturally. By early fall we're delighting in butternut squash and other root vegetables. Come early winter, it's time for non-equatorial humans to start packing in the high-fat, high-protein nourishment, including all those thin, deranged Vatas running around the Rocky Mountains in fifteen degree weather, slurping cold raspberry-carrot smoothies.

THE PHONE CALL TO ILLINOIS came late at night. Less than a year into her raw vegan diet and not that many months into her college career, Gabrielle sounded so deeply unhappy that I jumped into our little black Honda and blasted across the lonesome prairie, 13-hours-straight to Colorado.

We had agreed to meet at the rec center on the CU campus. As I hurried in that direction, someone who vaguely resembled my lovely, auburn-haired daughter came walking toward me on the woodsy path. Whoever this young woman was, and at that point I wasn't sure, she seemed to be moving on splintery colt legs, holding her books with emaciated stick arms. Her face was so changed, so lacking in flesh, I didn't at first recognize my own child. Later that evening, catching a glimpse as she stepped out of the shower, I cried to see her naked body as thin and bony as an anorexic.

272

That's exactly what the doctor assumed, of course, insisting that Gabe enroll in a free class on eating disorders with all the other sad, gaunt females showing up at the student health center. This made us angry. We both knew she loved to eat and kept everything down, having a healthy regard for food and no desire to be sickly skinny. Yet despite her three meals a day, plus snacks, Gabe had lost far too much weight since leaving home. Her strength was diminishing and her brain was constantly racing. She couldn't turn off her thoughts, she told me, couldn't focus, couldn't sleep. Overcome with anxiety, she would lie awake for hours, watching her mind madly zipping around on fast forward. From a calm, healthy, curvy high school senior of 128 pounds, she was now a scrawny, nervous, sleepless wreck, weighing a scant 102. First she was diagnosed with thyroid dysfunction. Then her periods went missing.

I now rue the day my daughter found *Diet for a New America* in a bookstore at age 17, especially since I paid for it. As I flipped through the pages, its message seemed innocent enough: eat lower on the food chain, save animals, get healthy. But like so many other teens, Gabe became an overnight vegan zealot, despite the fact that she knew almost nothing about nutrition. Instantly renouncing all animal products, she began eating soy as her primary protein source every day. One year later, she became an aficionado of raw as well, heavily influenced by the influx of raw celebrities and "go raw" cookbooks everywhere she looked. After graduating and moving away to college, she joined a local support group for weekly raw potlucks. Buying her own food processor, juicer and dehydrator came next, followed by long hours in her itty-bitty kitchen trying to prepare wholesome, uncooked all-plant meals.

You'd think not having to cook would be less time consuming. Think again as you imagine creating "cheese" out of blue-green algae and almonds; or "chicken salad" out of pecans, cashews, and sunflower seeds. At least Gabe was no longer eating soy, and I must admit her raw key-lime pie was delectable. Yet she rapidly started shedding weight from her gorgeously proportioned body and no matter how much she ate, which was like a race horse all day long, she got skinnier and skinnier and it became scarier and scarier to watch.

Just as she was about to hit a new low of 100 pounds, looking and feeling like an eating disordered wreck, Gabrielle made her own smart decision to get off the trendy, politically-correct raw vegan diet, which had corresponded with all the destructive changes. Slowly she gained back much-needed muscle and fat, her strong feminine body, her appropriately paced thoughts, her new appreciation for

273

a good night's sleep and—with the help of a gifted nutritionist—her monthly periods. A year later she met and subsequently married a Frenchman who's not only a first-rate chef but thinks all-raw and all-vegan diets are *barbarian!* (Highly opinionated, yes, but then again he *is* French). Yohan cooks her warm, moist, nourishing meals with thick creamy soups, buttery sauces, and daily portions of high-quality meat. Gabe is now a mother, a runner, and health counselor who overflows with energy and well-being.

I can already hear the shrill voices of activists: "A rare exception! Raw and vegan work perfectly for me!" And that is exactly my point. This diet might work fine for you at the onset, for David "Avocado" Wolfe, for all those sun-kissed models offering glowing testimony in every new tome—but not for my daughter, not for my best friend, not for all. There it is again, that unwarranted presumption that because my raw/vegan/paleo/Atkins/Ornish/whatever diet works well for me, it will therefore work well for you. And for everyone. "So buy my book!"

To their credit, most raw campaigners offer some sound dietary advice amidst the extremism: eat more organic greens and vegetables, ditch addictive substances like coffee/sugar, and gather wild foods for enhanced nutrition. David Wolfe also mentions types of meat he considers preferable as you move toward your goal of total raw vegan. His overall philosophy, however, is anti-animal food because flesh-eating creates "a very negative effect" on one's innermost consciousness. What a foolish assumption and one that the Buddha, Jesus, Muhammad and other enlightened humans throughout the ages have rejected.

Wolfe, self-proclaimed "rock star of the superfoods world," also suggests that everyone go raw at his or her own pace. Try eating all-raw throughout the day, he advises new recruits, then go ahead and cook your evening meal. Too bad he didn't leave it at that. Certainly, eating more fresh, uncooked plants would benefit all Americans. It's clear, however, where Wolfe and other crusaders prefer we all eventually go: to the extreme. This is the diet they promote and make their money from: 100% raw vegan every day of the year, presumably for the rest of your life. After attaining all-raw, fasting on juice or water one day each week is the "next step" that Mr. Wolfe would like you to consider. And after that?

EXTREME IS THE NAME of the game when it comes to the raw and vegan lifestyles. Let's face it: novel diets—100% plants, 100% raw, all raw with fasting—generate more excitement and sell more books and seminars than the same old call to eat more fresh fruit and vegetables. We can get that advice from our moms for free. Moreover, radical new ideas create a cult following of believers, many of them hoping to change their lives and self-identities as quickly as possible. In following an unorthodox dietary path, some also relish the idea of setting themselves apart from the masses in a virtuous way.

After meeting hundreds of such individuals, Steven Bratman, MD, coined a word for this obsession to follow a diet of "perfect" foods: *orthorexia nervosa*. According to Bratman, dietary extremism occurs when the individual "becomes obsessed, not with the *quantity* of food eaten, but the *quality*. What starts as a devotion to healthy eating can evolve into a pattern of incredibly strict diets." Bratman calls these people not victors, but victims. Ultimately, they become so dogmatic, so focused on eating a "pure diet" of plants only—or raw only or fruit only—that preparing, eating, preaching and defending their diet begins to dominate their lives.

Currently a physician in Colorado, Bratman knows all about food fanaticism. For twenty years he loyally followed and advocated a restrictive diet of one sort or another: macrobiotics, veganism, raw. For a good chunk of those years he was an organic farmer and, later, a cook at a large commune in upstate New York which attracted, as he calls them, "food idealists" whose obstinate demands he had to satisfy at every meal. As he recounts in his book *Health Food Junkies*, the vegetarians refused any food prepared in pots and pans "contaminated by fleshy vibrations," however thoroughly washed. They insisted as well on a separate kitchen for the fallen meat eaters, whose food had to be placed on a distant table.

> The cooks also had to satisfy the vegans.....who looked on cheese as poison, as well as the non-garlic, non-onion, Hindu-influenced crowd, who believed [all] onion-family foods provoked sexual desire. For the raw-foodists we laid out sliced raw vegetables in endless rows. Once, when a particularly enthusiastic visitor tried to convince me that slicing a vegetable would destroy its energy field, I felt so hassled that I ran at him wildly with a flat Chinese cleaver until he fled. Meanwhile, the macrobiotic followers condemned the raw vegetables for different theoretical reasons, and also set up a hue and cry over the serving of any "deadly nightshade" plants such as potatoes, tomatoes, and eggplants.

It finally dawned on Dr. Bratman that dietary goodness has a dark side. When eating healthy turns into an obsession, it's no longer all that healthy. In writing his book, the doctor's goal was to help pure-diet obsessed folks admit that they even have a problem. He then helps them explore the ultra-tight grip these dietary gurus and theories have on their minds and how such philosophies may be built on faulty logic rather than sound nutritional advice, working against their health over the long haul.

Truth be told, the raw foodies I personally know don't look all that healthy to me, including the woman who spearheaded the group my daughter joined and has been doing raw the longest. She's also the one who ate her newborn's placenta, added to a green salad after light steaming. Not to exceed 114 degrees, of course, the raw limit of acceptability before "an enormous percentage" of enzymes, vitamins, and minerals are "destroyed" by cooking, wherein the food becomes "more difficult to digest," leading to "overeating, cravings and disease"—or so the raw literature expounds.

Weirdly, science tells us nearly the opposite. So what's going on here? A profound disconnect from reality? Or simply wishful, child-like thinking? Research from Cornell and Harvard Medical School, among others, clearly indicates nutritional advantages to cooking our vegetables. Cabbage, peppers, zucchini, spinach, mushrooms and asparagus, for instance, supply more antioxidants when steamed or boiled than their raw counterparts. By breaking down the plants' thick cell walls, cooking *more than doubles* the amount of lycopene in tomatoes, a potent antioxidant that's linked to lowered risk for heart disease and cancer. Research confirms that individuals on a strict raw food diet do indeed test low in lycopene. A separate study discovered that the longer corn is cooked, the more cancer-battling compounds are released. Cooking likewise increases the availability of beta-carotene in carrots, while broccoli is healthier served raw. Vitamin C levels also stay higher in raw produce. The simple lesson here? Eat a variety of cooked and raw veggies for optimal nutrition. And educate yourself on the facts before flinging your blind beliefs across the Internet.

A former raw foodist from the greater Denver area spoke to me on condition of anonymity, citing egos she didn't want to bruise and friendships she didn't want to fracture (raw groups tend to be small and passionately bonded). A conventional vegan for a decade before going raw, "Deirdre" was greatly influenced by the Boutenkos, internationally known as The Raw Family. After permanently shutting down their oven and curing themselves of various serious illnesses, this proud Russian immigrant family—mother, father, son and daughter—began to preach the power of 100% raw, packing seminars and retreats while churning out

276

bestsellers like *Green Smoothie Revolution*. About one year into her own live food experiment, however, Deirdre started feeling not so alive. She started feeling very depressed. "It was like a winter depression, only it was July," she told me. "I was doing the diet really well, too. I read all the books, did all the trainings, but I knew something wasn't right. At that point I was going to stop, but I went to another workshop put on by the Boutenkos and they convinced me to go back on the raw diet."

Just like overnight vegans, rawdies often rapidly transform their lives after listening spellbound to authority figures possessing powers of passion and persuasion. So despite her growing doubts, the enchantment of forceful testimonials once again proved too strong for Deidre, especially when repeated mantra-like to sensitive and susceptible individuals searching for the golden key to health and happiness. *Eat raw vegan to be super healthy. Eat raw forever! Eat all raw!*

That winter, Deirdre's own body-wisdom finally broke through her protracted mind trance. Arriving home one evening, exhausted as usual, she darted indoors, out of the bitter mountain winds, and said in disgust to herself: "I am NOT eating cold vegetables again tonight!" Instead she cooked some hot minestrone soup and oven-roasted sweet potatoes. For the first time in many months, she felt warm and nourished inside and out—and she never turned back. Of the local raw group she once faithfully attended, Deirdre now claims, "Hardly anybody looked healthy. I would look around the room and see all these pale, emaciated-looking people with bad skin tones. They were like poster children for *Don't Eat This Way!*"

When she was still part of the group, however, Deirdre figured they simply hadn't been on the diet long enough. She even remembers reading Dr. Bratman's book on health food junkies and being completely revolted by it. "I thought he was ignorant and self-righteous. Who the fuck is this guy to disparage all these great ethical diets?" Now a healthy omnivore who eats both raw and cooked, Deirdre maintains that Bratman's chapter on raw foodies "just nails it." Today she firmly believes "the majority of people at the raw gatherings I attended had eating disorders. They were obsessed with food. It's all they ever talked about."

It's a purifying obsession for many, Deirdre believes, attempting to be purer, cleaner, and "more evolved" than the ignorant among us who continue to eat meat or cook food. "Some of them end up on the edge," she laments, having witnessed tragedy in her own raw group. It seems several female members became infatuated with Domanhur, an artistic cult based in northern Italy and accused by the government of secretly excavating a vast underground temple. Calling itself a spiritual eco-community, the Federation of Domanhur boasts its own constitution and currency, sleeps 20 people to a house, and encourages neo-paganism and marriage renewals, along with auspiciously timed conceptions. Their charismatic citizens also travel to far-flung places like Colorado, preaching raw veganism and extended fasting. "One man in particular, handsome and arrogant, swept them off their feet," Deirdre recounted to me, her face pinched with anger and sorrow. Following him to California, a young practitioner, Deirdre's good friend, died during a raw juice fast of 10 days, concurrent with intense breathwork and hot mineral soaks.

IT WOULDN'T BE the only time Deirdre witnessed what she calls "a foodie going over the edge with the whole diet trip, the whole spiritual trip, and losing touch with reality." Another woman she personally knows was practicing Natural Hygiene (an early form of raw veganism) while assisting and traveling with one of its top proponents, Dr. Douglas Graham. In a lifestyle choice strikingly similar to the flesh mortifications of the Orphics and Pythagoreans—attempting to separate spirit as far as possible from the human body—this woman had refined her eating habits more and more to the point of ingesting raw fruit only. (Some fruitarians will eat nothing but fallen produce, refusing to swallow even the seeds for fear of killing a future plant.) However, when pears and pomegranates didn't rocket her into Everland, Deirdre's friend decided to try living on breath alone (breatharian). By the time her frantic parents did an intervention and had her hospitalized, she was down to 68 pounds. "Emotionally she was not at all stable," Deirdre relayed to me, shaking her head. "She was screaming at her parents. She was furious at them *and* the hospital for putting 'poison' in her body. She was so brainwashed with the idea that cooked food is poison. We were all brainwashed with that."

Doctor Bratman regretfully confirms that diet devoutness can lead to physical danger, even death, if weight drops too low. "Emaciation is common among followers of certain health food diets, such as raw foodism, and this can at times reach the extremes seen in anorexia nervosa," he concludes on *orthorexia.com*. "However, the underlying motivation is quite different." An anorexic wants to lose more weight to look good, while an orthorexic wants to feel light, pure, and other worldly. Kate, Bratman's patient, was experiencing only minor health issues when she first tried Natural Hygiene. "I figured in order for this to work I needed to do it fully and eat all my foods raw," she wrote on *Beyond Vegetarianism*. "I did this for about two weeks and experienced the light euphoric feeling....I felt clearer, much less bloated and lethargic, but I was getting weaker in terms of muscle strength." Five years later, still eating raw, Kate's weight dropped so low that she died from malnutrition.

Deirdre knows just one person from her original group of about two dozen who seems to be doing alright on a raw vegan diet, up to this point at least. "His constitution appears to be able to handle it," she says of the sturdy Pitta-type man. However, she doesn't know if he sticks to all-raw in private. Who actually knows this about ANYBODY who preaches a constrained diet? *Vegans sneaking cheese like skittish mice in an empty house....Rawdies clamping their aching jaws into wood-fired pizzas.* Tired of the deceit, a growing number of well-known vegans and rawdies are outing themselves to their fans. Unable to sustain their health over the years on these monkish diets, they are no longer willing to live a public lie. *Ex-vegan's admission of 14 eggs a week to rebalance her nervous system and abolish anxiety...Online confessions of ecstatic first bites of cooked meat followed by long-absent outpourings of energy.*

Others heavily invested in the business or celebrity side of raw veganism are apparently sticking it out. When they're not fighting it out, that is, or sticking it to us, as evidenced by public reports and testimonials: *Raw vegan gurus sue each other for millions....aggressive promotion of overpriced, not-so-raw supplements ....$10,000 for supervised fasting....more deaths at fasting retreats....California Medical Board disciplines raw-advocate MD for his unprofessional conduct and incompetence....more reports of "superfit" raw vegan gurus getting pudgy and rapidly aging....80-10-10 believers who look like meth addicts.*

Modest and sincere, the Queen of Raw, Victoria Boutenko, gives us hope there is a better way: the path of moderation. After a difficult period of self-inquiry, she acknowledged that the first edition of her book, *12 Steps to Raw Foods*, contained fanaticism about 100% raw, when many were struggling to adhere to just 60%. After publishing a "much kinder.....more useful" edition, Boutenko shredded and recycled all remaining copies of the original and announced she was resigning from her all-raw position. While her own diet remains just shy of that status, she now admits "it can be healthier to eat a bowl of cooked green vegetables than a whole jar of raw nutbutter."

The all-raw regimen certainly is, as David Wolfe claims, a food "frontier"— yet another unproven diet being gobbled up by our trusting and idealistic young people. Yet just like strict vegans who have taken life-long vows, 100% raw food-ies are participating in a new human experiment. What will their long-term health results be? Kaleigh from Ontario did feel better during the first four months of her raw vegan diet. After that, she felt "progressively worse for the next seven years," she confesses in *Let Them Eat Meat*. But she stayed model-skinny and never touched media-disdained animal fat and cholesterol, so she convinced herself that she was healthy. Today Kaleigh freely admits gravitating toward raw veganism at a young age "because it's not a balanced diet and I was not a balanced person."

> Harvey Diamond, David Wolfe, and Paul Bragg would like you to believe you can get everything you need from a raw food vegan diet, but try it out for 10 years and watch yourself turn into a neurotic, nervous, hyper-sensitive, and adrenally burnt-out mess.

Do yourself a big favor and dispense of any diet that 1) has 100% in its title; 2) offers no valid long-term nutrition research with positive outcomes; and 3) disregards the life situation and unique dietary needs of the individual. You might also consider the wisdom of ignoring all food gurus who depend on extreme diets to market their products, sell books, and make a boatload of money.

As my friend Annie, the skilled Chinese Medicine practitioner, reminds us: "Radical diets like strict veganism and all-raw serve some people very well as *temporary* diets for purposes of detoxification, cleansing, or healing from disease or poor eating habits. Chinese Medicine and other honorable traditions prescribe them short-term for exactly these reasons. However, these diets were never, *ever* meant to become a permanent lifestyle."

34.

BODY OF EVIDENCE:
THE ONE AND ONLY YOU

Notice how everyone has just arrived here from a journey....
Look at the chefs preparing special plates for everyone,
according to what they need.

—Jalaluddin Rumi

IDEOLOGY IS GRAND but when it comes to the actual food you put inside your belly, reality intervenes: your individual genetic and biochemical reality. Forget the strident voices of vegan-paleo-low-fat-high-fat activists. Toss their books and banish their blogs. There is only one entity that knows the healthiest diet for you, day in and day out: your very own beautiful body.

Your body is not only intelligent and complex beyond measure, it's the most perfect biofeedback machine on the planet. It will tell you directly, unequivocally, which foods you should eat and which you should not, how much and during what season, even the best times of day. Most of us stopped listening to the very clear messages of our bodies long ago. And what did we do instead? We started plugging into the group mind. The moment you did that, the moment you stopped listening to your own embodied self—whether out of not-knowing or insecurity or youthful idealism—you abdicated your personal power and turned it over to an outside authority. That authority might be a diet guru, the popular media, your peer group, Vegans for Life, or Paleo Forever. It doesn't matter which you chose to follow because not one of them promotes your astonishing individuality.

What many of these ideologues and groups want you to believe is that they know more about your body than you do: what nourishes it, what it feels, what it needs. That's how they gain influence and self-admiration, make money and sell books: by stripping you of your own internal discernment, wisdom, and power.

281

Author and educator Caroline Myss writes frequently about getting wired into the group/tribal mind, especially when young and impressionable. Yet in order to mature and discover our own truths, we must *consciously unplug*. The tribe, as Myss affirms, doesn't want you to develop your individuality and break away from its code of beliefs. "It doesn't want to hear: I've got the most wonderful news! I'm not anything like you!" Whether it's PETA or the Tea Party, your tribe wants you to believe and act in one way, their way, and if you defect, shaming will ensue. Yet only by unplugging from group mind can you evolve and develop your own intuition and higher perception. Says Myss: "Every truth you finally understand will change the rules of your life."

To change the rules and begin to live your own truth, you have to renounce all pre-packaged, one-for-all philosophies about health and diet. You have to look inward, to your in-house doctor, and take full responsibility for your food choices, every one of them. In so doing, you will become empowered to know your body in a new and visceral way, like the animal you are. You will learn to be present, to pay attention, to become a superb listener to the most obvious *and* the most subtle language of your physical being. In turn, your body will become an intimate friend that supports and sustains you—not some seeming foe that attacks you with constant hunger, digestive problems, or relentless fatigue.

Sadly, every author of every pro-veg'n book or blog I have ever read fails to recommend self-inquiry. *Pay attention. Be fully conscious of the short and long-term results to your health when you eat this way.* As well, I have yet to see the caveat that should preface every single book enticing readers to follow a new diet regime. *This diet may not be appropriate for all persons. Your body is unique.* Proponents seem to think their diet is the absolute best for all without exception. Just cast off your pathetic ignorance and do as I do!

For ethical advocates like Rod Preece, vegetarianism is largely a philosophical choice based on a laudable ideal: non-suffering for animals, domesticated animals anyway. He doesn't want all those animal deaths on his karmic debit card and insists you shouldn't either. Tellingly, I have not found one passage, not one word in his nearly 400-page book, *Sins of the Flesh*, not even in his more personal prologue, where Preece refers to *his body*—his ingesting, digesting, metabolizing, corporal self. Sure, this is a scholarly tome but it's also a not-so subtle put-down of "sinful" omnivores and a rapturous tribute to his own dietary stance. He refers briefly to the same blatantly biased health stats we've all heard before, comparing vegetarianism to a diet heavy in processed meat, as if there were no other way to include animal-sourced food. But how does his veg diet make him *feel?* How is it affecting his *energy* and *stamina* as the years accumulate, his *cognition*, his overall sense of *health* and *well-being?* None of these essential physiological markers are even addressed. How can you recommend a diet to the entire world and not share your own body's long-term health results? (Vegan zealots: I'm talking to you. Let's put those 20-year lab results online for all to see.)

The philosophy is admirable; therefore, the practical results will be admirable—a logical fallacy if ever I read one. In a book about food history and the supremacy of the vegetarian way, this lack of reference to personal bodily results strikes me as strange, even sad, a perpetuation of the mind/body disconnect that has battered the western psyche all the way back to the mechanistic philosophy of Descartes.

By contrast, contemporary philosopher Alva Noë teaches that consciousness is not a state of mind inhabiting the brain; it's a dynamic interaction between your mind, body, and the world. Indeed, science now confirms that "brain cells" are in no way limited to your brain. From esophagus to anus, your gut alone contains 100 million neurons, more than your entire spinal cord, plus a complex network of neurotransmitters that gives orders to your brain more often than it takes them. Tens of thousands of neurons exist in your heart as well, delivering messages that affect your emotions, memories, and decisions. Healers and the more kinesthetic among us have known this all along: intelligence resides in our bodies as much as our minds. There is no firm separation between the two. And if ever there existed a terrific reason to consult the wise body/mind, it's regarding our daily food choices. Note to vegan ethicists: eating is not an intellectual process.

The academic argument that veganism is morally required because all of us can find full health eating plants-only is not grounded in corporal reality. As Linda Eastburn, medical intuitive, gently chided me regarding my till-the-death ethical diet, "Don't try to figure out an answer with your mind alone." Let your decisions be guided by how your body feels, by what nurtures you, by what exhilarates and brightens you. When you eat a diet that fails to nourish, however scrupulously planned, your body will signal this in no uncertain terms: faltering health. And when you find the foods that do nourish your body, you will know it—and this applies to all choices in life—because you'll find yourself spontaneously saying day after day, year after year: *This feels good. This feels right.*

Yet systemic intelligence is not the same as cognition, and language does arise in the physical brain, talking us into all sorts of actions and beliefs that are not necessarily good for us. Speaking of which, I've been hanging out almost exclusively in my word-drenched cerebral cortex this morning, intently working on this chapter and in no way listening to my body (one of the hazards of a language-heavy profession) which is now transmitting its unambiguous message via sudden overwhelming fatigue and my brain careening to a halt. *You haven't had your 25 grams of essential animal protein this morning,* it's hollering—my virtual guarantee of lucid thinking, kick-ass energy, and ongoing stamina for hours on end.

Instead, I've been grazing on plentiful plant food, as was my habit for decades. Lots of good organic fare, of course: whole grains, flax, blueberries, cashews, etc. (I gave soy the boot years ago.) Yet clearly, all this plant energy isn't supplying the synergistic nutrition my body needs. Once again I am reminded in unarguable terms what it took me years to finally admit: if I fail to eat enough animal protein by late morning, I start to feel puny, *really puny.* Lethargic and unmotivated, incapable of complex thoughts, my synapses shrinking instead of extending. What a useless state and one that happened to me frequently as a martyr veg'n. In this condition I had absolutely nothing to give to my family, nor to my students or friends. I had favored the fish and chickens instead.

Ahhh, now that's better, tremendously better. I just feasted on six ounces of delectable wild salmon, plus a kale salad with raw veggies and a hard-boiled egg. Within 20 minutes of that first fishy bite, no lie, I feel fabulous—as if every cell started singing on cue—and my brain is humming again on all eight cylinders. I am perpetually amazed just how swiftly and completely the correct portions *for me* of animal protein and fat, plus complex plant carbs, replenish my grateful body. I will digest this same meal perfectly, with no sense of heaviness, and I will be soundly, sweetly energized for a good 4-5 hours. With plants-only, including high-protein/fat fare, I do a fast-fade and need to eat every 90 minutes, indicative of inadequate cellular fuel and not even possible in many work situations. And the energy I receive is nowhere near the same as a meal anchored by fish, fowl, bison or eggs—muted and lackluster instead of brilliant and potent. It's like a light pop ditty that's quickly forgotten, versus a full-on Beethoven symphony that resonates through the cells of my body for hours on end.

I forgot what it was like to even feel this way as my no-meat years started to add up and I was laid low by a crippling lack of energy. By then I was feeling old in my 40s. Fortunately, that's also when my frustrated body accelerated its gentle whispers into a shriek. *Nourish me!*

284

SO OUT WITH GROUP MIND and in with bio-individuality. What a difference embracing this truth has made in the lives of so many who struggled with restricted or one-size-fits-all diets. The concept of bio-individuality—also called customized nutrition—derives from the perfectly rational principle, supported by 21st century biomedicine and DNA profiling, that each human is unique and fares best on a personalized diet. Nature loves diversity, and not solely for beauty's sake— although its selection for increased functionality has certainly created a planet of wildly varied beauty. Nature loves diversity because it's a really smart insurance policy for each species' continuance.

So if some of us humans, for example, get knocked out by killer bacteria in the alfalfa sprouts, we non-sprout eaters can soldier on. Same in reverse for a tainted-meat scenario. Yes, *some* of us fare quite well as vegetarians and thank goodness. Many centuries of successful lacto-vegetarianism in the East verify this reality. Unfortunately, we don't yet know how strict vegans will fare in the grand evolutionary scheme. Since biochemistry and metabolism vary considerably among individuals, I suspect that some diligently supplemented vegans will do alright on their restrictive diet, while others will die sooner than necessary.

The idea of bio-individuality is not new. American biochemist Dr. Roger J. Williams was among the first to recognize that humans differ biochemically from one another, sometimes remarkably so. And just who is this influential Williams guy you never heard of? First off, his credentials are impeccable. A member of the National Academy of Sciences, President of the American Chemical Society and Emeritus Professor of Chemistry at the University of Texas until age 92, Dr. Williams founded the prestigious Biochemical Institute in Austin, where more vitamins and their variants have been discovered than anywhere else in the world. In this day of mega-supplementing, has anyone *not* heard of folic acid or vitamin B5 (pantothenic acid)? Williams named the first and discovered the second.

In his 1956 groundbreaking book, *Biochemical Individuality: The Basis for the Genetotrophic Concept*, Williams clarifies how each of us has specific nutritional needs due to our "unique biochemical profiles," shaped by both genetics and the environment. Understanding and meeting these individual needs will encourage health and combat disease. In other words, there is no "normal person" and no "correct diet." As Williams points out: "While the same physical mechanisms and the same metabolic processes are operating in all human bodies, the structures are sufficiently diverse [that] the sum total of all the reactions taking place in one individual's body may be very different from those taking place in the body of another individual." This goes a long way in explaining why nutrition is so damn complex and confounding, and why we want to pull out our hair every time a new dietary study comes out contradicting the last. Industry-tweaked studies aside, it's likely that researchers studied metabolically diverse individuals or ethnic groups, with different or even opposing genetically-inherited dietary requirements.

Digging into the nutrition literature these days is like tumbling into the proverbial rabbit hole: it's convoluted and confusing. For every study finding a link between low-carb/high-fat and increased health, another pops up favoring more carbs/lower-fat. So after decades of debate and political backbiting, especially among diet gurus and heavily-invested food institutes, the light has clicked on and the right question is finally being asked: *Could they both be true?*

Stanford School of Medicine is taking a close look at this key question. In 2014 researchers started their second round of recruiting men and women in good health, randomly assigning them to a very low-carb or very low-fat diet of high nutritional quality. Their objective? To discover if there's a genetic component determining which individuals lose weight while increasing their health on these radically different diets. About time.

TRASHING ONE-FOR-ALL DIETS

I first encountered the concept of bio-individuality nearly ten years ago when my daughter Gabe thrust some in-depth, metabolic-typing tests in my face, following her truly bad experiences on both the raw and vegan diets. "You gotta take these tests!" she insisted, her cat-green eyes emanating excitement and vindication. "Ha! I'm not even remotely cut out to be a vegan. No wonder I felt like total crap the whole time."

In perfecting the science of metabolic typing, researchers like Dr. George Watson, Dr. Henry Bieler, and William Wolcott picked up where the gifted Dr. Williams left off. They were frustrated with the conflicting, constantly changing information streaming from the food and diet industry, always flaunting the newest and "healthiest" diet. It turns out there's no such thing as the healthiest diet. There's only *the healthiest diet for you*. And in its particulars, that "best diet" is likely different for your neighbor, your best friend, even your spouse or children.

We all take for granted that humans are measurably different on the outside, right? From facial features to skin color to body structure, the evidence is oh-so obvious. Yet we are largely ignorant of the biological diversity that exists within.

286

Just as no two people share the same fingerprints or DNA, from a physiological/metabolic perspective humans are also markedly varied and our dietary choices need to reflect this. That's why waking up one morning and thinking "I'm going to be a vegan!" is not all that rational.

Due to our individual genetic blueprint—a product of ancient and more recent adaptations by our ancestors—humans can be measurably distinctive in the way our bodies process different food and derive energy from it. When Dr. Williams studied the anatomy of real humans vs. an idealized textbook version, he discovered astounding variations in vital organs like the heart and stomach—differences in size, shape, and precise location.

The variety found in our gut is even more striking. The average length of an adult's small intestine varies enormously, from 15 to 32 feet, with disparities in diameter as well. And since its primary function is the digestion, absorption and transfer of nutrients, length and diameter are major factors when it comes to efficiency. One investigation revealed that human colon size also varies immensely, particularly among ethnic groups (Miloslavich). The average Russian studied had a colon *twice as long* as the average Turk! No surprise then: their traditional diets are drastically different as well, the former heavy on grains and the latter big on fish and olive oil.

Our gut microbes—up to a thousand different species of bacteria essential to our health—likewise vary greatly among individuals and populations groups. Food choices affect the quality of these crucial microbes (high fiber promotes diversity; high-protein reduces the bacteria associated with obesity), but how and where we live, even how we were born, also affect microflora quality. The Hadza of Tanzania, who still hunt and forage most of their food, may have the healthiest and most varied microbiome on the planet. So claims anthropologist Dr. Jeff Leach who lived among them to study their "dirty" world. Here's what the Hadza have going for them that most of us sanitized urbanites do not: they live outdoors; they don't use antibiotics; they don't drink treated water; and they were breastfed for the first two to three years of life. Every Hadza also experienced a natural birth. Moving down that narrow, harrowing birth canal is where we pick up our first good dose of healthy microbes.

Did you even know that you are more bacterial than human? Depending on the individual, your body is inhabited by anywhere from 3 to 10 times more bacterial cells than the human kind. This makes for another disparity among us because a higher number and variety of healthy gut bacteria translates to more efficient

287

digestion. "Because of the differences in our colons (and ultimately the number of bacteria in them)," writes biologist Robb Dunn for *Scientific American*, "we must also vary in how effectively we turn....hard-to-break-down plant material into fatty acids." Plant eater alert! Just how much do you know about your ancestry, colon size, and intestinal flora?

Due to our unique anatomy and biochemistry, some of us are decidedly less efficient at digesting and utilizing high-fiber foods like cruciferous vegetables, especially raw ones, as our equally unique farts display in notes of high and low, lyrical and staccato. And every one of us lacks the correct enzyme to digest plant cellulose—but watch out! Our ever-clever food industries are taking human cellulose consumption to the next evolutionary level, moving us from plant stems to tree trunks. That's right: commercial foods now contain an unprecedented amount of chemically-processed *wood pulp* as cheap filler and questionable fiber. Finely powdered trees in your morning yogurt, anyone? How about ground-up cotton stalks, i.e., industrial "gin trash," for added fiber in your salad dressing? Naturally, the USDA and Big Ag are quick to assure us that ingesting GM cotton rubbish and chemically-bleached wood pulp is perfectly safe.

Pulp fiction and mass ignorance aside, how do we know which foods are best for the individual? Specifically the irreplaceable, incomparable, one and only *you*. The best method is extensive self-observation coupled with brutal honesty. This is where a beloved ethical philosophy may need to get the boot, allowing functional physiology to take its proper place at the table. Studying the long-term health outcomes of populations eating a specific diet over many generations is also worth your time—especially if it's your own ethnic group's traditional diet.

This is the message being broadcast by the burgeoning science of nutritional genomics: your genetic inheritance plays a significant role in determining which foods will optimize your health and your life, and which are more likely to prematurely end it. That's because nutrition is one of the environmental factors—called a selective pressure—that influences gene expression. It's a complex field but the upshot is this: you are the proud owner of an individualized nutritional profile, thanks in part to your near *and* distant ancestors' food selections.

Dr. Patrick Stover of Cornell University confirms that identifying genetic variations that arose as a consequence of diet as a selective pressure "helps identify gene alleles that affect nutrient utilization." Along with the Institute of Medicine, Stover predicts a coming revolution in both public and private nutrition practices. The time will soon arrive when you will submit a saliva sample to a local lab for genetic typing and receive a detailed analysis explaining how to tailor a custom diet that aligns with your individual DNA and metabolic needs. The trouble here for ethical vegans is, of course, it may not be what they want to hear.

FOR NOW WE HAVE a cruder, cheaper, still valuable tool: metabolic typing. With this method, nutritionists are able to "type" a person's pronounced metabolic tendencies and recommend an appropriate diet. Looking at the macronutrients is one way to accomplish this. (Oxidation rates are another way; we'll look at that shortly.) Our individual needs fall along a continuum, according to the macronutrient theory. At one end of the spectrum are individuals who thrive on abundant amounts of high-protein/fatty foods like meat, fish, and dairy. At the other end are those who function at their very best when eating plenty of high-carb, low-fat foods such as fruits and grains. The nutritional needs of others are more moderate and fall somewhere in between. And if you've been paying close attention to your body's responses to different food inputs over the years, *you already know this.*

That's why all do-it-my-way dietary dogma needs to be trashed. With our new, expanding knowledge of nutrigenetics and bio-individuality, any goading toward a universal diet should now be viewed as unethical. The very same foods that fuel some diet guru's metabolic engine in a gloriously efficient manner may gradually weaken and debilitate yours. (I'm lookin' at you, Dr. Doug "Banana" Graham.) You can be eating all "healthy" foods, taking all the "right" supplements and still be undernourished and fatigued if you are deficient in the specific foods and correct proportion of macronutrients that your metabolism requires to operate at its best.

Bingo! This helps explain why the vegetarian and vegan diets so spectacularly failed me and my daughter, plus so many others I know, while some individuals are cruising right along after 15, even 20 years. Raw Vegan Man, for instance, continues to flourish on raw plants only—or so he says. Thus, for some unknown reason (altruism? egoism? desiring me-clones around the world?), he and other very vocal proponents want *all of us* to be low-protein Vegan Man or Woman. Likewise with certain high-protein Paleo Cave Men who assert that the rest of us would be smart to eat like they do. It all makes for captivating blog-fare and best-selling books, but none of them gets it exactly right: *You are an original.*

Every "one for all" diet fails to recognize this basic truth, to the detriment of many faithful followers. When you blindly jump aboard the veg, paleo, raw or

Atkins Express and fail to follow the optimal diet for your unique biochemistry—your nutritional requirements on a cellular level—you are courting likely future dysfunction. Consequently, all the ethical priests and low-protein promoters who indiscriminately encourage a vegan diet for all comers, may be sending young, naïve, high-protein types on the road to suffering and compromised health. Let's look closely at the ethics of *that,* shall we?

My daughter and I got to the dysfunction stage but thankfully, instinctively changed course before any disease process set in, pounding fish and other animal protein as if we were malnourished which, undoubtedly, we were. Regrettably, early female vegans who ate low-protein and now suffer from osteoporosis were not so fortunate. As vegan activist Reed Mangels commented online:

> I've been troubled for some time by emails from long-term vegans who are now in their 60s and have (to their shock) osteoporosis, despite weight bearing exercise and plenty of fruits and vegetables (but very low calcium, protein, and vitamin D).

This is a brave admittance on the part of Mangels because two decades prior she advised all vegans *not to worry* about their lower calcium and protein intake. "The RDAs for calcium were made for people consuming typical American high-protein diets," Mangels made clear in a 1991 *Vegetarian Times* article (Wiley). "For those whose protein intake is lower but adequate, or whose protein is from non-animal sources, calcium intakes below the RDAs are probably adequate."

Actually, probably not. But it's far too late for all those women who believed this kind of "not really sure, but just do it!" pro-vegan advice and now suffer from osteoporosis, a serious condition that thins bones, greatly increases fracture risk, and decimates lives.

THIS IS WHAT HAPPENS with novel, nonhistorical diets: biased optimism, wholly inadequate research, and potentially terrible long-term outcomes. The exact same thing happened with vitamin B12, the most complex vitamin currently known. Early vegans were told *now don't you worry your pretty head* about B12's total lack in a plant diet. Your body's stores are sufficient, advocates assured everyone: they last a long time. Uh, *no.*

Stores of vitamin B12 in a healthy liver last just a few years, according to the Linus Pauling Institute. So deficiencies began appearing en masse—over half the vegans in EPIC-Oxford suffered a B12 deficiency—and even a mild deficiency increases risk for depression, confusion, fatigue and anemia. That's because without sufficient amounts of this essential vitamin your body can't make enough red blood cells to deliver all the oxygen needed. Inadequate B12 also raises your risk for stroke, low bone mineral density and, for women, giving birth to a baby with neural tube defects. It results in high homocysteine levels as well, linked to heart disease. Even more ominous, ongoing B12 deficiency can cause permanent damage to your brain and nervous system. We are talking serious dementia.

Dismayed by the accumulating evidence, intractable vegans starting coming up with some truly bizarre proposals to reinforce their claim that humans can thrive on plants alone. *Since B12 is produced by bacteria in the colon, your body can simply absorb all that it needs!* When this inventive theory proved false, they came up with an even more peculiar/repulsive solution. *We can obtain all the necessary B12 from ingesting our feces—some animals do this, you know!* (Just be sure to kill all the bacteria and viruses first.) Anything to avoid synthetic supplementation, thereby admitting strict veganism is unnatural to humans.

Unfortunately/fortunately, the amount of active B12 from your own poop is far too limited to be of benefit. Ditto unwashed plants plucked from manure-treated soils. You would need 24+ cups of dirty spinach every day to meet your RDA. *Alright, so there's nutritional yeast!* Besides the fact that yeast is phylogenetically more related to animals than plants (researchers are using the yeast genome as a potent tool to learn more about human genes), the B12 in yeast is in the form of a non-bioavailable analogue. Ditto for fermented soy and sea vegetables: insufficient amounts of absorbable B12. Vegans, you mustn't be hard-headed about this. Without proper supplementation, you—along with your breastfed infants—are at high risk for depression and, down the road, brain damage.

Really, modern humans have two choices to ensure adequate B12 and a shot at a healthy long life. Regularly take a synthetic supplement, orally or in fortified food, or eat the natural vitamin B12 found in eggs, dairy, and animal flesh. Fish and shellfish offer it in abundance. *Again, we must ask ourselves: Is our primary responsibility to other species or to our own? To salmon or to self?* Most rational humans will arrive at the same, sane conclusion. And for those who fail to thrive on the vegan diet, this response makes more sense than ever now that we have access to 100% pastured, humanely-raised animal protein.

So if you *are* taking all the right supplements, doing everything right and still crashing on a vegan diet—while your best friend on the same regime appears to be thriving—this is likely the result of your metabolic individuality. Maybe it's time to get to know your body on a more intimate level.

WISE CHOICES OR ETHICAL COP-OUT?

"The missing link" in nutrition knowledge is what today's scientists are calling the concept of bio-individuality, the culmination of over 80 years of pioneering work by outstanding medical researchers, biochemists, physicians, and dentists. Among the early visionaries, Doctors George Watson, Weston A. Price, Roger Williams, and Francis Pottenger stand out. Watson, in particular, brilliantly diagnosed metabolically incompatible nutrition as a critical factor in not just physical health but psychological disorders. Hard to believe but in the 1960s the idea that food can affect our moods and behavior was revolutionary, even laughed at.

Valuable as their work is, these dedicated individuals are building on ancient ancestral wisdom. Every classical and enduring medical tradition recognizes the importance of human bio-individuality. Over 2,000 years ago, the Roman healer Lucretius pithily noted the obvious: "One man's food is another man's poison." For powerful proof of this concept, just look at food allergies. One person can wolf down an entire jar of Justin's yummy Honey Peanut Butter but another, inadvertently consuming a single drop of peanut oil at Jii's Thai restaurant, will go into anaphylaxis shock and may die. Poison indeed. On a less dangerous level, when my friend Jean eats exclusively plant food for her first meal of the day, she quickly fades and flounders. (No coffee to disguise the effect; caffeine gives her the jangles.) Yet my friend Trishmarie noshes on fruit and little else for breakfast but swears she feels great all morning. (Oh yeah, and she washes down four cups of coffee by noon, *no problemo*.)

When it comes to exacting dietary needs and how we process and utilize our food, intraspecies variation is so common among modern humans that it's baffling how anyone could believe that one type of diet will work for all. Here are just a few examples among hundreds: Of the six genotypes of the APOE gene, those who inherit E2 benefit most from high-fat, low-carb diets, while E4 carriers do best with low-fat, high-carb. People who inherit multiple copies of the AMY1 gene are easily able to break down bulky starch molecules into simple sugars due to abundant amylase in their saliva; others inherit *zero* AMY1 genes, making the breakdown of carbs both metabolically difficult and physiologically stressful. (Easy quiz: which of these groups will most likely suffer as vegans?)

292

Some of us are not able to absorb B12 normally, while others can't make our own taurine or carnitine and *must* derive them from animal food. Still others among us—especially those with coastal-dwelling, fish-eating ancestors—lack the proper enzymes to synthesize very-long-chain fatty acids from plants. We too must obtain them directly from animals.

While most humans produce sufficient glycine and tyrosine, specific populations are unable to synthesize these amino acids in adequate amounts. Up to 25% of us have a genetic variant that boosts our need for folate, and some individuals carry a gene variation that increases their need for choline, an essential nutrient that's already tougher to get in a vegan diet. Approximately 15% of us are allergic to nickel—abundant in nuts, soybeans and grains—while up to 50% suffer from fructose malabsorption, making many fruits taboo. *Moreover, half of us aren't able to convert plant beta-carotene into vitamin A, available only from animals.*

Individuals also vary in their ability to absorb dietary calcium, and we respond differently to dietary cholesterol as well. For a minority, total serum cholesterol rises just slightly after eating cholesterol but so does the "good" HDL cholesterol, along with a mild increase in the benign "fluffy" type of LDL. The majority of us, a solid 70%, show a rise in beneficial HDL cholesterol and no increase in LDL or total cholesterol, even if we polish off three whole eggs per day!

And those glycemic index numbers you thought were set in stone? Each is merely *an average* of hundreds of individual glycemic responses, high and low, to specific foods, e.g., some of us are much more reactive to carbohydrates. The high end of this is "carbohydrate intolerance" which induces, ironically, intense sugar cravings. Genetic polymorphisms determine this and any would-be vegan would be very wise to find out if he/she is carb intolerant. Insulin sensitivity also varies from person to person and can fluctuate over time.

There's a huge disparity in our digestive enzymes as well, greatly influencing nutrient intake values (pepsin content of gastric juice can vary a thousand fold). Food allergies and sensitivities are likewise very individual and widespread. As computational biologist Tim Triche Jr. astutely concludes, "The breadth of human genetic variation, as well as the vast amount that we simply don't know regarding metabolic intermediaries and hormonal signaling, throws an enormous monkey wrench into any blanket diet recommendation for a diverse society."

Not just food, modern pharmaceuticals also confirm Lucretius' early views on bio-individuality. The chemistry of these drugs is precise, yet they can affect individuals in completely different ways, working just fine for one while sending another, in convulsions, to the emergency room. Years ago, searching in vain for a natural sleep aid, I told my pharmacist that melatonin keeps me awake all night, as if I'd just been injected with 500 mg of caffeine. She let loose with a splendid laugh and confided that her boyfriend takes No-Doze to fall asleep.

AYURVEDIC MEDICINE HAS prescribed bio-individual nutrition for over fifty centuries—because it works. Dr. Marc Halpern, founder of the California College of Ayurveda, adamantly believes that it's erroneous and potentially harmful to offer one-diet-for-all advice to the masses. "In Ayurveda, each person is seen as an individual with unique genetics and biochemistry," he writes in *Journey into Ayurveda*. Based on the complexities of your constitution, or *dosha*, Ayurveda advises a specific diet regime to help bring you into full health.

"This avoids the Everybody Must syndrome that infiltrates many systems of healing," Halpern claims. "Ayurveda vehemently disagrees with this notion and subscribes to the philosophy that 'nothing is right for everyone and everything is right for someone'....some benefit from hot, spicy food while others from milder or bland foods. Some people need the nourishment of sweet-tasting grains and others the cleansing qualities of bitters....some people benefit from meat while others thrive as vegetarians."

For over 2,500 years, Traditional Chinese Medicine has similarly advocated individualized nutrition counseling. Animal flesh is recognized for its healing and strengthening properties, while a raw or plants-only diet may be prescribed during illness or for brief periods of cleansing. Eat in harmony with your constitution and life situation, this ancient tradition teaches, and your body will respond with increased health. Balance is the goal and flexibility is the key.

"Let your food be your medicine," Hippocrates affirmed more than 2,000 years ago and in 13th century Persia, the poet Rumi tells us, citizens were served "special plates" according to their unique dietary needs. Modern humans, by contrast, consume whatever has the slickest advertising and hottest babe promoting it. Meanwhile, our medical doctors rarely even inquire about diet because they know so very little. Yet as Hippocrates admonished, "Foolish the doctor who despises knowledge acquired by the ancients."

From ancient healing wisdom to the emerging field of nutritional genomics, the empirical evidence supporting individualized nutrition versus mob diets is unassailable. Regrettably, I was still in the rigid throes of ethical vegetarianism when I first heard about bio-individuality, not yet ready to break loose and self-explore. Years later, healed by animal-sourced food, I took the metabolic tests out of curiosity, wondering if the results would match up with my own hard-earned, real-life conclusions. They did—uncannily so.

The tests confirmed what I had painstakingly deduced over the years by finally listening to my body: I am a high-protein, fast-oxidizing type. For optimal health I need to eat approximately 35% protein at every meal. That's a lot for a small woman, but that's who I am and that's what I need. My health is now excellent. My cup runneth over with energy and love. My blood panels are impressive and I maintain my ideal weight through the years. The best proteins for me are high in purine, available only in animal flesh and organs. As a veg'n, I was doing myself great harm, eating *the exact opposite* of a healthy diet for my biochemistry.

Everything rapidly shifted from "did I cop out of my ethics?" to its legitimate, comprehensible place. Suddenly explicable was the inhaling of salmon that went down like honey from the gods, the lavish spreading of bright yellow ghee. When I learned the ancestral diet of the Irish has always been high in buttermilk, cheese, and fatty fish, everything clicked: my Celtic ancestry, my body's affirmative response to fish and dairy, and my high-fat/low-carb needs.* (The Irish also have high celiac rates as their ancestors ate oats, not wheat.) "They have a hereditary need for more fat than other populations," confirms William Wolcott in *The Metabolic Typing Diet*, further noting that, remarkably, the low-fat diet that lowers heart disease in the Bantu tribes of Africa can *increase* risk for people of Anglo-Saxon descent. It was at that moment I sorely wished I had known about my ancestral influences and genetic dictates as an idealistic, albeit ignorant teen.

Diving into vegetarianism at a young age and continuing this carb-dominant diet for two decades was the worst dietary choice I could have possibly made—except, of course, if I had become a vegan instead. I did it for the animals. I did it for their dignity, for their rights and their lives. I didn't realize that in so doing, I was sacrificing my own right to cellular efficiency and a long and healthy life.

THE WARM ENGINE OF YOUR BODY

So you take a metabolic-typing test and discover you're a carb type. Fabulous! This means you are a slow oxidizer who might do fine as a vegetarian—or even a

---

*"Each one of our genetic ancestors faced the same challenge—survival," states Sharon Moalem, MD, author of *The DNA Restart: Eat for Your Genes*. "The results of each of these struggles are encoded in our genes today. A simple example is if you can enjoy dairy products as an adult, then it's a sign that your ancestors kept animals in order to drink their milk and they gave you the genetics to do so as well."

vegan—maybe for the rest of your life if you eat broadly and supplement wisely. But you already know this because you feel great on a high-carb plant diet. Since you metabolize food slowly, you have a natural aversion to sizeable amounts of protein and fat. Perchance that's why you keep insisting that *everybody* should switch to a vegan diet? Yes yes, it works for you and others like you with low-protein/high-carb needs; now stifle the sermonizing and read on.

Categorizing individuals by oxidation rate—the speed at which you convert food into energy—was first accomplished by Dr. George Watson, a distinguished UCLA researcher who discovered two major metabolic types among humans, fast and slow oxidizers. (Normal and under-oxidizers are out there but less common.) In addition to finding a disparity in CO_2 levels, Watson discovered that the blood pH of these two major types differ greatly, fast-oxidizers being more acidic. He also realized that the kinds of food benefiting each type were radically different. Once his subjects began eating the correct food and macronutrient proportions for their type, physical and emotional improvements were dramatic—much like Drs. Douillard and Klaper discovered when their "failing to thrive" vegan patients started ingesting animal sourced food.

Those ex-vegans were no doubt fast-oxidizers, exactly like my daughter and myself. This means we burn through food *fast*, tend to be thin and can lose weight very easily—even when we don't want to. Research reveals that it's fatty foods and the more dense proteins that effectively slow our rapid oxidative rates, so we need a high proportion of both at every meal. Good sources of fat like coconut and avocados are out there, so why can't fast-oxidizers just fulfill their high-protein requirements with plants as well?

Here's why: despite what vegans want to believe, there are fundamental differences between animal and plant proteins that affect us at the cellular level, and it's our individual metabolic activity at the cellular level that delivers us to full health or condemns us to dysfunction and disease. Besides the fact that animal proteins contain all the essential amino acids in the correct ratios, high-purine proteins are available from animals only, and protein types require high-purine foods due to our rapid cellular oxidation rates. Aha! During all those draggy, over-supplemented veg'n years, I always felt there *must* exist yet another mysterious X factor in animal food that just isn't in plants. And now I know for certain.

So what's this purine stuff anyway, you rightly ask, and why is it so critical? In brief, purines are aromatic organic compounds and the building-blocks of DNA and RNA, nucleoproteins carefully encoded with our genetic information.

Purine-containing nucleoproteins play a vital role in energy production and the upshot is this: those of us who metabolize food quickly need *a whole lot* of high-purine protein, along with plentiful fat, to slow down this conversion and produce sustained energy. We do poorly with high-carb meals. In fact, they are terrible for us; we can't handle how speedily this food is converted into energy. Fast oxidizers race through carbs so rapidly we're very soon hungry again, and eating this way translates into swiftly plummeting levels of energy, strength, and stamina.

Fast oxidizers need to *minimize* consumption of foods like fruits, veggies, and grains. Drink a glass of orange juice first thing in the morning and we feel like going back to bed. A bowl of fresh strawberries mid-afternoon and we're ready for a nap. Even the low-glycemic carbs should be eaten in moderation and never alone. Instead, we need to focus on high-purine protein, found only in animal sources. This is a metabolic truth that took years, even decades for fast-oxidizing ex-veg'ns to comprehend: *high-purine animal foods are converted into energy at the proper rate for our metabolic engines.*

These unique proteins work to build and sustain our health in a way that low-purine plant proteins simply cannot. This explains the feeling of raging appetite and listless energy many of us feel as we try to go about our day eating primarily plant foods, however high in quality, quantity, and variety. It's a very real hunger of the body at a cellular level, a hunger that never seems to go away. As "Kali" affirms, when she switched to a high-protein, high-fat diet she established her ideal weight and felt tremendous.

> But all my friends and family would yell at me that I was going to die of a heart attack because of how I ate. They believe in a low-fat diet because that's what they've always been told. But when I eat like that I'm starving all day long. When I eat high protein, high fat, the starvation goes away and so does the brain fog, insomnia, and aches and pains. I have tons more energy and can prove to my family that my way of eating is right for me!

Individuals who oxidize food quickly like Kali need a high-purine protein at almost every meal. Low-purine proteins like dairy and legumes are okay but not a substitute. These people will notice that when lower-purine foods are the primary protein source, their performance and energy will start to drag. On the other hand, incorporating the higher-purines into their meals on a daily basis will supercharge their body with the ideal fuel for their metabolic engines. Vroom! Vroom!

Here are the protein foods high in purine, every one of them from animals: sardines, herring, mussel, anchovy, caviar, kidney, liver, all organ meats, bison and wild game. *There are no high-purine plant foods.* Medium-purine foods from animals include beef, chicken, turkey, duck, geese, salmon, mackerel, shrimp, abalone, oyster, scallops and dark tuna. The only medium-purine plant foods are beans and lentils. However, protein types who can handle legumes should eat them in addition to, not as a substitute for, the high purine in animal food.

Low-purine plant foods include tofu and tempeh (more legumes), while low-purine animal foods are eggs and dairy. All these are good protein sources but ineffective compared to high-purine animal food in providing sustained, vibrant energy to high oxidizers. Ample amounts of nuts, seeds, butter and healthy oils work well for this metabolic type also, due to its high-fat requirements. But for a top-quality, all-in-one fat/protein/high-purine package, wild fish, wild game, and pastured bison deliver like nothing else.

To sum it all up: fast-oxidizing protein types have strong appetites; metabolize food rapidly; require meals that deliver high-purine animal protein and ample fat for sustained energy; tend to do well in cool climates; *and have no good business being a vegan.* We have a lower tolerance for carbs—even healthy complex carbs—and a dismal tolerance for sweets, alcohol, and caffeine. When fast oxidizers drink alcohol, a simple sugar, it's like tossing gasoline on your metabolic fire, according to William Wolcott, due to its "superfast conversion to energy instead of steady and prolonged like you need." (Although a few sips at your cousin's wedding won't kill you.) Your ideal macronutrient ratio is approximately 35% protein, 30% fat, and just 35% carbs.

And that daily shot or two of coffee? If you're addicted, let's hope you're not a fast-burning protein type. Turns out that caffeine speeds up oxidation rates even further, creating additional imbalance. Furthermore, your caffeine-excited brain triggers your adrenal glands to produce more adrenalin, a pleasurable stimulation for sure, but over time your adrenals will become exhausted—and so will you.

WHAT ABOUT CARB TYPES? This is the ideal metabolic type for all you vegans out there still reading this book. (The rest have shredded it into a pulpy additive.) Carb types tend to be slower oxidizers with lighter appetites. You're the kind who can go all morning on a granola bar and a cup of thick, black coffee. My ex, the ever adventurous, globe-trotting Larry, used to drive me nuts with all the dried fruit and grains he'd pack for our wilderness trips, meals that revved him for hours but sent me promptly crashing. Eventually I started bringing mini-cans of salmon and sardines to begin each day. Then, and only then, did I enjoy abundant and sustained energy on our long canoe journeys.

If you're a high-carb type like Larry and metabolize food slowly, you need to *avoid* meals heavy in protein and fat, which will knock you off-balance and make you feel sluggish. You should also stay away from purine-rich foods because they will further slow your oxidation rate. Choose proteins like garbanzo beans, seeds, trout, and white meat poultry. Avoid dark and red meats with their higher purine content. (Anyone with kidney stones or gout should avoid high purine foods as well.) Good fats for slow oxidizers include olive, flax, coconut, and unsalted nuts. Leaving out high-fat dairy also works to your advantage.

The ideal meal proportions for a slow-oxidizer are approximately 20% protein, 20% fat and 60% carbs, with a high tolerance for sweets and caffeine. You're the lucky folks who can gobble up cherry cheesecake and swill Kahlua-spiked coffee post-dinner and still sleep sweetly through the night. You look at us funny when we divulge that we had to quit caffeine because it drained our energy by day and tore up our sleep by night.

Because high-carb types can more easily handle increased carb loads, they are credible candidates for the veg'n lifestyle. And like Raw Vegan Man tending his orchids in Hawaii, they're apt to do well in warm climates. *Is this all starting to make sense or what?*

Mixed types fall somewhere between carb and protein types on the metabolic spectrum. Your dietary needs exist betwixt and between as well, depending on your ancestry (which is often mixed) and unique biochemistry. You might do alright as a vegetarian or vegan, but then again, you might not. Mixed types need to monitor the physiological and emotional effects of a chosen diet very closely.

It gets fairly complicated but four key systems determine your metabolic type and whether you will thrive or take a dive as a vegan: oxidation rate; catabolic and anabolic balance; autonomic nervous system; and endocrine system. Differences in these systems among individuals are by and large genetically inherited and not a matter of choice. Lifestyle, aging, and the environment also factor in. Read Williams' and Watson's superb books if you're intrigued by the science and clinical research behind metabolic typing, but here's the bottom line for all you fast-burning, high-protein types out there trying to survive on a veg'n diet: If you consistently feel lethargic and flat, or hungry and restless after a "nutritious" high-plant meal, your corporal self is straight away trying to tell you: *Sorry babe, you're pumping the wrong kind of fuel into your body's warm engine.*

Your metabolic engine doesn't care about your animal ethics or environmental philosophy; it just needs the right fuel to efficiently convert food into energy. So whether you need more protein, higher purine, more fat or more carbs, when you finally figure out the proper type and blend of fuel for your unique self, you will 100% sure-fire know it! You'll feel energized and emotionally balanced, maintain your proper weight, enjoy strong immunity, and age slowly and beautifully.

Continue to eat the wrong diet for your constitution and you risk a slow spiraling downward into the low-energy dumps: increasing fatigue, slower cognition, faster aging, and decreased quality of life. Will you be as capable of giving back to the world in this compromised state? No you will not. By learning about my metabolic type earlier, I could have saved myself years of fading energy and self-absorption as a righteous vegetarian who had shut herself off from deeper inquiry. Yet in figuring out this hard-earned knowledge by myself—which foods fuel me, lift me and sustain me—what I gained was invaluable and liberating: an intuitive, finely-tuned body/mind which now listens very closely, conscious of the least whispering that something is off, and shrewdly recognizing when everything is humming along in perfect balance.

So go ahead and take a professional nutritionist's metabolic-typing test (plus DNA testing if available), but it won't tell you everything. What's also important is to start listening to your own discerning body and its ancient, ancestral wisdom. For you are much more than a type—be it high-protein, high-carb, or something in between—you are an extraordinary individual whose genetic inheritance and dietary needs are complex and multi-faceted, and no vegan preacher or paleo pusher should be telling you how to eat.

35.

SNIFFING LIKE A BLACK BEAR

Intuitive eating is as sweet as it gets. Nourishing the body
with the best version of what it is asking for.

—Sara Courter

To INSTINCTIVELY KNOW the healthiest foods for you, how much to consume and in what proportions, you must do one simple thing: *pay attention*. You must transform into the perceptive human animal that you were always meant to be, employing your full awareness and entire palette of glorious senses. Just like the curious black bear sniffing and woofing outside our wilderness cabin, knowing which high-carb berries to pluck with her nimble lips and the precise afternoon they'll be perfectly ripe. Just like this same canyon's solitary cougar, stalking his mobile, protein-dense feast just after dusk when the pickings are best.

Wild animals don't need some diet guru or flashy Madison Avenue ad to tell them what to eat, which foods will build their strength and make their metabolic engines purr with delight. Their shrewd bodies don't develop insulin resistance, diabetes, or cardiovascular disease either. Animals are so much smarter food-wise than we are because there aren't any head trips or belief systems getting in the way of their intuitive choices. As well, they know instinctively which foods to avoid because they are weakening, poisoning, or simply lacking in the correct nutrients to fuel their powerful engines.

Are you ready to pay attention to your own intelligent body, your own animal wisdom? To discover the best foods for your specific nutritional needs? It's really just one smooth instinctual process: mindfulness, observation, and assessment (yea or nay). But far too many of us in this head-led culture of dietary priests and glossy advertising have simply stopped paying attention to our very own body's clear messages. But guess what? The guru is you.

Mindfulness means being fully and silently present to the moment, with a non-judgmental, non-dogmatic mind. Even if it's your thousandth pea-protein burger or first bite of red meat in 30 years, you must be present: from your initial curious sniff all the way to that food's final elimination, and everything that lies between: tongue, mouth, esophagus, stomach, gut, and obliging arsehole. Your instinctual body will tell you everything that you need to know. *Listen to what your body is telling you.*

However, the more passionate a vegan, vegetarian, or beef eater you are, the more you will need to ratchet up your courage and get your meddling mind out of the way. Bring curiosity to your observations. Bring kindness. Your body is its own miniature ecosystem, complicated in its workings and specific in its needs. Choose to be an impartial witness to what is being revealed.

FIRST OFF, ASK YOURSELF: Am I even hungry? Is the food I've selected fresh? Is it as whole, sustainably produced, and cruelty-free as possible? If you can answer yes to all these questions, you are ready to proceed with the remarkable spiritual experience that occurs—whether you are aware of it or not—every single time you partake of the gift of earthly food to nourish your body and extend your life.

Start your new experience of food with something simple but full-throttle, like high-fat sour yogurt or an orange-fleshed potato splattered with pungent ginger. How about fresh-caught, salt-crusted trout with some face-skewing bitter kale? Observe everything you can about this compact life force you are about to ingest: its aroma, color, shape, texture and temperature, even its sounds (hissing like a stew or silent as an eggplant). Use your nose, eyes, ears and supple hands to revel in the sustenance before you. Contemplate its source, plant or animal, and express genuine thankfulness for the gift of its life.

Now close your eyes to sharpen your sense of smell as you bring the chosen edible to your discriminating nose. Already, there will be clear signals of pleasure or distaste. But if everything feels just right and in no way wrong, notice your excited salivating glands, your attentive inner mouth, teeth and soft palate, all patiently waiting to do service. As you grind, sip, or rip into that dead plant or animal, notice everything you can about this particular victual now inside your corporal being. Push it around your oral cavity with an assiduous tongue as you start to masticate—10,000 receptive taste buds zooming vital information to the gustatory cortex area of your brain.

Unless you just got shot up by the dentist, chew evenly on both sides of your mouth, noticing the sense of imbalance when you use one side only. Observe your speed. *Now slow it down!* Savor this food's unique flavor; let it insinuate, flow, explode into your awareness. Gnaw each morsel so thoroughly, it's rendered soft or even liquefied, increasing nutrient intake and aiding digestion. Now bring this pliant mush, once a sturdy living thing, to the very back of your jawbone, to your open throat, the gateway to your inner body—the very same entryway that caused Krishna's mother to gasp in divine awe as she gazed into her baby's open mouth and glimpsed the entire universe, the earth and stars and all creation.

Your mouth is a sacred cavity, a holy hollow, the place where eater and eaten first mingle before merging as one. And we could all use some of that divine awe when it comes to contemplating the plants and animals that nourish us every day of our lives. So go ahead, mindfully swallow this soft, life-giving tissue. Then ask yourself two essential questions: Do I feel good about eating this life form? Is my astute body still flashing the all-go signal?

As you become your own authority in food awareness, you will begin to notice more and more subtleties of sensation, hints, and disclosures. Pay attention to anything not feeling "just right" during the entire process. Your body will tell you when something is wrong, but almost all of us chug-a-lug so quickly, even whole chunks of food, that we miss every cue.

Eat, therefore, like a practicing Buddhist. Zen Master Thich Nhat Hanh recommends 30 chews per bite, done in silence. Do this and you'll notice anything off-base in terms of taste, ripeness, and compatibility. Possible negative reactions include a sudden drop in energy, burping, spontaneous halting of the chomping, even a strong desire to spit the food out. This sounds incredibly obvious, and it is. Yet we tend to eat our food so mindlessly in this culture—while blog-surfing or talking non-stop—that we're often oblivious to our body's most primal messages.

I've seen people gulp down spoiled or tainted food, or just way too much food, with great regret when the result was indigestion or even food poisoning. My ex, skinny Larry, who always eats crazy-fast, once scarfed down highly poisonous mushrooms, unwittingly served with dinner during a trekking trip in Kenya. He was deathly sick for days, not sure if he would even make it. Yet the campers who first smelled, slowly chewed, and then promptly spit the toxic mushrooms out were wisely listening to their bodies' first critical signals of "somethin' ain't right here." So the first act of mindfulness in all areas of life is this: *Slow Down.* Smell the roses *and* the mushrooms.

Once swallowed, your food will continue to communicate all along the gut, in obvious language, whether it serves or disserves you. Your metabolic experience will be silent, satisfying and empowering—or wholly unsatisfying and weakening—or something in between. These messages can be discerned for many hours after a meal, *if* you are present and listening. Do you feel an exhilarating sense of rising energy after eating certain foods? Or a power suck instead? Or maybe it's a fantastic rush that doesn't last and ends with an energy drain, a punch of lethargy. Do you feel cognitively sharp after eating that high-carb or high-protein meal? Or spacey and dull?

Check your body's response to a single food or meal after a few minutes, 30 minutes, and every hour thereafter. Pay attention to any negative reactions like bloating, fatigue, depression, muscle weakness, or your brain evaporating. If you've eaten the right food and correct amount for your unique metabolism, you should experience none of these impairments—just excellent, sustained energy for a good 3-5 hours after a meal. Because you've selected the right fuel mix for your metabolism, this translates into a growing sense of calmness and well-being, a strong motivation to get to work or play, and a keen desire to live your life to the fullest, *starting right now*.

Consider keeping a daily journal so you can pinpoint the exact foods and combinations that fail you. If you feel hungry or tired remarkably less than four hours after a complete meal, you are eating the wrong food. The ex-veg'ns that I interviewed felt hungry nearly all the time, or within an hour of every meal, and often jaggedly hungry—no matter the types of plant foods eaten, what combo, or how much. When the hunger set in, most of them didn't feel motivated to do anything until they ate yet again.

ONCE YOU BEAR WITNESS to your body's personal truth that you should or shouldn't be a meat or dairy consumer, vegan or vegetarian, don't think that's the end of the story. Your body is always changing with time and the shifting circumstances of your life. On an atomic level, your body changes very quickly. "Notice how each particle moves," Rumi uncannily intuited eight centuries before science discovered that your body's atoms are constantly on the go, from skin cells to blood cells, 98% of them replaced every year. Did you know your stomach lining lasts just five days? That you grow a new skin every month? Even your bones are constantly being broken down and replaced. Extreme makeover indeed.

"The body is maintained in a dynamic equilibrium between in-built destructive and constructive processes," contends science writer Steve Grand. "If it weren't, then it couldn't adapt, and adaptation is the name of the game." Who knows? I might be able to revisit my lacto-veg diet in later years, and by the time he hits fifty, Vegan Thug may be eating wild game every night for supper. "Although you were born with a specific set of dietary requirements dictated by your genetic heritage, your needs can shift," concurs William Wolcott, citing aging, stress and lifestyle changes as reasons you may need to modify a well-loved diet. "Where metabolism is concerned, everything is highly individualized and continually in flux." This is where paying close attention to the wisdom of your own body—and being willing to adapt and change—will serve you well as you move gracefully through the years. A fixed idea about the "right" diet will not.

Some might view this self-responsibility, this unplugging from group mind as a liability, not a liberation. Isn't there enough existential burden of choice in our hyped-up 21st century lives? Why not make everything so much easier and just go with the latest diet obsession or whatever's trending? *Why not?* Why not abdicate your personal power? Why not ignore your own insights when it comes to food and all your choices in life? Here's why not: because your health will likely falter and your spirit will surely die.

Wise choices lead to self-empowerment in all areas of life and your diet is no exception. Understanding your body's marvelous individuality, including how it metabolizes food, will bring you increased energy and stamina—and a greater shot at happiness. Therefore, be flexible through the changes in your life and steer away from righteous, uncompromising philosophies and "everybody must" diets. A rigid perfectionism is not a healthy way to eat, live, or die.

Sages throughout the ages—Aristotle, Confucius, Buddha—understood that extremism destroys health, happiness, and harmony. In his first discourse of the Pali Canon, the Buddha describes the concept of The Middle Way: a path that leads to self-awakening and the cessation of suffering. By encouraging moderation in how we live, The Middle Way rejects the extremes of both austerity and sensual indulgence. Austerity, in particular, the Buddha called addictive, painful, and unworthy. Long-suffering vegans who finally quit would surely agree.

Early Chinese civilization was able to absorb Buddhism due to its stability and maturity, according to philosopher Alan Watts, who describes this society as reasonable, non-fanatical, and humanistic: "Humanness or human-heartedness was always felt to be superior to righteousness." Reasonable men and women are capable of compromise, Watts affirms; however, those "who have dehumanized themselves by becoming the blind worshipers of an idea or an ideal are fanatics whose devotion to abstractions makes them the enemies of life."

As we mature and become more attuned to our body/mind and increasingly smart in our life choices—including food and diet—we embrace functional truth versus beautiful theories and ideals. We go with what delivers full health and happiness. We go with what works.

36.

THE BUDDHA ATE MEAT

ETHICAL VEGANS ARE PROUD of their non-participation in the suffering of animals. Non-harm, *ahimsa,* is the principle that they live by. *Nothing had to die for my dinner.* They are fooling themselves, of course. It's a big purer-than-thou vegan lie. To do no harm on this earthly plane is not possible. If you live, you kill. If you eat, you kill. Either that or you let others do the killing for you. It's part of the bargain you struck the moment you were born into physical form. Welcome to samsara.

Practicing Buddhists understand and accept that our fleeting world contains much suffering, with each of us both giver and taker of sorrow. They don't try to hedge or tiptoe around this earthly reality. The Sanskrit word *samsara* means "continuous flow," the cycle of birth, death, and rebirth to which all of us in the material world are bound. Pain and distress attend our biological existence on this spinning planet, and according to Buddhist thought we will revisit existence again and again in ever new and fascinating forms until we are finally conscious of our true nature. Participating in this organic stew of life, these transmutations from one life form into another—eater into eaten—means exactly this: one creature's suffering and death is another's sustenance and joy.

Satisfaction is what a crab feels as it hunts down and devours those adorable just-hatched turtles frantically scuttling toward the sea. Likewise when the eagle or the fisherman eat lustily of this same crab to build the marrow of their bones and the platelets of their blood. "Life is everything eating everything else," as James Joyce succinctly reminds us. This fundamental truth may explain why most Buddhists are not vegetarians. They are realists who see life clearly, including our own transitory existence in the all creating, all destroying web of life.

Years ago, still loathing animal flesh, I attended a Tibetan Buddhist retreat high in the Rockies and was stunned to discover beef or chicken as the primary dish for lunch and dinner, without exception—and with no contrition. The smiling Tibetan monks in spice-colored robes were digging in with gusto. Venerable Shravasti Dhammika explains:

> Vegetarianism was not a part of the early Buddhist tradition and the Buddha himself was not a vegetarian. The Buddha got his food either by going on alms rounds or by being invited to the houses of his supporters, and in both cases he ate what he was given. Before his enlightenment he had experimented with various diets including a meatless diet, but he eventually abandoned them believing that they did not contribute to spiritual development.

The Sutta Nipata scripture, part of the Pali Canon of Theravada Buddhism, speaks to this, declaring it is spiritual immorality that makes one impure, not the eating of meat. "The Buddha is often described as eating meat," Dhammika confirms. "He recommended meat broth as a cure for certain types of illness and advised monks for practical reasons to avoid certain types of meat, implying that other types were quite acceptable."

But I am not Buddhist, you say, nor a misguided monk. Believe me, I understand your refusal to contribute to the killing of sentient creatures. But even if you repudiate the eating of animals, you are killing animals by proxy at every meal. Consider the field mice, pheasants, snakes and tender young rabbits—all of the innocent wild beings diced and sliced by the tiller that prepares the soil for your favorite grains, vegetables, and legumes. Or shredded and beheaded by the giant harvester that helps to deliver your beloved blue corn chips and basmati rice.

Do these smaller creatures not feel pain and suffering? Describing "the green waterfall" of frogs and anoles desperately trying to escape his combine, one farmer states that on some days the verdant cascade of animal bodies is just a shower. Other days, especially during the wet season, it turns into "a deluge," total carnage, estimated at a few thousand dead bodies per acre. Frog pâté.

In *Prodigal Summer,* Barbara Kingsolver chillingly describes more killings: "I've watched enough harvests to know that cutting a wheat field amounts to more decapitated bunnies under the combine than you would believe." Vividly she depicts "the matted grey fur, the gleaming jaw bone and shock of scattered teeth" of the raccoon she found chopped up by the mower. It's impossible to know exactly how many wild animals are slain in our fields of crops for human consumption. Historically these creatures have been viewed as expendable and no one bothered to count. Recent research, however, reveals a bloodbath.

"Meat eating is murder!" the self-delusional PETA gangs cry out, hiding their own blood-stained hands from the public. According to their own rules, you don't have to be present at the killings that put food in your belly—or even be aware of them—to be morally implicated. Steven Davis, who grew up on a farm, is very aware of the animal sacrifices involved in bringing plant food to our tables. "I remember riding on farm equipment and seeing mice, gophers, and pheasants that were injured or killed every time we worked the fields," writes Davis, former head of Animal Husbandry at Oregon State University.

Although we can't know the exact number wiped out, we do know that the more times a crop field is visited, as in today's intensive Big Ag operations— plowing, disking, harrowing, planting, cultivating, recurring pesticide/herbicide applications, and harvesting—the more animals are fatally thrashed. Estimated mortality rate is 52% to 77% for all vertebrate animals present during *just one* of these farm operations, harvesting (Tew and Macdonald; S. Davis; Edge; Nass). Based on these and other studies, Davis conservatively estimates 1.8 billion wild animals would be killed annually if all our currently cultivated US croplands were used to grow plants to feed people only, Big Ag-style.

This is where vegans who are even aware of these mass killings want to talk "least harm." They want to talk numbers. Ethics devolved into arithmetic. Alright, alright, some vegans are now willing to admit, we're ALL killing animals in order to eat, but who is killing the MOST? Omnivores are responsible for an estimated 10.2 billion domestic land animal deaths per year in the States alone, plant eaters point out. Therefore, in accord with the principle of least harm, the morally correct path will always be veganism.

Not necessarily. First off, none of those billion-plus wild animals slaughtered in industrial plant fields feed hungry humans; domesticated farm animals do. Second, 98% of our current US food animals are poultry. If we gradually moved to the larger foraging mammals only, as proposed by Davis, and raised them on their natural diet of 100% grass using a no-till, pasture-forage model, this might mean *fewer* total animals killed (domestic and wild) than in the all-vegan model. Let's give this intriguing idea a closer look.

ACCORDING TO THE USDA, 31.9 *million* cattle (not billion) were killed for food in the US in 2013. This amounts to 25.8 billion pounds of food available to 320 million Americans, or over 80 pounds of protein-dense beef per individual. As most beef cuts offer 7 grams protein per ounce, this translates to over 9,000 grams of complete protein for every man, woman, and child in the US, thus allowing 25 grams of daily animal protein for every American all year long—more for adults, actually, as infants and children require 20-50% less. (Additional protein could be obtained from organic, non-industrial plants, plus locally pastured eggs/dairy when available.) Again, this diet is achieved with *32 million* domestic animals vs. 1.8 *billion* wild animals killed in our commercial croplands. (Around 1.2 billion, minus acreage presently used for animal feed.) Because a typical grass-fed steer offers more than 400 pounds of quality meat, this diet represents just 1/5 of *one* large foraging animal per person per year.

In the US and worldwide, a huge amount of grazing land for these foragers is already available (even factory animals spend the first 40% of their lives in open fields), and it's often the steeper terrain and drylands that aren't suitable for crop production anyway. In addition, grasslands currently razed to grow animal feed could convert back to their healthy natural state—which historically has always included large herbivores—allowing for additional human-targeted protein. And because no-till land grazed by herbivores means minimal collateral deaths as compared to Big Ag's intensive crop production, in this model the more industrial plant food a person consumes, the more animal deaths are represented.

No-till grazing, in fact, *increases* wild animal populations. Suzanne, who lived on a small farm in South Africa unsuitable for cultivation (shallow soil, hardpan, marginal rainfall), put her efforts into restoring the natural grassland. Eventually it provided "an amazing amount of food in the form of eggs, milk, and meat," she testifies in *Flesh is Grass*. Moreover, "there's very little collateral killing when land is in perennial pasture [and] year by year I saw the wildlife on my property increase both in numbers and in variety." Ecologists are in accord: "The predominant feeling among wildlife ecologists is that no-till agriculture will have broadly positive effects on mammalian wildlife" populations (Wooley).

The vegan claim to least harm also presumes that Davis's original collateral death estimates for Big Ag food production are on target, numbers gathered by a few academics from a limited number of studies of short duration, often involving just rodents and only one operation (harvesting). Talk to real farmers who are out in the industrial fields day in and day out, year after year, and we begin to comprehend that these wild animal deaths have been largely underestimated. "When I inquired about the lives lost on a mechanized farm, I realized what costs we all pay at the supermarket," laments Ted Kerasote in *Bloodties*. "One Oregon farmer told me that half the cottontail rabbits went into his combine when he cut a wheat field, that virtually all the small mammals, ground birds, and reptiles were killed when he harvested his crops."

Another experienced farmer responds to veg'ns who believe their diet saves animals or is less cruel than an omnivore's diet: "Modern, large-scale cereal grain production comes at a minimum cost of several deaths per pound, whereas grass-fed meat production, whether from production agriculture or hunting, is counted at several pounds per death," contends this veteran Texas agriculturist. "Anyone who believes that by eating a pound of pasta instead of a pound of venison they are 'saving a life' is delusional." (Aware of threats of violence to individuals who question the moral supremacy of veganism, this farmer and others chose not to publicize their names.) These conclusions are based on years of on-the-ground observations and data collection while driving tractors, combines, and harvesters many thousands of miles for plant agribusiness (primarily rice operations), as well as personal interviews with other farmers. They represent an extension and refinement of an earlier case study and are offered to all consumers "who favor responsibility and information."

Rice feeds humans, not animals. It feeds a whole lot of vegans and vegetarians. The truth is we will never know the precise number of sentient beings killed in each machine-ready field of human-targeted rice, wheat, canola, veggies or legumes. Animal density varies considerably with the crop, location, and water availability. Even tractor-driving farmers cannot witness all the casualties from their high perch, but they witness plenty just the same.

SO WHO EXACTLY is suffering and dying for our easily acquired human plant foods? Take a deep breath and read on. Vertebrate deaths recorded by scientists and farmers include (but are not limited to): voles, shrews, turtles, frogs, snakes, lizards, hares, skunks, pigeons, pheasants, quails, muskrats, mice, rats, possums, raccoons, egrets, sparrows and starlings—these comprise "the regulars"—along with the less frequent mallards, coots, teals, ducks, herons, crows and hawks. Also reported minced are the occasional fawns and lost dogs and cats. The majority are amphibians, rodents, and insectivores (insect-eating carnivores), with the last two in particular getting badly hammered.

311

Sorry to further shake vegans awake but, if you insist on playing the numbers game, these billions of sliced-up deaths credited to plant eaters don't include all the animals crushed and blended into the dirt by the titanic tires of these rolling industrial machines. Don't believe it? Ever stood next to one of these monsters? Let alone climbed up and straddled one? (And in the wide-open US breadbasket, sorry, but there are no forests where animals "run and hide" as some vegans long to believe.) Nor do these figures include additional vertebrates killed by poisons, traps and other cruel methods, either in the field or during transportation and storage of our human-targeted food.

It's impossible to know how high the numbers. And for the moment, we will *dis*-count the billions of insects and other small invertebrates killed by pesticides or botanical sprays in order to gain our grains and greens, nuts and fruits, because most plant eaters maintain that these lives "don't count."

If you're doing it for the animals, you need to look at these enormous figures without shutting down your mind. We can't calculate the exact death toll for each pound of Big Ag food ingested by humans, but we can arrive at reasonable estimates. Just one pound of rice, according to an experienced cultivator, represents several sentient creatures killed over the course of its production, storage, and transport. Compare that to 200 pounds of nutrient-dense, boneless meat for just one sentient animal killed, a large game species such as an elk, or 400-500 pounds from a pasture-raised (no grains) beef cattle. Then add in all the nutrient-rich vital organs and bones, and you can feed *several hundred humans a meal of top-quality protein/fat/mineral-rich food from just one animal*—versus only five humans sharing a pound of rice, say one bowl each, representing several dead animals (and minimal protein). And since least-harm vegans are so into numbers, how about an entire Alaskan community being fed for a full year on the protein from a single bowhead whale?

What's more, unlike commercial plant agriculture, wild mammals and 100% pastured domestic herbivores entail no wholesale clearing/scraping of the land. Quite the opposite: these roaming animals *require* healthy landscapes to thrive. According to the least harm theory, it is clear what our moral choice should be. Is it time for ethical vegans to break out the bow instead of the bowl?

Behind every meaty meal is an absence, the death of an animal, writes Carol Adams in *The Sexual Politics of Meat*. But when will she and other vegetarians and vegans finally own up to their own "absent referent" each and every time they sit down to take nourishment and pleasure from a meal? When will they

312

acknowledge their own ignorance or daily disregard for all these invisible wild animals butchered in the fields?

These unseen beings have been passed over and discounted by plant eaters just as surely as they accuse meat eaters of discounting the lives of unseen chickens and cows. Unless these people get 100% of their nourishment from no-till organic gardens worked by hand (and no bone meal to amend the soil), it's time for veg'ns to face up to their own complicity in the violent animal deaths that ensure the food they depend on and enjoy.

For these billions of animals, victims of industrial plant agriculture, there are no animal rightists, no humane societies working on their behalf and close to zero accountability by plant eaters. As Adams proclaimed in *Neither Man nor Beast: Feminism and the Defense of Animals,* not realizing she was describing her own duplicity: "If the problem is invisible…there will be ethical invisibility."

Those veg'ns who are even aware of these immense numbers have switched the basis of their ethical choices in food yet again, anything to retain the moral high ground. Forget "least harm." It's now "intent" that rules the righteous. But once knowledge replaces ignorance (as happened to clueless factory meat eaters), plant consumers are fully responsible for their role in these deaths.

CONSIDER AS WELL the intricate ecosystems, millennia in the making, systematically destroyed by the coming of agriculture to the plains, prairies, woods and wetlands of America. "Is a vegetarian who eats products that originated from industrial monocrop agriculture, contributing to the well-being of the planet?" queries ex-vegan Kent Schoberle, countering a simplistic Vegetarian Society statement that veg'nism is the compassionate choice everyone must make for the benefit of animals and the environment.

The truth is industrial plant agriculture that directly feeds humans is extremely destructive to the environment, dependent on not only wild animal deaths for its existence but reduced biodiversity, massive land and water depletion, and intensive use of carbon-spewing fossil fuels. Avows Schoberle: "Every time you till or disturb the soil, you are wrecking ecosystems and organisms, releasing sequestered carbon into the atmosphere, and degrading the topsoil that's accumulated over many hundreds of years."

Ignorance? Cruelty? The root of the problem is not meat-eating. It is modern corporate agriculture in all its life-loathing, profit-driven forms. If you are sincere in your desire to reduce animal suffering and environmental destruction, then the most important question to ask yourself is *not* whether you are a vegan. It is this: Do my food choices support industrial agriculture?

The numbers game is getting us nowhere. Blaming and shaming are counter-productive. Give it up, vegans! We need to work together to change the way our food is produced in this world.

A NEW TYPE OF SPECIESIST

Ever since our nomadic hunting and gathering ancestors transformed into settled agrarians, *Homo sapiens* have been rapidly changing the face of the planet. It is agriculture that allowed humans to expand across the landscape and reproduce exponentially to our current 7 billion and counting, a rate of growth biologist E.O. Wilson calls "more bacterial than primate." Humans have now cleared 38% of the earth's ice-free land for crops and grazing, the largest use of land on our overused planet, and along with vast fields of monocrops come not just individual animal deaths, but species obliteration.

Here's but one example among hundreds: Since the arrival of the steel plow to our American grasslands, 98% of the black-tailed prairie dog population has been exterminated, often by farmers poisoning or blowing "that vile vermin" out of its burrows. But the suffering doesn't stop there because dozens of other species rely on this energetic rodent for their survival, including the ferruginous hawk, golden eagle, American badger, swift fox, mountain plover, and nearly extinct black-footed ferret. In all, more than 30 grassland species depend on or greatly benefit from this smart, inquisitive creature.

Prairie dogs are so intelligent that scientists have decoded in their rhythmic barks and squeaks a sophisticated language that warns of the direction, speed, even the color of invading predators: *A red fox is racing toward our colony from the north!* This gregarious but endangered mammal likely possesses the second most complex language on earth, bested only by humans. If agriculturists and suburban developers continue to get their way, however, it will be just another dead language in the decades to come.

It was crop farmers who tore up our Great Plains, a sea of fertile grasslands before their arrival, 32 million acres in all. Descending in droves during the Great Plow-Up of 1909-1929, they dammed rivers, drained wetlands, and sucked up water sources for irrigation, decimating prime habitat for once-abundant wildlife species like the now endangered pallid sturgeon, a 70-million year-old survivor of the dinosaur era that might not make it through a mere 100 years of destructive modern agriculture. The whooping crane is yet another endangered species from our American breadbasket, down to 16 birds at one point and still on the brink of extinction. Hundreds more imperiled plains and prairie species are languishing, waiting to be listed for protection.

Today, 75% of our nation's wheat, a cereal grain fed to humans not livestock, comes from the animal-depleted Great Plains. And ethanol to fill our gas tanks has now surpassed animal feed in corn usage, the number one US crop in acreage. This is not to deny that this region also supports half of our beef cattle, nor that 36% of US crop acreage feeds livestock, 95% of it corn (Brester). Rather, this is to remind finger-pointing vegans that unless they consume zero industrial food, they are not exempt from the raping of the land and the slaughter of innocents in order to eat their sweet potato pancakes and tamale-polenta pie. Omnie or veggie, there's a silent stream of wild animal blood running straight to our dinner plates.

AMERICA'S BIOLOGICALLY RICH prairie ecosystem suffered a similar fate at the hands of agriculture. It is now 99.8% gone, scraped nearly bare of native grass and wildlife to make room for monocrops, including the grains and legumes on which plant eaters thrive. Vegans, are you willing to stop eating your preferred foods, as you are demanding of omnivores? To allow the prairie to slowly return and the long-suffering animals to reclaim their indigenous rights?

Before cultivation, my own native Illinois teemed with biodiversity in the form of 22 million acres of luxuriant tallgrass prairie. Grass so high you could ride out on horseback and not see over it. Vegetation so lush parents were fearful of their children getting lost in it. Today, just 2,000 acres remain, *less than one-hundredth of one percent.*

All our prairie-woodland states—once home to plentiful black bears, fishers, martens, cougars, wolves and bison—have been radically altered by first the steel plow and now the combine, transformed from biodiverse abundance into homogenous superfields of soy, canola, and corn that end up not only in gasoline and animal feed, but protein bars, ice cream, and veggie burgers.

Have you been fighting to save Brazil's rainforests? Then fight for America's prairies too, the second most endangered ecosystem on earth and nearly as rich in diversity of species, many of them threatened with extinction or already gone.

315

"Don't forget to add them to the death toll of your vegetarian meal," Lierre Keith admonishes us in *The Vegetarian Myth: Food, Justice, and Sustainability.* "They count and they died for your dinner, along with all the animals that have dwindled past the point of genetic feasibility. 'You can look a cow in the eye' reads an ad for soy burgers. What about a buffalo?"

In order to grow human food and keep Big Ag stock rising, our native animals continue to be destroyed to create the commercial farms and orchards on which all of us depend. And wherever wild animals remain in conflict with agriculturists, planned extermination by government agencies is commonplace. If not gunned down on the spot, these animals must flee in terror the tiller, the reaper, and the colossal Caterpillar, finding tenuous lives elsewhere—or more likely, starvation and death. And let us never forget the millions of animal-honoring native people in the Americas who were also extirpated and annihilated to gain the agricultural lands that all of us rely on to fill our aching-for-food bellies.

Even today, the escalating demand for quinoa by vegans and others translates into native Bolivians suffering from reduced nutrition and diminished health. No longer able to afford their traditional food, they've reluctantly switched to cheap, processed carbs. Yes, when it comes to our food choices, the suffering arrives in surprising ways. Agriculture isn't exactly a war, asserts Keith, because the soil, water, animals and natives can't fight back. "Agriculture is really more like ethnic cleansing, wiping out the indigenous dwellers so the invaders can take the land."

Industrial agriculture is our modern Shiva, the terrifying pre-Buddhist/Hindu god of destruction and creation, one feeding the other in an endless cycle of death begetting food begetting life. Vegans love to talk about the creation (nut cheese/ rice cakes) but not the annihilation that precedes it (vanishing wetlands/extinct songbirds).

Those who aren't afraid to look deeply into this contradiction insist, yet again, that in this imperfect world we must harm as few sentient animals as possible. But even beyond all the wild animals in agricultural fields, what these plant eaters neglect to include in their "least harm" policy is human animals. And clearly—the evidence is mounting—veganism is causing harm to those humans who fail to thrive, who outright suffer, whose bodies are weakened by this restrictive diet.

Yet animal rightists refuse to tolerate any must-eat-meat "excuses," thus excluding members of their own species from the matrix of sentient beings with intrinsic rights to a healthy and fulfilling life.

"NO EXEMPTIONS!" the more extreme bloggers shout out. "The only defensible option is to go vegan!" Most are more than ready to slam omnivores into their morally inferior place. "Patty Jo, you are an ignorant childish bitch," brays one online moralist. "Humans aren't meant to eat meat, you selfish girl. I bet you look like death warmed over and nothing like all those beautiful people who eat only plants." Others go graphic. "Here are some great videos for all of you corpse-crunching, puss-slurping, bestiality enthusiasts out there whining that vegans are too preachy and judgmental," writes Eric Dubay on his global conspiracy site. The only reason omnivores feel judged, his followers agree, is because "they're doing the wrong thing!"

Not only hypocrites—by excluding billions of field-slaughtered animals from the discussion—these radical animal rightists are speciesists of an entirely new order: favoring other species over their own. In the animal kingdom, this has no precedent. Every species on the planet gives preference to its own kind for reasons of survival, bonding, and perpetuation. It's the way of all nature and to deny this is to attempt to stand outside of nature, a hopeless and absurd venture if you inhabit human skin.

Yet ethical vegans who exist outside this species standard, this inviolable code, believe we should not show partiality to humans over any other sentient creature. We are of equal moral standing, the animal rightists avow; the life of a human being is of no more inherent worth than that of a pig or a rat or a cow—or a headless mollusk for that matter.

They keep proclaiming, *without offering any valid evidence,* that any and all humans can thrive on plants alone. Thus, according to their in-house mythology, an individual's so-called "need" for meat to lead a productive and healthy life is invalid, and knowingly taking the life of an animal is immoral. Yet I'm willing to bet they'd make instant exception for a rampaging grizzly about to take them out. So why doesn't their compassion extend to their own fellow creatures whose plants-only diet is gradually, relentlessly taking them out?

After four years of misery and faltering health as a vegan, despite doing everything right, competitive athlete Jade reluctantly started putting animal food back into her diet, including wild game, pastured bison meat, and bone marrow. She was shocked by her rapid return to health. Yet the transition was psychologically difficult because her own vegan community was harshly judgmental and non-supportive. Most were appalled or disgusted. She felt like a bad person simply for seeking good health. The guilt was overwhelming.

> It was hard at first. Very hard. Especially being that I was dating a very righteous vegan zealot and immersed in a community of others on the same page. I was utterly frightened when I went to buy some eggs at the local co-op. I was waiting for the vegan police to come and get me. I seriously felt like I was committing a crime. My ex wouldn't even enter the store with me.

"Ex" because Jade finally ditched the guy after he told her *he'd rather she was a sick and unhealthy vegan than a healthy meat eater*. And you thought I was making up that reverse speciesism claim? No, this is how far off the compassion map some vegans will veer in favoring other animals over their fellow humans. They are incapable of stepping out of their severely contracted paradigm to help a friend or lover. Even Gandhi refused a doctor's orders to give his daughter-in-law eggs when she was dying, yes dying, of malnutrition. This is where veganism gets weird, even perverse. An unborn chicken over a daughter? Only when he learned the eggs were unfertilized did he finally give permission. She swiftly regained her health.

Here's Jade describing her vegan boyfriend's behavior in *Let Them Eat Meat*: "He went back and forth whether he wanted to continue our relationship or not. Every time I ate he tried to make me feel guilty and dinner always ended with me crying. I decided I needed to leave and so I did." This isn't an isolated case. Shaming and shunning invariably ensue when someone leaves a close-knit community which considers itself morally superior to the rest of society and whose beliefs border on fanaticism.

Publicly ridiculing apostates is all over the online veg community, with celeb types especially mocked and derided, raked over the feverish coals of contempt. *How dare you criticize our perfect ideology!* Ex-vegan chef Alex Jamieson still wants to promote plant-based living, but as she told *The Current Review*: "The only problem is that I'm no longer welcomed back into that vegan community. I've been shut out of that conversation to help people be healthier in that way ….because I'm somehow a heretic." But you don't have to be a famous chef or public figure to be shunned. Many ex-vegans describe instant banishment by their former friends.

Jessica recounted to blogger Rhys Southan how she and a group of non-veg friends were sitting around a glowing campfire one night when she revealed that she'd been "craving eggs like a crazy woman. I was having a mild identity crisis and actually said to them, *Who am I if I am not vegan?* They all said that I should 'listen' to my body. When I told them my vegan friends were going to disown me, they said the obvious, 'then they're not really your friends.' Looking back, I don't think I needed too much coaching, just reassurance that I wasn't a terrible, evil person if I decided to eat eggs."

Her former vegan community now snubs her, including her ex-boyfriend: "I told him that I was eating eggs and dairy and he flipped shit— he was genuinely angry with me. Eventually he flat-out told me that he was distancing himself from me....I knew that news would travel fast, and it did. I walked into a vegan restaurant I used to eat at frequently and the guy ringing me up was wearing a shirt that said *Never Trust an Ex-Vegan*. That same day I walked up to a table of vegans I knew and one dude wouldn't even talk to me. It was sad because he looked like he had to try so hard to not be friendly. He felt he was doing the right thing by shunning me."

Audrey, 12 years a vegetarian, primarily vegan, states that many plants-only proselytes talk and act the way cult members do, living in fear of being rejected by their community and losing their identity should they swerve off the straight and narrow. "I lived in a vegan community for half a year," she boldly comments on a pro-vegan site, "and there was one guy who was getting very ill and needed to eat meat (which immediately improved his health). He had to secretly cook it at night, and when he was discovered it was like the Salem Witch Trials."

Some extremists go even further. When Jade went public with her decision to leave veganism due to failing health, she received death threats. Very specific death threats: they wanted her animal companions killed first, in front of her. "There were also threats of sexual violence made against me," she reveals in *Let Them Eat Meat*, "a common silencing tactic used against women." Some even insisted she was the fictional creation of the meat industry. "The paranoia and total break from reality that I witnessed among the people making these accusations was astounding," concludes Jade, who was equally disturbed that "not one prominent vegan blogger....came out to stand against this and call for a reasonable, respectful dialogue." She was very disappointed as well that "two very well known and much loved members of the vegan and animals rights community, who admitted to me they were not vegan behind the scenes due to health reasons," did not come forth with this information in support of her.

Yes, a great many "compassionate" veg'ns will callously dismiss the plight of ex-veggies who have learned the long, hard, suffering way that due to genetic or metabolic dictates, they must eat some quantity of animal products to be healthy.

They're called lazy or gluttonous or lacking in true moral fiber: *No one REALLY needs animal-sourced food in order to thrive. You just crave the taste of meat and won't admit it!*

Social psychologist Melanie Joy even coined a word, *carnism*, to describe the delusion of meat-eating, claiming that omnivores follow an immoral, if unconscious belief system comparable to the violent mythology of Nazism. We do this, declares Joy, because we've been indoctrinated from a young age to believe it is natural and necessary to eat animal flesh. None of us eat meat because we have to, she continues; we do so only because we want to.

These sanctimonious sermonizers—either in denial or simply ignorant of the multitudes who have opted out of veg'nism following years of noble struggle and worsening health—point to themselves as shining examples of fit and committed veg'ns who stick to their morals. Other virtuous crusaders, not looking all that in the pink, their heads in the rarefied clouds of pure philosophy, may reflexively ignore their own bodies' subtle to pressing signals, sacrificing their health on the veg'n altar of selflessness. Thus, their moral principles remain intact over the years, even as their bodies may not. Filmmaker and writer Rhys Southan muses:

> One of the revelations I had as I was quitting veganism was that for me, veganism was a sacrifice. I hadn't ever thought of it that way and excitedly announced this insight to one of my roommates at the time. She was an ex-vegan too, and her response was something along the lines of "duh." But it was news to me, and once I realized that being vegan was abdicating responsibility to my own well-being and happiness, I felt much better about quitting it.

INTERSPECIES SACRIFICE is atypical but it does exist. *Female gorilla protects human toddler fallen into zoo enclosure. Dog locates child in burning building.* And ancient lore has long whispered of dolphins saving drowning sailors, lifting them out of the churning sea to carry their limp bodies back to shore. Even today we read accounts of dolphins rescuing swimmers from shark attacks, smacking the water with their tails and flippers while forming a protective ring around the flailing human. These animals are practicing empathy as we know it, but not one of them surrendered their innate drive for health and longevity. These same caring dolphins will continue to chomp mackerel and squid for dinner.

As for species predilection in humans, some seem to care more for their cats than their own kind (they don't talk back; they love you unconditionally). Like-

320

wise for Buddy or Samantha, the dog who's like their very own child. Yet how many of us would surrender our own health and well-being for the greater good of a canine or kitty? Or *any* non-human animal? Many vegans seem to think this kind of sacrifice is morally required of everyone, even those who emerge weak and damaged on their brand of restrictive diet, *even if those suffering persons turn out, down the veg road, to be themselves.* At best, a steadfast altruism is operating here; at worst, a pious martyrdom wherein one puts the good of others, in this case other species, before the good of oneself and one's own. For the more fanatic ascetic-types, this reverse speciesism may spring from an unconscious loathing of the human condition, i.e., spirits unbearably trapped in material bodies that need to be fed, fed, constantly fed! That our food must be other life forms is "unfortunate." That our food, for some, must be other animals is "intolerable."

Thankfully, favoring another species' well-being over one's own is the rare exception; otherwise, species would die out, planetary diversity would crash, and the 3.8 billion-year-old web of life would unravel. On the other hand, maybe this is what some vegans want. No more animals means no more animal suffering! Clear-headed ex-veg Southan argues that it is our notions of human responsibility and attachment, not values of sentience or intelligence, that really guide our decisions as to which creatures shall live and which shall die.

> There is no contradiction between liking animals and eating them if rights come from responsibility and you feel a greater responsibility for yourself and have found that you cannot thrive without animal products. The same values that make us concerned about animals can make us concerned about ourselves.

In *Introduction to Animal Rights*, scholar Gary Francione offers the burning house scenario as proof that we would choose to save ourselves over a pet bird, for instance, and our own child over a baboon. "[We] would save our own child even if the other being in the fiery house were someone else's child, or Mother Teresa, or some other human whom we valued. Indeed, if we are willing to be honest about it, most of us would choose to save our own child over a dozen other people's children." Yet if other beings shouldn't suffer based on sentience alone, as animal rightists maintain, any decision about whom to save from the burning house, given there's time to save only one, should be completely random.

It is not. When the Nazis tried to starve Leningrad into submission in 1941, blockading all supply routes to the city for 900 days, the hierarchy of life that we are genetically encoded to live by was inexorably exposed. Not a single hungry human put an animal's life before his or her own. With up to 100,000 Leningraders dying every month and even meager bread rations disappearing, the famished citizens resorted to eating rats, birds, zoo animals and, finally, their own beloved pets. As starvation took over—the streets of Leningrad strewn with the dead and dying—the still-living boiled their leather belts in a desperate search for nutrition, scratched off wallpaper paste made from potatoes, and ate joiner's glue derived from livestock hooves. In a final, frenzied attempt to secure protein and prolong their lives, they resorted to eating human body parts found in the streets. "What informed this hierarchy," asks Southan, "if everyone—aside from the leather and potato paste—was equally sentient?"

As this radical scenario illustrates, your instinct and responsibility as a human is first and foremost to your own survival and well-being. That is nature's rule, not mine. Unhealthy people lacking in energy and stamina make lousy reproducers, parents, and planetary advocates. Once your unique health requirements are met—whether that means being a vegan or eating a non-optional quantity of daily or weekly animal protein—only then are you free to look beyond yourself and assist in the well-being of others and the earth. Logically and inherently (no need to burn down the house to confirm), besides oneself, our concern will flow first to whatever inner circle of fellow humans we feel most responsible and attached—likely our own children, partner, parents and siblings—followed by other humans, followed by other animal species. If this were not the ground rule, nature as we know it would not exist.

Frankly, this seems to be the extreme vegan agenda: twist nature around so that speciesism, favoring one's own species, is no longer the norm, is repudiated, and thus the grateful use of other species for sustenance can be stamped out. We will accomplish this, they affirm, by becoming One World Vegans, spiritually evolved beings who are no longer slavishly bound to our biological instincts. As the rest of the world eventually and wisely joins us, we will be able to gradually eliminate all food animals through sterilization and diminishing demand—thus halting the exploitation. This will include *all* domesticated food animals, not just those from factory farms, for it is the use of animals at all that is immoral in the all-vegan world.

Sighs one blogger, dreaming of a planet where suffering does not exist: "If everyone went vegan, what a wonderful world that would be. I think a lot of the animals that we 'created' for food purposes would slowly disappear because they

322

were not designed to live in a natural setting—they would for sure die a peaceful death."

So gaining essential nourishment from animals is not okay—and yes, for many of us it is essential—but animal genocide is? ("Peaceful death," by the way, jibes perfectly with romantic vegan mythology.) According to this same folklore, to prevent possible future suffering we must deny all farm animals their existence, phasing them out for eternity. So how about *human animals* that live in crowded, filthy, inhumane, politically terrifying conditions? Who suffer horrendous emotional and physical pain and die far younger than they should? Do these god-like vegans want to deny them existence as well? Will that help to deliver the gilded, perfect world of non-suffering they so fervently seek?

Anyone with a heart understands that the factory model of meat production is stupid and immoral, but ethical vegans also oppose the raising of free-roaming animals on small family farms. (Some demand that all our pets be phased out of existence as well.) Once these billions of oppressed animals are finally gone, they breathlessly proclaim, we can devote the planet to 100% plant agriculture and feed a hungry world.

Aha! Industrial crop agriculture again: Shiva in disguise. This imposing deity of destruction—the River Ganges tumbling from his blue hair, the serpent of kundalini coiled around his neck—has transformed into a monstrous, multi-headed $400,000 blood-red combine, with whirring, shredding blades for teeth and crushing 42-inch tires for feet. All praise to Shiva! Annihilator of intact ecosystems! Destroyer of indigenous animals and plants!

37.

THE KILLING FIELDS

The road to hell is paved with good intentions.

—William Blake

IF WE REALLY want to get down and dirty about species equality, why are vegans directing most of their energy toward domesticated animals? How fascinating—and disturbing—that many have far less to say about the prior and ongoing wild animal suffering that ensures the continuation of our modern urban lifestyle. The bird-rich woodlands hacked up to erect the species-sterile cities and suburbs that most vegans, and the rest of us, inhabit. The amphibian-rich wetlands drained dry for supermarkets and health food stores where they purchase their quinoa, coffee, and kiwis from around the globe. The mammal-abounding fields ripped up and replaced by all those monstrous, monotonous fields of soy that ensure plentiful tofurkeys on their holiday tables.

They condemn the human privileges pursued by meat-eating speciesists, yet plant eaters pursue their own—and at great cost to animals. "Why are vegans accepting of agriculture and civilization when human expansion steals land from wild animals and kills them?" ex-vegan Rhys Southan wants to know in *Forget Sentience: Here's the Real Reason We Grant Right*s. "Though vegans don't like to admit it, even they can't believe that wild animals have rights because then civilization and agriculture become impossible." Viewing this moral conundrum through another lens, when wild animals inhabit land needed for human-bound vegetables, fruits and grains, they're getting in the way of our responsibility to ourselves. "Vegans should be happy," says Southan. "This responsibility explanation gets rid of the objection that if vegans really cared about suffering reduction, they would be more worried about wild animal suffering than factory farms."

Yet ethical vegans continue to cite qualities like sentience, intelligence, and higher social organization as the proper determinants for which animals they will fight hardest to protect. So why are most vegans focused on cows instead of, say, wolves? Humans don't eat these wild canids but they sure do love to exterminate them in shamefully cruel ways, like blasting them from low-flying helicopters or ensnaring them in steel traps that deliver slow, agonizing death.

Yet these animals are highly-intelligent social beings, possessed of remarkable focus, drive, and pack loyalty. By contrast, cows mull around looking bored, brainless, and lost—the reason cow bells were invented. Every species must be honored and cows do express moodiness and maternal caring, but let's get real, these aren't the brightest beings on the planet, especially compared to their rowdy auroch ancestors. Go stroll out on farmer John's pasture sometime and look long and deep into those liquid, vacant, bovine eyes. Then, if you dare, go look into a wild wolf's eyes (this may take decades but the patient and adventurous will be rewarded). You'll be startled, nay *electrified* by the orange fire blazing in those vibrant canine eyes, emanating vigor and keen awareness. Inside those cunning, light-giving eyes, you may even catch a glimmer of your own wild, forgotten self.

But vegans are largely city folk who've never glimpsed the shadow of a wolf in their lives, and urban dwellers relate more easily to docile domestic animals than their increasingly marginalized, wild and unpredictable cousins—including all the scurrying, slithering ones that inhabit fields of grain. "Intuitively, something does feel different about killing a wild animal with a wheat thresher, than killing a goat by knocking him out and slitting his throat," admits Southan, *even if both experience the same amount of pain.*

Here's the difference: domestic goats, sheep, and cows are as beloved and familiar as our childhood story books, their intentional deaths brought about by bloodied human hands. This kind of killing, according to vegans, is unacceptable. Slinky, creeping, feral animals, however, may be alien to one's sensibilities, their demise accomplished by cold, mechanical farm machines. That's one of the many luxuries of urban living: daily estrangement from invisible dying beasts in our agricultural fields. Alienation, or sometimes ignorance, thus allows for the desired vegan end: tofu scramble and corn tortillas. Moreover, wild animals feed on other sentient animals, the more out-there vegans remind us: deplorable!

Ideally, according to this same aberrant anti-nature agenda, we will live in a future world where wild animals don't do this, i.e., don't eat each other. Ditto for meat-eating household pets, evidently, as a certain clan of kale eaters insists that your cat—a claw-wielding, rodent-stomping carnivore that relies on nutrients from animal tissues to survive—should go vegan. Does anyone else smell rank anthropomorphism in the air?

It's all part of a child-like fantasy that all humans, indeed all creatures, will revert to an Edenic state of all-plants nutrition. Like Odysseus, these people have been blown off-course from reality and arrived in the land of the Lotus-eaters. They are modern-day Lotophages, subsisting on the fruits of the field while succumbing to the narcotic of self-delusion that every human and every animal, regardless of their position on the food chain, should eat just like they do. If they had their way, this New Earth would hang out signposts for all of its beasts: NO HUNTING ALLOWED! What a soothing sedative to believe such a pretty myth. Never mind the hordes of rabbits and rodents, uneaten and unchecked, that would wreak havoc to our food crops, many of which vegans like to eat for supper.

This oft-seen vegan preference for humanizing our pets and saving domestic farm animals does seem strangely misguided, given that it is wild animals who carry the gene pools that create the stunning biodiversity of our planet's fauna—a diversity that is rapidly diminishing day by day. Over 1,000 times quicker than natural extinction—that's how fast our earth's diverse species are vanishing, with one very arrogant species almost wholly culpable for this brisk diminishment. If vegans really care about animals, their continued existence and their suffering, let's see a whole lot more of them forcefully speak up for the wild ones. Bravo for condemning factory farms but let's direct equal amounts of that righteous passion to the rights of wild species to exist in healthy, intact ecosystems.

AS INDIVIDUALS, WILD ANIMALS are also suffering, left to die as bloody smears on our highways or, if incredibly lucky, hustled to the nearest wildlife recovery center. Whether they got there due to shotgun, poison or speeding car, rehab work with wild critters is labor intensive and heart wrenching. How much more appealing to commit to gourmet veggie pizzas and blueberry smoothies for the next 30 years than to spend even 30 hours in "Scrapeland" at your local wildlife center. Make that 30 minutes, which is all I lasted at this nausea-inducing outdoor work station, where you grab extendable tools and scrape dried feces mixed with vomit off hordes of sheets and blankets yanked from the cages of wounded animals. Traumatized, mangled, bleeding animals arriving in a never-ending stream.

Luckily, I was more urgently needed in the Bird Room, where I vigilantly tweezers-fed sluggish grubs, squirming earthworms, and chopped-up crickets (all of whom, no doubt, would have preferred to live) to bullet-wounded robins, broken-winged bluebirds, and naked, voracious baby swallows. During my non-stop five hour shifts, I felt just like a sleep-deprived new mother with perpetually depleted breasts, desperately trying to nourish multitudes of squawking, pleading, bawling babies all at once, many of whom would never make it out alive. After every volunteer stint, I collapsed in utter exhaustion.

Across the land, thousands of devoted animal lovers do this arduous, messy work up to ten hours a day, five to six days a week. I can't help but contrast these dedicated workers with that subset of scornful vegans who sit in front of laptops and rant against omnivores, blogging about saving animals but rarely interacting with the wild ones, rarely sleeping on the earth like a true animal, the wild earth that nurtures us, sustains us, and shaped us into humans: every finger, toe, and far-seeing eye. Removed from the reality of biological interdependence that dictates our short stay on this fertile, erotic planet, urbanites live in a largely sterile environment of concrete and glass, softened by pockets of municipal parks but far from the fierce ambivalence of Nature. For those humans who truly live in nature or share their lives on an intimate basis with animals—farmers, ranchers, forest residents, wilderness dwellers—non-harm and veganism are naïve ideals which have no grounding in biological truth.

THE WORLD WE WERE BORN TO

Typical of the prototype, when I fast-tracked into a teen vegetarian I'd been living in cities my entire life, shielded from the wild's coarse, unruly passions. Nature meant imported pink tulips, Kentucky bluegrass, and pruned arborvitae. Even the irrepressible weeds—"the ugly of the universe; the rough, the wicked, and the wild" as poet Theodore Roethke affectionately calls them—were largely absent, evicted in the name of orderly sameness.

Animals were either the Desired, i.e., domestic pets, or the Undesired: spiders, skunks, jiggers, and all those damn mosquitoes. Anything exotic as a field mouse that dared venture indoors, elicited shrieks of protest. And snakes? Secretive and otherworldly: desiccated skin the disquieting evidence of their slithery existence. My sole snippet of "real" nature was a nearby urban creek, pulsating with buggy, watery life and overhung with dense green willows and black alders. To this flowing paean to Life, I found myself drawn again and again in a kind of blissful reverie, as if remembering something we had long ago lost, a community of un-tamed beings in which we had participated fully and fervently.

Comparatively little animal suffering and death are witnessed in a cityscape, leading some vegans to the ludicrous conclusion that wild animals live in some kind of low-stress Happy Land compared to livestock that are fed daily and eventually, one day, led to their death. Yes, even pastured quadrupeds left free to wander will know fear and suffering on that final day—as will most of us. But, wild animals, the largest predators excepted, live on that razor's edge of fear and death every night and day of their lives. That's why they freeze in terror at the least rustle in the brush or sudden shadow out of the sky, why their eyes loom large on the side of their heads and their ears are constantly quivering antennae. Yes, go live in a wild setting where nature is largely intact and you will witness animal fear and suffering on a regular basis. All you have to do is walk around with open eyes. Some days you don't even have to do that because the suffering comes and finds you.

JUST THIS WEEK a female mule deer came walking down the dirt road that dead-ends at our mountain cabin. Slow and unsteady, she seemed confused to see me on the front porch in the early morning light, but her doleful eyes said everything: "I'm not here for *you*." Skirting the small pond, she mounted a grassy hill and wandered round and round the tall, scattered ponderosa pines with no apparent purpose, not grazing, not at all wary. An hour later the silent doe seemed ready to leave and tentatively started to head out. Instead, she circled back, climbed the hill again and repeated her strange behavior before wearily departing on the dusty road that led her in. Climbing that same hill, I spotted her handsome mate on a nearby gentle slope. His severed thigh was a long way from his ravaged and bloody body—its soft, tawny fur lifting and falling in the light morning breeze. I've come upon such killings before in these mountains. You'd think I would get used to them but never do, and I cried out at sight of the mangled head, the white starkness of the ribcage recently stripped of all muscle. And I felt deeply for his mate and what she had encountered at the far end of her lonely trek. I also knew, animal that I am, that I needed to leave this death scene immediately.

It snowed all that night, a good five inches of fine dry powder. Stepping out after breakfast, I discovered the hungry executioner. Shockingly fresh, five-inch-wide imprints of 4-toed cat paws tracked past our cabin and across the frozen creek—each step spanking new and perfectly imprinted. And they filled me not with fear but awe. In the glittering sunshine, in the crystalline snow, they shone like brilliant embossed jewels, hundreds of them, stretching into the field before me and miles beyond. Clearly, this mountain lion had followed my own favorite walking trail from distant meadows, treading within a few yards of our front door. His stride was leisurely, confident. He had found good fortune here and hoped to find it again. In a few weeks he'd be back, looking for another hot nourishing meal to sustain his life force and get him through this harsh Colorado winter.

Within these foothill canyons of granite outcroppings, juniper and pine, the original inhabitants still assemble: cougar, black bear, elk, deer, coyote, bobcat and bison, even a few humans. And Lobo is moving closer every year, getting ready to reclaim his share of the sustenance. Each spring a pair of Canada geese returns to our pond's little island to lay their yolk-wrapped progeny, and each spring a lean black bear swims out there in the dead middle of the night to snatch his fair portion of nutrition.

My first year here, seven out of ten babies made it out of their gooey pre-birth and into the light, an absolute miracle I was told. But by the second week, two goslings were gone; next day, three; day after, four. Then the father mysteriously disappeared and a lame male goose took over, limping faithfully behind the other survivors: mom and three very nervous goslings. Geese don't like being left alone. A gosling will sob uncontrollably should this happen; there is more safety in numbers. But the hobbling surrogate male had to be left behind to certain death when mother and siblings flew off in search of a "safer" spot—no such thing in the wild.

The following spring, nine baby geese were hatched and nine baby geese were eaten. Not one survived the essential needs of coyote, wily fox, and brother bear. "Good day, Peter!" I would call out to the trembling young rabbit hiding in the brush, exact same spot on my hike every afternoon. "Be careful out here!" The next day Peter was spread all over my walking path, his delicate spine scattered among yellow wildflowers, his silky grey fur pierced by the daggered leaves of yucca. April is the cruelest month, the London poet told us, but out here in the wild, April through March is the cruelest month.

The infant raccoons hiding in the tall cottonwood never made it through last summer either, nor the baby turtles, nor the solitary deer my neighbors Craig and Leslie identified by the four-chambered stomach left behind, full of undigested shoots and tender green grass. Everything else, every bone, every tendon, every scrap had been dragged off by an exultant pack of ravenous coyotes.

On and on....you can't hide from the animal suffering here, the anguish and the satisfaction, the feeder and the fed, the ongoing cycle of life eating life. You

329

can hide in the city, in the yoga studio, or your comfortable condo but not here. When you truly live in nature and take your rightful place therein, just one very insignificant creature among your fellows, you will witness animal suffering and death on a daily basis. You will also find yourself as the unwitting perpetrator.

The indigo bunting violently killed as it crashes against the picture window installed for your wildlife viewing pleasure....the tiny unidentifiable bird that flew down your stovepipe in the middle of the night, her blackened body found buried in the ashes. Oh hey, white-footed mouse, why did you climb into my watering can to drown in an inch of water? And you, muted sparrow? Dying your slow death in the abandoned outhouse—unable to fly out of the crescent moon cut into its door, the one I forgot to cover—a golden worm crawling out of your now-vacant eye.

And then there are the even smaller animals discovered dead or dying as a result of our choices. Monarch butterflies smirched across our windshields. *Death by speed.* Wolf spiders in the bathtub; ants in the hummingbird feeder; beetles flying into open paint cans. *Death by drowning.* Grain moths dancing inside our porch lights, hundreds of disintegrating bodies found meshed together the next morning in one all-devouring life-net. *Death by fire.*

MOST ANIMAL RIGHTISTS don't consider invertebrates like spiders and insects to possess sentience, let alone intelligence, letting themselves off the ethical hook for their squashed sufferings and underfoot deaths. Yet how do we know what these animals feel and sense? We don't. What we know for certain is that many invertebrates release endorphins in response to pain, opioid peptides that function as neurotransmitters and once believed exclusive to vertebrates. The nervous system of the "lowly" earthworm, for example, releases an opiate that reduces the perception of pain, just as in humans, and they certainly do squirm, wiggle, and writhe like mad when hooked or otherwise messed with. Why display suffering behavior if not suffering?

Soon to die anyway, you say? How long is an invertebrate's life? The smallest butterfly may live only a week, while female tarantulas can live 30 or 40 years, longer than many humans. Just what does it mean to say these "lesser" beings live short lives? So is yours compared to a Rougheye Rockfish or a Bowhead Whale. Both live on average over 200 years. And why do size and duration matter anyway? This is just more human-comparing, similar to the speciesism that animal rightists condemn. Call it sizeism, durationism, or whatever you please, is the life of an 8-ton African elephant more valuable than that of a .00001-ounce emerald dragonfly fried to death in your car grille?

Ecologically, both are important, dragonflies perhaps even more so in the overall balance of nature, for without insects and their vital role in the food chain, life as we know it would cease to exist. Yet many animal rightists leave insects out of their innermost circle of concern. Why? Because it's impossible not to kill them on a regular basis just by living your life.

HUNG UP ON HIERARCHY

We really don't know if insects possess sentience. However, with their ganglionic nervous system—consisting of a brain, central nerve cord, and neurotransmitters (sound familiar?)—just like other invertebrates they are quite capable of complex learning. And since we're talking food here, let's zoom in for a look at their diet.

Remember those poisonous African mushrooms that nearly killed my ex? Most insects exhibit a keen ability to associate specific food qualities with unsuitability for consumption, a certainty that demands precise observations which lead to definite conclusions. (My human mate failed on both counts.) Wasps and grasshoppers, for instance, are able to associate the sensory qualities of food—like taste and odor—with toxicity or even (pay attention here) nutrient deficiency. One species of grasshopper, *Schistocerca americana,* quickly learned to reject the fresh spinach offered by researchers because it lacked the specific sterols required for optimal functionality (Behmer). They simply stopped eating the green goods altogether. Once the correct sterol was added, the hoppers munched the spinach with enthusiasm. They learned a positive association with this new food because it fulfilled a nutritional deficit. Wisely, they also stopped eating when satiated.

Would that humans were as smart as grasshoppers in rejecting foods which don't meet our nutritional needs. And to stop stuffing ourselves like idiots when already full! Far from being as perceptive as the humble *S. americana,* modern *Homo sapiens* are known to consume non-nutritional foods in gargantuan batches, damaging our health and shortening our lives.

Meanwhile, we often reject foods that are nutrient-rich—like spinach. We fail to intuitively distinguish between real foods that provide, say, the essential fatty acid DHA, from lab-concocted foods that provide none. Unlike other animals, we willingly and regularly eat foods that are anti-nutrient and seriously harmful—pass the Doritos and diet soda, please! In many cases there appears to be no asso-

331

ciative learning. So which one is the more observant and intelligent species? The grasshopper purposefully selecting healthy foods that provide essential nutrients, refusing to eat unhealthy offerings and stopping altogether when satiated? Or the sugar-sucking, trans-fat inhaling human who selects junk—basically dead food—and overeats to oblivion?

Is it possible the insects of this planet are more evolved than we are, in the Buddhist sense? They seem to relish their existence, selecting nourishment that extends their lives. They don't turn pain into suffering the way humans do and then attach to the suffering. Nor are they attached to their individual bodies and personalities—perhaps because they somehow realize, through all the myriad and rapid transformations, that they will swiftly morph into food for some other living being. They recognize their place in the consumptive web of life.

Think of those shimmering dragonflies zipping across rivers and ponds. Notice how light their bodies, how purposeful their movements, how void of confusion and angst. We humans, meanwhile, are intensely attached to our bodies: to the point of obsession over appearance, to the point of fixation on youthfulness, a denial of change and aging, a refusal to ponder our own death. Cutting through the attachment and the clinging is what enlightenment is all about. *Insects are light in mind and body, quick to transform, dazzling to consider.*

Writing in "Confusion Arises as Wisdom," Ringu Tulku Rinpoche clarifies the path to our deepest understanding as taught by the 12th century Buddhist monk, Gampopa. "In reality, there is nothing absolute; everything can be many different ways. The more deeply you understand this, the more lightly you take things. When you directly know this, you have recognized the nature of your mind."

YET INSECTS ARE LARGELY ignored in the animal ethics debate, long regarded as tiny reflex machines, all buzzing hardware and no discerning software. Modern research is proving otherwise, radically altering our perception of these petite invertebrates and their capacity to learn and perhaps even delight in life.

Insects are capable of cognitive feats once credited to "higher" vertebrates only, animal behaviorists now tell us, like ants and wasps recognizing the individual faces of their fellows. Honeybees possess even more remarkable visual, memory, and communication skills. These busy, buzzy, well-studied pollinators not only learn all the various colors, fragrances, and exact locations of specific flowers but are able to count, memorize human faces, and understand abstract concepts like "sameness" versus "differences."

salt-of-the-earth farmer could have predicted. Soil is dynamic and alive. It takes years to build organic carbon and fertility, decades to recover from abuse.

When our great grandparents were born, roughly 120 years ago, our croplands averaged 24 inches of topsoil. Today that number is six. *Six inches*, the length of your outstretched hand, separates humanity from the non-organic subsoil in which nothing will grow. *Nothing*. Professor John Crawford, University of Sydney, calculates that at current loss rates we will run out of topsoil worldwide in less than 60 years. You're worried about global warming taking us out? The collapse of our soil may do it sooner. "I find it quite ironic," Crawford told the World Economic Forum, "that while the Mars Curiosity Rover is poking around looking for life in Martian soil, we're in the process of extinguishing life in our own."

Could there exist in the human imagination a more bountiful and beautiful habitation than our own planet? It gives and gives and we take and take, rarely giving back, systematically degrading the earth's body, along with our own, via exhausted soil and nutrient-depleted food. Billion-dollar takings from industrial palm oil that's ubiquitous in our processed foods and snacks, but toxic to our kidneys, lungs, liver and heart. What ignorant folly is this? Clear-cutting Indonesia and Malaysia; decimating the lives of native forest people; slaughtering endangered tigers and orangutans with guns and machetes so profiteers can sell more Bagel Bites and Oreo cookies. Is this intelligence at work? Maybe we really are a big-brained fluke. No other species adulterates its own food and systematically destroys its own home. Our wise earth will slowly repair, transform, and survive in altered form, but humanity may not. Given the severe consequences of climate disruption already starting to slam us, the planet itself may be in the process of sloughing off its indulgent, incompetent caretakers.

In *The Unsettling of America,* Wendell Berry describes the difference between a nurturer and an exploiter: "The exploiter typically serves an institution or organization; the nurturer serves the land, household, community, place. The exploiter thinks in terms of numbers, quantities, hard facts; the nurturer in terms of character, condition, quality." The benchmark for an exploiter is efficiency, but for a nurturer it is good care. Everyone who eats industrial food—and that's just about all of us—participates in the exploitation of the earth. We're only six decades into this global corporate food experiment and not only is our topsoil disappearing but much of what's left is worn-out and inferior.

Sure, oil-based fertilizers have freed farmers to plant more often, but at terrible cost to the integrity of our soil. Misuse of chemical fertilizers, along with over-plowing, has dangerously depleted our agricultural lands. The Great Satan is what some enviros call the 19th century German chemist who reduced a complex renewable organic system, as ancient as life on earth, into the abbreviated synthetic science of NPK: nitrogen, phosphorus, and potassium. Liebig was his name and how very appropriate. (Yes, the same chemist who falsely declared plant and animal protein to be equivalent.) In undervaluing the natural process of decay and soil building, Justus von Liebig committed a fatal error and enshrined a big fib. He thought we could outsmart nature, and for awhile, with Big Ag's preliminary high yields, it looked like we had. Our degraded topsoil and diminishing returns now tell a different story, a trajectory not unlike the unfolding scenario of far too many vegans: an initial terrific outcome, followed by less than promising results, followed by declining health. Straying from nature's successfully evolved systems, we learn the hard way, has consequences.

Civilizations rise or fall with the fertility of their soil, yet corporate agriculture is oblivious, dumping ever more synthetic chemicals on our cropfields, trying to make an end-run around nature's rot and renew process. In the US alone, Big Ag unloads 24 million tons of chemicals every year, worth $37 billion. With this kind of short-circuited profit mentality, the soil becomes just like the imprisoned animals: another economic factor on a spreadsheet, to be dealt with as artificially and efficiently as possible on the way to the corporate bank. In reality, every grassy field, every loamy patch of soil embraces the very foundation of life and we humans ignore this truth at our peril.

"ENVISION A LANDSCAPE OF ABUNDANCE"

Next time you're out in the garden, anybody's garden, bow down and scoop up a fistful of dirt, then inhale long and deep. It's vigorous, fast-evolving microorganisms creating that feral fragrance. The very one that excited the Dionysian crowd to acts of procreation in the fields; the same heady scent that propelled me and my boyfriend deep into the Northwest forest to create our own earthly bliss. Over two billion years ago, these pungent nutrient recyclers were among the first life on earth, yet modern agribusiness pays them no respect.

Now pull up a rampaging weed in that same garden, soil still clinging to its tangled roots. Close your eyes and hold its intricate, intertwining mycelia next to your discerning nose for more of that *oh my god* primordial perfume, that moist carbon-dense bouquet of decay and creation *mmm* that nearly knocks you over with its fecundity and richness. It's like inhaling the earth itself and reminds us in an always powerful way, who we are at the most elemental level and where we shall return.

On my hands and knees in my own summer garden, somewhere between the okra and zucchini, I have found paradise. It's humus that I'm sniffing out there like a happy beast in the sun and rain, the dark and truly opulent organic stuff that remains after animal and vegetable matter undergo radical decomposition—a transmutation accomplished by many billions of micro-creatures inhabiting every scoopful of soil. The word *humus* derives from the Latin for earth, and it's etymologically related to *humble*, low or modest. Out there crawling in the dirt with the grubs and earthworms, gardeners can certainly attest to feeling humble. And it's humility that's sorely needed in our world today, a recognition of humanity's complete dependence on the fertility of the soil. Without humility, without a high regard for the soil and the life forms there abounding, we are doomed to a future of diminishing earthly returns, an arrogant fall from grace.

The failure of the Green Revolution exhibits exactly this. Lauded in the 1960s as the answer to global hunger, this high-tech Ag system supplanted local farmers and diverse indigenous crops in favor of monocultures: a few high-yielding varieties dependent upon fossil fuels, chemical fertilizers, and tons of pesticides to kill the swarms of rapacious pests that flock to single-crop fields. Initial results were highly praised and then the shock of reality set in as humans once again ignored ecological principles in favor of fast technology and obese profits. Over time, the ratio of production to energy input keeps dropping and third-world people are still starving, unable to afford the high-tech grains produced in their own countries. Ultimately, those who benefited were Big Ag and Big Oil, along with machine manufacturers and large landowners. Those who lost—and lost big—were the millions of small farmers displaced from their land, leading to impoverishment, reduced food security, and an upwelling of discontent and violence.

Now the aggressive global corporations are at it again, thrusting their GM seeds onto farmers in developing nations. Any wonder why there's vehement opposition when these same cultivators witnessed failing crops, soaring debt, and mass-suicide among their Green Revolution neighbors? In India alone, over 300,000 farmers have killed themselves since 1995. The poison of choice is often the very same miracle liquid that was supposed to save them—pesticide. What's more, these family farmers were already doing it right: practicing seed-saving and seed-breeding techniques that ensure the genotype diversity that's adaptable to local soils and diseases and more resilient to climate change. These farmers also understood healthy soil ecology, something that appears to be over the heads of high-tech and GM pushers, whose industry practices have resulted in radically reduced soil fertility, increased erosion, water shortages, and micro-nutrient deficiencies in our food.

"OUR MODERN FOOD SYSTEM seems to want to disembody itself from the soil," Joel Salatin warns a swelling crowd that same warm August evening at our local Chautauqua, an 1898 historical meeting place resembling a cavernous barn. "Yet healthy soil is fundamental to our existence! The soil holds a profound world of beings that we don't see, and it is a physical and spiritual truth that all of life is utterly dependent on this invisible world."

Joel, late-fifties, very sturdy and healthy-looking from his fresh-air life in the Virginia countryside, is standing alone on stage, dressed in white khakis and a *Polyface*-emblazoned maroon shirt. Did I say standing? This man never stops moving! Whimsical gestures are his trademark, and right now he's gently holding out his two fists to the audience. Slowly and dramatically he opens them, palms up. "In this double-handful of soil exist more beings than all the humans who have ever lived on this planet," Joel calmly tells us. "It's a community of beings that's been around for a long time and we're responsible for this community," he continues, lamenting that our modern culture doesn't value and honor the Carbon Cycle, the very foundation of life: the sun and photosynthesis; decomposition of animals and plants; the whole never-ending shebang of nutrient cycling and recycling. Past cultures have honored, even venerated this life-giving process, but other than biologists, gardeners, and comatose sun worshipers in Daytona Beach, nay, not ours. "We have broken our ecological umbilical cord," Joel admonishes us, our connection to the Carbon Cycle, to the Soil and the Sun.

So instead of animal droppings being spread and recycled, enriching the soil as in the diversified farming of our ancestors, that manure has turned into a curse: a stinking, polluting, global-warming curse. That's because in Big Ag operations—20,000 cattle slammed into miserable confines, ankle-deep in their own parasitic waste—all manure is turned into toxic sludge, instead of the magic soil elixir it was always meant to be. But an earth-wise farmer, Joel insists, "doesn't bury his very own community in excrement and toxicity in order to grow government-subsidized food for someplace halfway around the world!"

Here's what happens to that same manure on a grass-based family farm. On each pasture, on every fertile field, it is recycled and put to excellent use nourishing the land and the animals, which in turn nourish us. Depending on the season, chickens or perhaps turkeys are rotated to a pasture lightly grazed by cattle that have also moved on. In these "lush pastures supported by ecstatic copulating earthworms," as Joel calls them, these birds gladly carry out their vital ecological tasks: scratching through cow patties for nutritious grubs and larvae; spreading their own manure and essential nitrogen as they roam the verdant fields and dig away; all the while, enriching the grass which nourishes the cows whose droppings nourish the birds which nourish the humans (with protein-rich eggs created from worms and insects plucked from humus-rich soil). That's a whole lot of nourishing going on.

And then the cycle starts all over again because that's how nature works—birds clean up after the herbivores—and if you've ever witnessed white egrets hitching a ride on the broad backs of cattle, you know exactly what this smart farmer is talking about.

Unlike the abused, overgrazed land of industrial cattle operations, Joel's grass stays healthy and suitably trimmed because the herbivores are rotated daily. Their manure, because it's of proper scale on an appropriately sized farm, becomes not poisonous sludge entering our waterways, but a blessing on the land. Nor does it contribute to global warming because it's immediately recycled into the soil. Natural pest control is intrinsic to this operation, and fossil fuel-based chemicals aren't needed because grass farming relies on the energy of the sun. Mr. Salatin has never applied a single ounce of chemical fertilizer, pesticide, or herbicide to his soil or crops. Every vegan enviro argument is obliterated by Polyface and the thousands of earth-smart, family farms just like it, evaporated like dew by the solar energy which fuels all natural systems.

Emerging from behind the podium, Joel is super-animated now, cavorting around like a cut-loose filly, pantomiming all the creatures which live contentedly on his mixed-use family farm: soil organisms moving and munching; bovines leisurely wandering in the warming sun; hens prancing in the open air. Roaming the big stage, wildly gesticulating, passionately instructing, Joel can't spit out his finely-wrought words fast enough. This man's on fire! He's also hilarious in that keenly intelligent way of all truth-tellers: Jon Stewart in farm clothes.

Voice intensifying, gestures ever more flamboyant, this barnstorming natural thespian is in full swing. "Envision a landscape of abundance!" Joel thunders at us, sitting on the edge of our seats, not knowing whether to laugh at his zany antics, or cry at his poignant message. "Clean, attractive, non-polluting family farms growing a cornucopia of crops in deep rich soils, raising a variety of free-roaming beasts. Humans, plants, and animals together in one extraordinarily virile, biodiverse, symbiotic system! This is what the American landscape used to look like," he shouts out to us, "and we urgently need to call it back!"

THERE IS NOTHING NATURAL nor healthy about a monocrop industrial farm. It is a lonely, misplaced venture. Gone are the families, the children, the animals, the vegetable gardens, the lovingly tended roses. Typically, a formerly independent farmer has morphed into a corporate hired-hand, raising a single crop like genet-ically-altered soybeans on 5,000 stripped-bare acres behind closed metallic gates which warn: "No Trespassing. Biosecurity." This so-called farm does not honor the carbon cycle, does not maintain fertile soil via the humus-building process, and leaves animals out of the system. It is in a word, unsustainable. Does not hold water. On shaky ground.

"Almost all of the problems of our industrial food flow from the original sin of monoculture," writes Michael Pollan in his preface to Salatin's *Holy Cows and Hog Heaven.* Certainly, an enormous monoculture of soy, corn, wheat or cattle is an ultra-efficient business concept, but "it runs diametrically counter to the way nature works, which nothing in this world can do indefinitely," argues Pollan. "Insect resistance, agricultural pollution, food-borne illness, and antibiotic re-sistance are what happen when the logic of monoculture runs up against the logic of nature."

"Folks, this ain't normal!" Joel cries out to the wildly cheering crowd. We *need* free-roaming and well-cared for domestic animals on our farms because no natural system can function without animals. We *need* an exuberant mix of soil-enriching vegetation for these natural grazers who self-select for nutritional value. (At Polyface, Joel aims for 40 varieties of grasses, fescues, and clovers on every square yard, his "salad bar pastures" as he fondly calls them.) And we *need* the wild creatures that lurk in the fields and ravines, critters that provide food for the larger predators that in turn provide ecological balance.

It all comes down to appropriate scale and natural diversity. On the Salatin farm, four generations raise not only chickens and cattle but also turkeys, pigs and rabbits, alongside sweet corn, tomatoes, grapes, blackberries and more. On a mere 100 acres of grass, this family produces an astounding variety and quantity of earth-friendly organic food, serving more than 5,000 families, 10 retail outlets, and 50 restaurants, while earning a respectable living and spreading the bounty by shopping in their own community.

Locals arrive at the farm to buy their food directly. Why? Because they sense something radically different when they walk out on the land. Unlike chemical-dependent conglomerates, this farm looks and smells good, like earthy compost and sweet honeysuckle. The staff is upbeat and welcoming. And the animals, with access to 450 acres of adjoining forest, are treated with respect as they move, chew, chomp or peck away, according to their nature. "We need to honor the chickenness of the chicken!" Joel is practically pleading with us, reminding us that the horrors of factory farms need not exist and indeed did *not* exist for many thousands of years of traditional, honorable farming.

The beauty of the local organic food movement is its wholehearted respect for the plant/animal/soil cycle that enriches the biome and revitalizes our own bodies and communities. The hideousness of the corporate view of production is its complete disrespect for every one of these. It profits the few at the great expense of the many. So which of these systems are *your* food dollars supporting?

FIGHTING THE INDUSTRIAL BEAST

"We need a Food Emancipation Proclamation!" Joel hollers inside the mammoth old barn, and the overflow crowd roars back its approval. "Emancipate yourself from processed industrial food that floats on oil! Extricate yourself from the clutches of global corporations and rediscover your own yards and kitchens!" Food choice is more basic than religion, the good man tells us. It gives us the fuel, the energy, the strength to do everything in life. We must honor the sacredness of our food.

Ah, to have a life mission so tangible and honorable. But that is exactly Joel's point; this is *our* honorable mission, yours and mine. To take back our power, one meal at a time, with our daily choices. To regain our food sovereignty and restore nature to its rightful place. "We need a local food tsunami!" Joel counsels us with fervor. "Thousands of farmers see their work as a sacred trust between their land and the dinner plate. Those who take such a view should be patronized. They should be encouraged. You and I should buy their food!"

The local food revolution has taken off here in Boulder County, an exciting beehive of regenerative agriculture, entrepreneurial food products, chic locally-sourced restaurants, and an active supportive citizenry. To saunter through our Saturday farmer's market is to encounter village abundance: a profusion of fresh organic produce, honey, flowers, craft brews, grassy meats and artisan cheeses offered to elated humans moving shoulder to shoulder along a packed 13th Street. *Fresh peaches from Paonia! Please move to the back of the line! Just laid pastured eggs! Get 'em here!* Spiced with live drumming and freestyle dancing, this bustling market is so popular it hasn't missed a beat in 30 years and lasts as far into fall as we can push it before the really serious snow cuts loose.

From coast to coast, farmer's markets are booming. Nearly 8,300 now bring in over $7 billion annually and those numbers just keep rising. California leads the pack (pursued by New York and Michigan), with nearly 30 thriving markets in foodcentric San Francisco alone. Pint-sized Massachusetts boasts an impressive 300 markets statewide, while big wild Alaska, despite its condensed growing season, recently posted a 46% gain. That's because citizens everywhere delight to shop in the open air, mingle with resident farmers, and rediscover what real food tastes like straight from the soil. We also love thumbing our collective nose at too-big-to-care Industrial Ag.

With Community Supported Agriculture (CSA), eco-enthusiasts can go further and back their local farmers with up-front cash, getting an assortment of seasonal produce in return. Over 500,000 Americans already support their farmers in this honorable fashion. Our federal government certainly doesn't, dolling out billions in subsidies to jumbo agribusinesses which, like most corporate entities, have zero loyalty to people or place.

Writes Steven Gorelick in *The Ecologist,* "Today's economic 'winners' include trans-national corporations that locate wherever they are offered tax breaks, cheap labor, and lax environmental and workplace rules—and then move on when a better deal is offered elsewhere."

Sustainable, small family farms, by contrast, are rooted in allegiance to place. As Gary Snyder has always urged us: "Find your place on this earth and dig in." So at Cure Organic Farm, tucked into Colorado's prairie flatlands, Anne and Paul Cure are digging in deep and proud, raising over 100 varieties of organic herbs, vegetables, and flowers on a mere twelve acres of land. "We love having a relationship with the families that eat our food," they told me, "helping those families develop a relationship to the land." Their biodynamic farm is home to honeybee hives, heritage pigs, over 150 laying hens and ducks, plus Rambouillet sheep raised for their fiber and meat. "We are land stewards," Anne and Paul maintain,

358

"committed to educating future farmers and fostering a culture of giving, providing nourishment to those in need."

Sprinkled across these same grasslands are hundreds more family farms whose resourceful owners build roadside stalls or stand-alone mini stores right on their property—no middle man necessary, thank you very much. Instead of a mere 16 pennies of every food dollar trickling down to hard-laboring farmers, as in our current industrial system, 100% sounds just about right.

Miffed by the exploding local movement, corporates are now spreading the word that economies of scale make global products more eco-friendly than local food, but don't you believe it. Food products don't just suddenly appear inside all those oil-guzzling, long-haul freezer vans and cargo ships. Every item has to be trucked there from the farms or factories, and then those trucks must be driven back. People must also drive to grocery stores and then return. With local food, the entire middle, long-distance transport chain is eliminated. Corporate defenders also bring up the absurd example of someone driving 200 miles for "local" eggs, but the truth is a lot of us walk or bicycle to our centrally located farmer's market, eliminating that final fossil-fuel transport chain as well. And economies of efficiency and finance continue to be developed for small farmers, including the immensely successful Farm to School program which brings fresh, whole foods to our children, opening the door to a market worth billions.

With their creative culinary creations—not to mention enviro-politics—slow-food restaurants are also pulling in local foodies across the land. How about some Juxtaposition of Duck for tonight's dinner at the Black Cat in midtown Boulder? That's pastured local duck served with grapefruit mustard, tempura parsnips, and onion scape ragout. Veg'ns will surely revel in the Potato and Beet Napoleon, prepared with quinoa crust, elderberry gastrique, and baby spinach. Some restaurant owners are even living and laboring on their own family farms. Black Cat's award-winning chef Eric Skokan sources nearly 90% of *everything* from the 130-acre organic farm he created with wife Jill, just a few miles from town. "Because we harvest every day," Skokan states proudly, "we can select varieties for flavor, not storage and transportation—which is all too common these days."

From Providence, Rhode Island to Tillamook, Oregon, the 98% of Americans who don't live on farms are yearning to taste food hand-picked this very morning. Ours is a real hunger to see and smell fertile green fields, to commune with our neighbors—that's why attendance at elegant farm-to-table dinners is exploding. And in those long, leisurely evenings given over to camaraderie and the delights of the palate, we exemplify the best of the Slow Food movement and its peaceful resistance to the extremes of fast food and nutrient-stripped mass agriculture.

Fighting the industrial beast its own way, the Slow Money movement inspires community investment. "We are working in the soil of a new economy," founder Woody Tasch announced at Slow Money's recent nationwide gathering. Forget *venture* capital with its dependence on exploitation and excess consumption; that model is ruining our health and the planet's. The economy of the 21st century will be based on *nurture* capital, on sustainability at the farm and community levels.

THE WORK HAS BEGUN in earnest. After a steep decline, the number of US farms is up for the first time since 1935, and many of these farmers are young college grads, fresh-faced and eager. That's good news because our nation's food growers are getting up there; the average age is now 55. According to the USDA, we desperately need up to 100,000 new farmers. So even if you're a bored bank teller in spiked heels who's never lifted a pitchfork in your life, you can enroll in the Organic Farm Training program at Michigan State and start getting some real dirt under those manicured fingernails.

The first ripples of the coming food tsunami are sweeping across the nation, destroying not only corporate myths but vegan myths about omnivores and sustainability. In cities across America, urban farming is spreading like seeds in a windstorm. At Rohit Kumar's southern California home, 5,000 pounds of food are grown annually on a plot the size of a basketball court—enough to feed his family of four all year long—and in central Seattle, Lee Kindell harvests 50 pounds of edible fish every 3-4 months from his closed-loop hydroponics system, feeding their poop to strawberries and other crops he raises alongside chickens and bees. From Asheville to Albuquerque, school kids are growing their own lunch food, teaching the USDA about real nutrition, and citizens of Boston and Ann Arbor fought for their right to raise backyard goats and chickens. "This is a serious issue; it's no yolk." declared Mayor Dave Cieslewicz as Madison reversed its poultry ban. "Chickens are really bringing us together as a community."

And so much more is happening. International Slow Food aligning with the United Nations to advance farmers' livelihoods and animal welfare. Foundations like Weston Price promoting the nutrient-dense whole foods of our ancestors. Biodynamic farming—crops, animals and soil as one self-sustaining ecosystem— now taking off in 47 countries. Pasture cropping in Australia that's producing *three food sources* every year (sheep, cereal, and edible native grass seeds) from a single no-till parcel that mimics nature. Indigenous tribes fighting for restoration of their native hunting and fishing rights, turning their backs on disease-causing industrial food. As Amy George, Tsleil-Waututh Nation elder, chided the passive and reluctant men in her tribe: "Just when are you going to stand up for your children and their future? It's time to warrior up!"

THE LOCAL FOOD MOVEMENT has potential for explosive lateral growth, leaping from town to town. Even our largest urban areas are drawing up guidelines to foster vertical farming and regional cuisine, including heavy players like New York City—second only to the military in billions spent on food. Innovative city councils are also jumping into the food foray—when towering stalks of sweet corn kept showing up in Portland, Oregon front yards, the city switched from angry prosecution to active encouragement of urban agriculture.

Meanwhile, Portland, Maine is pushing for 50% local food in public schools within five years, and the Vermont Farm to Plate Network is working to double food production and build long-term viability in the entire New England region. Proclaimed a beaming Chuck Ross at the Network's annual gathering: "We are putting people back on the land to learn from it, work it, restore it, and steward it for subsequent generations!"

And then there's Sedgwick, Maine, population 1,200. The whole country is watching Sedgwick—everyone in the food-freedom movement, that is. In good old Yankee style, this tight-knit coastal community became the nation's first to declare food sovereignty. Voting *yes!* for their fundamental right to choose their own food and nutrition, the fair citizens of Sedgwick decreed it unlawful for both the state and feds to interfere. In so doing, this feisty Maine town borrows a great line from its neighbor to the west: *Live free or die!*

Other communities have followed Sedgwick's lead, adamantly declaring food sovereignty. Be it tart apples or sweet wedding cakes, raw milk or locally raised meat, these residents want to enter into buyer-seller agreements exactly like our grandparents did—and leave the meddling politicians out of it. They're tired of ever-expanding, costly regulations that keep them from making a decent living, especially since it's industrial products that are causing food borne illnesses, not theirs. It's tough enough making a go of it in rural communities, but up until the last few generations you didn't need a $10,000 facility for a handful of goats, nor a special license every time you want to sell cinnamon rolls to your neighbors.

You and I don't have control over our food: government and a mere handful of corporations do. Wander through America's crowded and adored farmers markets and it's difficult to fathom but, yes, even here in Boulder County, foodie capital of the Mountain West, only 3% of our food is locally sourced. Fully 97% arrives from around the world—and Colorado is a major agricultural state! Most Americans don't have a clue where their food comes from and live disconnected from the land, enslaved to a global system that wants to keep us powerless. Veggie or omnie, we buy the bulk of our food from superchains, much of it processed and imported, hiding genetically modified organisms and dependent on child labor, wild animal deaths, and soil-depleting practices to haul in fast profits.

The transition from thousands of small locally-owned stores to a few Goliath supermarkets was virtually complete by the 1950s. "That is not very long ago," Joel Salatin reminds his rapt audience in the old Chautauqua barn, his voice blending wistfulness with hope. "Until then, where was all the food? Dear folks, the food was in our kitchens and our gardens, our local fields and forests. It was in the pantry, the cellar, the backyard." It was in our hands; it was in our power. And it wasn't stripped of nutrition, sprayed with cancer-linked pesticides, and harvested in depleted soils. So unplug all the microwaves and toss the frozen frankenfood! It's time to rediscover our own kitchens. Time to start buying and, yes, growing some healthy food of our own!

"NATURE BATS LAST"

With the looming radical convergence of global heat-up, vanishing topsoil and evaporating water, creating self-sustaining communities is now imperative. Even the conservative accounting firm PricewaterhouseCoopers predicts widespread economic devastation and at-risk food production if humanity fails to avoid the catastrophic 2-degree-rise tipping point now on track for 2050. And beyond that? The difference between a two and four-degree rise, as one climate expert tersely informs us, is human civilization.

Yet the human race continues, pathologically, to pursue a limitless growth economy and to dig, drill, and frack for ever more fossil fuel—dumping carbon into the atmosphere at an aggressive rate. How will our children ever forgive us? Consider this: the average American city has only three days worth of food on its grocery shelves and the average industrial food product travels 1,500 miles via a vast international supply chain. If the supply line breaks at any point, or distant soil and water dry up, millions will be affected. The high-warp speed at which climate change is unfolding makes the shift from fossil fuels extremely urgent, and 1/3 of human-caused emissions are coming from our global food system.

We're not talking just cattle poop here. Updated new numbers more honestly include the entire process: crops for direct and indirect human consumption; storage and transportation; pesticide/fertilizer production and use; livestock factories; and plant/animal refrigeration. *Omnie or veggie, we are escalating climate change with our mindless industrial food habits.* "Our current global food economy is already showing signs of breakdown," Michael Brownlee, director of the Local Food Shift Group, informed me during a sobering summertime interview that had me shivering in the ninety degree heat. "If humans continue to deny that the way we live and eat is not sustainable—and only want to make slight lifestyle changes—it's like rearranging chairs on the Titanic."

Even relatively prosperous communities in Colorado and elsewhere will feel the heat of future food shortages. "When the world food crisis finally lands here, we need to be ready to respond," cautions Brownlee, whose mission is to foster a foodshed perspective. "When you see the river rising, you go down to the river and start piling up the sandbags. That's what you do, and the people who see it are already moving on it." New strategies for intensive agriculture are now in place, like greenhouse cultivation on 40 acres at Denver International Airport's Agri-park. And new workers are being enlisted, as in the Veterans to Farmers program which places unemployed Iraq War veterans in local farming ventures. Our Local Food Shift's goal for the Rocky Mountain Front Range and its eight million people? At least 25% local food within the next 10 years.

Get real, the cynics say. It can't be done. Big Ag is too entrenched, humans too ensnared by their no-brain habits. But that's exactly what the naysayers said about the now-exploding organic movement. Just a few decades ago, people were laughing out loud at the crazy farmer-hippies! In their wildest dreams, no one thought organic would move beyond a few romantic back-to-the-landers who despised chemicals and kept faith in nature's truths. Customers lampooned the overpriced greens wilting in the back of funky little stores, and the pesticide industry predicted low yields and market collapse. Laugh no more at a rock-solid idea whose time has come. Or rather, come again. Only a few generations ago, *all* our food was organic.

Now the fastest-growing sector in food sales, organic has more than proven its viability against agribusiness. It's far more efficient, using 45% less energy and emitting 60% less greenhouse gases. Moreover, much-anticipated long-term study results from Iowa (Delate et al) confirm what those not-so-crazy farmers believed and what common sense has always suggested: organic farming, with its natural soil amendments and crop rotations, does a far better job of building the fertility of the soil and retaining water, all the while producing high healthy yields. Corn and soybean yields were found to be "statistically equivalent" to their chemically-doused counterparts, while oat and alfalfa yields surpassed county averages. Organic also out-produced conventional during times of drought and excessive rainfall, a critical advantage as climate change pounds us with wilder and wilder weather.

And here's the real kick in our collective planetary face. Despite the world-wide application of five billion pounds of endocrine-disrupting, animal-slaying pesticides every single year, "no significant difference" was found in the number of pests visiting conventional versus organic plots. Skilled management practices, researchers conclude, override the need for any synthetics or pesticides. *All that poison, all those deaths, for nothing.*

The economic news for organic farmers is equally startling: worldwide sales have tripled, with a projected 20% annual growth rate. Many organic ventures of the 1970s have, in fact, been bought out by major food corporations. "Exactly!" retort the skeptics. "The originally movement has been co-opted." Yet the current farm movement is intrinsically and marvelously different. Small-scale, diversi-fied, local agriculture must by definition remain small, diverse and neighborly. Nothing in the word "organic" demands these same parameters.

Those of us who witnessed the farm seizures and foreclosures of the 1980s—when farmers were told to *get big or get out!*—have already seen what happens when family farms are bankrupted and brought to their knees by corporations which fuse them into giant monocultures: The cumulative loss of topsoil followed by chemical drenching in a futile effort to restore fertility. The ensuing toxic run-off that pollutes our streams and aquifers, destroying native fish and spawning grounds. The mass spraying of pesticides that endanger myriad species, including our own. The frightening growth of superweeds already resistant to these poisons. The creation of fake industrial food, empty calories and obese children, and the shoving of genetically altered food upon us without so much as an honest label. The grossly inhumane treatment of domesticated animals and the invisible slaying of wild ones. It's like bad science fiction. Perverse, idiot species devises methods to kill off the soil, water, plants and animals that sustain it.

Yes, we have seen what happens when small farms fade from our landscape and get big and then bigger. We have witnessed this calamity once and won't be fooled again. Or perhaps we should just wait to take back the land ourselves when these unsustainable super systems collapse, which collapse they will in due time. Chemical-dependent mono-agriculture and genetically-altered crops cannot long survive because they go directly against the way nature works. "Time has a way of weeding out the freaks," Joel Salatin reminds us. "In spite of everything that modern science can do, in spite of all the computer programs at our disposal," nature's design eventually emerges as the most appropriate and efficient.

Much like animal factories, industrial crop agriculture has been around a mere 50-60 years; sun-and-grass-dependent diversified farming a good 10,000 years. Dear readers who have come this far on the journey: in our guts we know which system will meet its eventual demise. And in our hearts we know which one will rejuvenate our damaged earth and endure through time, restoring dignity to our food animals, plants, and farmers. "For too long the food system has rewarded those who flaunt human cleverness and believe that human arrogance can trump nature's principles," Joel is close to whispering now in the echoing barn, insisting that each and every one of us listen. "But guess what, folks? Nature always bats last—and our food system is crying out for change."

IT'S NOT THE MEEK who shall inherit our compromised earth, it's the mindful. And the wide-awake among us have already begun to act, supporting organic local agriculture or even starting up our own pocket-sized urban farms. Actually, it's beginning to feel unconscionable to sit around and wait for our current food system to collapse, so here are some basic steps each one of us can take *today* to get this food tsunami moving full-force in our communities and worldwide:

- o Support local organic farmers with your food dollars; visit their farms and orchards: smell the soil; talk to them; *buy* from them.
- o STOP purchasing your food at box stores, chain restaurants and fast food outlets—and get yourself and the earth healthier in the process.
- o *Boycott ALL factory farmed meat and dairy for the rest of your life.*
- o Frequent your nearest farmer's market for family groceries—don't just make the rounds and nibble.
- o Buy in season, and if you can't always find local or regional food, at least buy from the USA vs. New Zealand or Ecuador, etc.

- Don't be fooled by those "cage-free" or "free-range" labels on eggs. No inspection system means fraud is common, so buy "Certified Humane" or from a local farmer whose birds you can observe.
- Purchase or catch your own fish from wild, sustainable fisheries.
- Grow your own food: an entire garden or simple pots of herbs and veggies on your front porch or deck.
- Purchase from local, organic, family dairies if your body does well with dairy products; raw or cultured are always best.
- *Become a Restaurant Vegan, whenever unsure of a food's origin.*
- Support local or regional ranches, buying 100% grass-raised, grass-finished meat only—and be brave and eat crickets!

Of course, becoming a locavore veg'n is an admirable goal and not out of the question for some individuals. Depending on your genetic and metabolic makeup, and where in the world you live, this might be possible. As a home-based vegan or vegetarian, however, your protein sources will likely be limited and unless you live in a year-round warm climate, only seasonally available. A minimal-meat or lacto-ovo diet, locally sourced, may be a wiser choice for your health. Pay close attention and you'll discover what is right for you.

IF YOUR QUARREL is not just with factory animals but the eating of animals at all, however humanely raised in an earth-sustaining manner, then I suggest you look long and deep at your revulsions concerning pain and death, including your own, and your denial of the laws of nature and the food chain of which you—yes, you, an animal in blue jeans and clogs—are an integral, organic part. For these laws, which bind each and every one of us to this splendid earth, demand the symbiotic nourishing of life with life. And it's evolutionary biology, not the individual, that gets to dictate which life forms best nourish another.

The vegan argument displays a lot of heart, we can all admit to that, but hardly any evolutionary logic.

40.

ANCESTRAL HUNTERS:
THE ANIMAL AS SACRED

"Our diet consists entirely of souls."

—Inuit expression

WHO BETTER UNDERSTOOD than our distant ancestors, the sacred, scary food exchange between humans and other animals? Over a million years ago, early humans on the sere African plains gazed often and deeply into the eyes of wild animals. Hunter-gatherers, *Homo erectus* understood their kindred creatures in profound and intimate ways. They had to. Their very existence depended upon it. Something that we risk-free, drive-up, all-you-can-shove-in-your-mouth moderns cannot even begin to fathom.

Few dispute our natural hunting heritage except, of course, lotus-eating vegans who want very badly for our ancient ancestors to have been plant-munchers only. They want this so badly, they will devote lengthy articles and endless blogs to the subject, attempting to prove the Golden Age of Idyllic Veganism really did exist, indicative of humanity's true nature.

So let's, for the moment, indulge in the possibility of this ancestral paradise before our flesh-eating fall. To do this we must time-travel all the way back to the Miocene, 15-25 million years ago, and ponder the leaf-eating monkeys and apes whose populations exploded during this period. When your habitat is treetops, that's what you grab and eat: leaves, nuts, and fruits in abundance. Yet even these primordial apes searched for substantial protein sources beyond plants. As much as the sweet juicy fruit, our primitive ancestors were after the larvae, grubs, and maggots gnawing away inside. To this day, wild monkeys often display more interest in the weevil than the infested fig, the grub than the creamy butterfruit.

Anthropologists used to spend a lot of time trying to figure out all the uneaten, discarded fruit on a tropical forest floor. "Monkeys do a lot of sniffing, feeling, exploratory nibbling and spitting out before they pick the fruit they want," Marvin Harris explains in *Good to Eat: Riddles of Food and Culture.* "But they are not looking for the perfect, ripe, unblemished Garden of Eden apple; they are trying to find the ones with the worm inside."

And let's not forget that these tree-flying hominoids arrived at their easy-pickings plant-and-insect diet alongside a wet, warm continent smothered in rain-forest. How then, dear vegans, does this cat-sized, teensy-brained, far-distant ancestor in any way *equate* to the bipedal human whose body and diet evolved in the face of a vastly different environment? And let's not fail to ponder standoffs with the fiercest and fastest predators on the planet—something that tree-dwellers rarely had to face. Two million years ago, when a changing climate forced these ancient hominoids to live on a dry, treeless grassland with all its dangers, thrills and unknowns, a whole new set of physical and mental skills was required. And the diet, morphology, and physiology of our ancestors began to differentiate in response to these fresh challenges.

"Animal foods play a special role in the nutritional physiology of our species," confirms anthropologist Harris. The hominoid that rigidly stuck to plants, the big-jawed vegetarian with massive molars, *Paranthropus robustus,* did not in the end turn out to be so robust. Its line went extinct. The *Homo erectus* line survived in large part due to a varied diet that included meat, resulting in a large, complex, problem-solving brain. Meanwhile, the docile, plant-eating *P. robustus* vanished into the African mist.

Still, a good number of vegans appear fixated on the quite charming idea that the hominoid species from which modern humans evolved was a passive plants-only eater, thereby proudly asserting that this is our natural diet and thus everyone would be very smart to follow it. It's a singularly strange obsession on several counts. Most obviously, to evolve means exactly that, to transform into something different over time. Furthermore, even those colossal-jawed, extinct plant-eaters feasted on termites now and then for their rich protein stores. Hammering the final nail in the coffin of the peaceful ape theory were Jane Goodall's 1960s field discoveries that rocked the anthropological world.

As it turns out, the modern chimpanzee, our closest relative with an estimated 98.5% shared DNA, is not the docile vegetarian once assumed. Rather, he is a very efficient and calculating hunter of mammals, including bushpigs, juvenile baboons and small antelopes, with a clear fondness for red colobus monkeys—35 vertebrate species in all. Although flesh constitutes a limited proportion of their diet—chimpanzees are omnivores, remember, not carnivores—it is a seasonally regular and deliberate choice. Researchers estimate per capita meat intake at 65 grams a day per adult during the dry season—about the same, actually, as a 130-pound protein-craving human.

This amount "approaches the meat intake by the members of some human foraging societies in the lean months of the year," according to renowned primate expert Dr. Craig B. Stanford, who agrees with other evolutionary biologists that predation by chimps is both socially and nutritionally based. "After all, meat from monkeys and other prey would be a package of protein, fat, and calories hard to equal from any plant food."

Further research reveals that female Gombe chimps who receive generous shares of flesh following a hunt have more surviving offspring, indicating a powerful reproductive benefit to meat-eating. "When we ask the question *when did meat become an important part of the human diet?*" continues Stanford, "we must look well before the evolutionary split between apes and humans in our own family tree."

Basically, if the nutritional rewards of a certain food are large enough compared to calorie output and risk—smart animals will go for it. That leaves out junk-eating humans, of course. Wild chimpanzees, by contrast, carefully plan their group ambushes to secure high nutrient benefits. Once all escape routes are covered, the surprised prey is swiftly grabbed and instantly flailed to death against a tree or rock. The fresh meat is then eaten alone or shared with the group. The brain is prized above all else because chimpanzees *are* intelligent. They not only know when extra stores of protein and fat are required, but realize there's something special in brain food.

It's called phosphatidylserine (PS), a superstar nutrient for cognitive function, and animal brains are loaded with it. While the human body produces some PS, athletes, the elderly, and the depressed among us may need more as it is the single best nutrient for revitalizing the brain and boosting energy at the cellular level. The highest-level safe sources are organ meats, like the liver and kidney. Organs also happen to be densely packed with the nutrients most commonly deficient in a plants-only diet: complete protein, riboflavin, co-enzyme Q10, zinc, selenium, the vitamins A, B12, D3 and K2, plus high amounts of DHA.

369

YET THE MYTH of our ancestral paradise dies hard. The iconic image of a pretty, peaceful Eden—the blameless lion reclining beside the innocent lamb, claws eternally retracted—has long haunted the human psyche yearning for a non-violent world. And today's passionate plant-eaters have taken up the cause with a ferocity that would do their wild-pig hunting ancestors proud.

Standing apart from these believers—who want so badly for our ancient kin to have been flesh abstainers that they look at all the paleontological evidence with what appears to be closed eyes—Harvard anthropologist and vegetarian Randall Collura readily admits that "we evolved eating a wide variety of diets containing both plants and animal food [and] the first thing we need to do is abandon the Garden of Eden mythology." It's not as sexy or saccharine a prehistory, but our ancestors were neither ferocious carnivores straight out of mythical Arcadia, nor docile fruit-pickers kicked out of a vegan Eden. They were resourceful omnivores and tenacious hustlers, both predator and prey, as likely to stalk as be stalked.

Adjusting to a lack of protective cover and vegetative abundance wasn't easy. As the fruitful, easy livin' forests disappeared, our hungry ancestors needed to sharpen their senses and learn to predict outcomes. Ambushing weaker creatures became the norm—lizards, birds, fish and small mammals were all candidates for consumption—but our distant kin also shadowed bigger, burlier animals in patient attendance of scraps. "Hunting for meat and marrow out on the naked spaces, the odd, two-legged newcomers learned to scan the horizon for descending vultures, to listen for the roar of lions, to track spoor on the run," declares William Stolzenburg in *Where the Wild Things Were.* "Lacking brawn, the apes needed pluck and hustle to succeed at what would become a pirating life in plain view.... If they could not subdue it, they would scavenge it."

It wasn't all flesh food by any means. The women gathered seasonal plant foods, probably endlessly. By some estimates, females in hunting societies did 80% of the family work compared to males. (Sound familiar, ladies?) Whenever available, edible plants constituted a notable portion of our ancestors' mixed diet; anthropologists are in agreement about this. However, including a lot of valuable plant food in one's diet does not a vegan or vegetarian make. Are we all finally clear on this fundamental point?

Enter *Australopithecus africanus* 2.5 million years ago, a contemporary of the extinct vegetarian *P. robustus* and possibly our true ancestor—the final verdict is still out. Bipedal tool users, these creatures were curious and adaptive, willing to work with the changing environment in ever inventive ways. This ability to be

370

creative and flexible in problem solving, including how and what to eat, turned early humans into very successful hunters. Reasoning power, foresight, and finely honed observational skills were all developed with one goal in mind: to survive.

The ever changing elements of nature—climate, topography, vegetation—and the presence of other animals—pursued, pursuing—these are the forces that created our fleet-footed ancestors, their nimble fingers, keen vision, and exploding brains. These are the forces that turned us into human beings. "In the relative heartbeat of a million years, between the chimp-like *Australopithecines* and the human form of *Homo sapiens*, the size of the brain tripled," affirms Stolzenburg. "It had become the fastest-growing organ in the history of life." So go ahead and disdain animal eating if you wish, but it's your meat-eating ancestors who gave you the capacity to think rationally, plan ahead, create beautiful art, and argue vegan philosophy.

It is biologically implausible that humans evolved our large brain on a plants-only diet. Our ancestors needed meat in order to obtain all of the nutrient-dense calories, proteins, fatty acids, and vitamin B12 required for large-brain evolution and maintenance, confirms researcher Suzana Herculano-Houzel of the Institute of Biomedical Sciences. Later, the invention of cooking allowed more foods to be eaten year-round, while releasing additional nutrients from plants and animals.

It's for all these reasons that big-bodied, raw-plant eaters, such as cows, have diminished brains. Even hulking gorillas possess just 1/3 the neurons of our hefty, neuron-rich human brains. Despite almost non-stop grazing—up to 80% of a 12-hour tropical day—large herbivores simply cannot get enough calories and essential nutrients on their vegan diet to support a large, complicated, labyrinth brain. Our smaller body size compared to other large mammals is an evolutionary trade-off. We got a bigger brain instead.

To feed the 86 billion neurons of our energy-hungry brains—2% of our body mass demanding 20% of the fuel—humans need regular, nutrient-dense packets of food that don't entail near-constant gathering, i.e., meat. With their miserable tales of non-stop grazing and unremitting hunger, ex-vegans tell me that they are so much happier, healthier and engaged, now that they're no longer enslaved to their stomachs.

Need more proof of our meaty evolution toward higher intelligence? In the Great Rift Valley of eastern Africa, archeologists discovered the enlarged, more spherical hominin craniums of *Homo habilis*, 1.5 million years old and evidence of greatly increased brain size and cognitive function. Sharp-edged butchering tools were found there as well, along with copious remains of devoured animals, from birds and fish to antelopes, pigs, and bovids. It's still hotly debated whether those human cut marks came before or after the chew marks of carnivores on those same bones. The upshot, however, is the same: early humans ate plenty of animals—and used ever more sophisticated tools to do so.

Modern vegans who grudgingly accept the overwhelming scientific evidence often refer to our human ancestors as partial vegetarians. If that moniker makes you feel better, go for it, but our human ancestors were omnivores just like us. We're certainly not carnivores with grasping claws, formidable jaws, and a highly elastic stomach for holding bulky amounts of hide, meat, organs and bones. Meat eaters aren't making the carnivore claim, as too many veggies falsely maintain. Nor are we herbivores, strict plant-eaters with large food sacs for fermentation and long digestive systems for handling profuse fiber.

Happily, we are right in between, with the specialized teeth, digestive capabilities, and adaptive skills to intake a healthy mix of both plant and animal foods, allowing us to survive just about any climate, topography, or challenging circumstance. Flexitarian is a fine 21st century word to describe humanity's original and ongoing eating behavior.

What's more, traditional methods of hunting and gathering went easy on the natural world compared to that grim reaper, modern corporate agriculture. Beets or beef, all industrial-scale food production leaves death and destruction in its wake. Given all this environmental havoc to keep our bloated refrigerators fully stocked, humankind's few surviving hunting-foraging societies may well be the wisest patrons of our planet's remaining resources.

"The last free people on earth" is what some of us call the hundred or so self-sufficient tribes still living in total isolation from the larger world, uncontacted and supremely content. Unbelievably, yes, they still exist. From the Amazon rainforest to the highlands of New Guinea, these indigenous people live in solidarity with the land and their communities, still hunting with spears and arrows, still gathering roots and shoots. On their forested Indian Ocean island, the Sentinelese have been "let be" to live continuously and sustainably for over 50,000 years—an island of self-sufficiency, a safe harbor from exploitation. Traditional hunting tribes in North America, including the Inuit of modern-day Canada, have not been so lucky.

372

PATIENTLY WAITING FOR THE CURRENTS

One of the primary virtues the Inuit teach their children is silence. Along with patience and gratitude, silence is a condition of high-quality living, a condition of the hunt. Deeply connected to the natural world, good hunters practice a form of meditation that doesn't require chanting, mantras, or imported Zen pillows. What it does require is stillness and presence. *Hunt the animal that comes to you.*

I am reminded here of a yoga retreat I attended on California's north coast a few years back. Gathering in a circle that first morning to share stories of purpose and place, one wise middle-age woman with light-giving eyes—I'll never forget those eyes—told us about the forest-dwelling people who've lived for generations in her native Appalachian region. "They don't need yoga or meditation," she informed the disbelieving young yogis. "They have nature."

Spread thinly across the high Arctic regions of our planet, the Inuit likewise possess intimate knowledge of their natural environment and its inhabitants, a product of quiet observation, direct inquiry, and nutritional necessity. How many of us, yogis included, can cite all the native animals—thriving, threatened and extinct—of our own bioregion? How far fewer of us actually spend our days in the humbling company of these vibrant, vanishing, co-evolving beings?

In contrast, the Inuit breathe, touch and wrap themselves in animals, dependent on them for their very existence. Until recently, these semi-nomadic people moved wherever the arctic creatures led them in this harsh, unforgiving landscape at the top of the world. Hunting sea mammals in the dark days of winter; tracking herds of caribou or muskoxen during the brief, intense spark of summer. Out of sealskins they created *gajaqs*, kayaks, and from animal bones, baleen and wood, they fashioned their *qamutiks*, sturdy sleds. Befriending wolves, they entered into symbiotic relationship, feeding them in exchange for being led to food. These people slept with animals, shared food with animals, respected them, worshipped them and, yes, ate them as needed to prolong their own lives.

The great peril of our existence lies in the fact that our diet consists entirely of souls. So goes a profound Inuit expression, echoing their ancestors' strong belief in animal souls, while acknowledging the fear and anxiety that are part and parcel of living in the Far North, never knowing when a whole village might starve if the animals didn't appear. In the shifting, flaming aurora borealis, Inuit hunters saw the ecstatic movements of animal spirits and prayed to them for guidance. Walking out to the sea's edge they invoked Sedna, the Old Woman who dwells among the watery beings of the deep. And guided by *angakkuit,* their powerful shaman—possessed of the ability to fly and transform into other beings—they appealed to the animals to be merciful in their giving to humans.

Inuit art, stunning in its beauty and mysticism, abounds with images of animals and the hunt. Their sculptures are freely created from wild beasts: whalebone and caribou pelvis; antlers and horns. Jagged teeth. And their vivid textiles and prints depict humans constantly surrounded, even inhabited by animals. Walruses reach out with human arms; men dance in white bear bodies; women metamorphose into shiny ravens.

This constant human-animal interchange—one playfully swapping with the other—is echoed in the art of the Inuit's neighbors, the Inupiaq of the Bering Sea. Look closely at their animal icons and you will find tiny human faces carved or sewn into them, peering out at you with inquiring, benevolent eyes. While Buddhists often symbolize our condition with images of a "gentle, meditating human figure seated in the midst of the world of phenomena, the Inupiaq would present a panoply of different creatures, each with a little hidden human face," writes Gary Snyder in *The Practice of the Wild.* "It is a way of saying that each creature is a spirit with an intelligence as brilliant as our own."

Today many Inuit continue to hunt and fish in the traditional way, creating their own sleds and gear while adapting to modern rifles, spears and snowmobiles as needed. The rich nutrition of walrus, whale, salmon, seal and musk-oxen is gladly shared with everyone, creating strong communal bonds. The idea of an individual owning food is foreign to this tribe. Hunting is done for all The People, and community freezers store any surplus meat, eaten both raw and cooked.

From the flesh and blubber of one bowhead whale, an entire village and all relations can be fed many times over. As Ronald Brower, Sr. of Barrow, Alaska, proudly states, "The bowhead whale for the Inuit people has been the center of our cultural, nutritional, and spiritual well-being for over 3,800 years." Before the disease of speed took over modern lives everywhere, the Inuit did not pursue a whale across open water, but patiently waited for the currents, winds, and animal spirits to bring one close to shore.

To ensure that liberated souls stay happy, the Inuit show respect to every food animal, expressing prayers of gratitude for its munificent gifts. And few gifts are as cherished as the dense, high-fat, high-protein flesh of *nattiq,* the ringed seal, whose wide-ranging abundance is very welcomed by natives (and polar bears) in this windswept land of scarce resources. The drinking of seal blood is traditional, symbolizing the spiritual unity of humans and animals and believed to fortify the consumer's own blood.

Compared to modern food from the *qallunaat*, "white people from the south" (food which many Inuit claim makes them weak and sick), their high-animal diet delivers bounteous energy, strength, stamina and lasting warmth. Hugely different from the vegan worldview of "exploitation," in the Inuit belief system the animals consider it a privilege to serve the great cycle of Life. And the Inuit consider it a privilege to serve as well, when their own time arrives to give back.

The Inuit do not sentimentalize death. They do honor and celebrate the endless cycles of birth, death, and interspecies nourishment in which all of earth's beings must participate. As one village elder prayed aloud during a recent hunt: "We give thanks to the seals for their lives in order that our world be sustained!" The deep-gift economy is what poet Snyder calls it, the ongoing, evolutionary, sacred energy exchange of life for life. If you view this sacrament of eating other life forms as a "ripping off" process, he gently reminds us, your metaphysics are hopelessly messed up.

YET CERTAIN LATTE-SIPPING vegans in temperate climes demand we ship tofu and grains to these same natives, denying them the hunt. And it's the Inuit that animal rights groups have tried to publicly shame and strip of their ancestral diet and livelihood in yet another crass example of reverse speciesism. For one of its more deceptive anti-sealing tirades, PETA borrowed the mascot of the 2010 Vancouver Olympics, the *inuksuk*—an iconic Inuit symbol of their ancestors—then defaced it for a campaign image: above the Olympic rings, drenched in blood, the inuksuk pummels to death a baby seal. Never mind that these people practice sustainable harvests for food and economic survival; do not kill seal pups; do not kill by beating; have nothing to do with the notorious, industrial mass slaughter of seals off Canada's east coast and publicly condemn it. In a perfect word-twist, Canadian journalist Aaron Spitzer aptly renames this reverse-speciesism group: People for the Un-Ethical Treatment of the Inuit.

"It doesn't matter where you live or what your ancestors ate!" assert the more fanatical animal liberationists. "Now that we can transport hemp, flax, and myriad processed plant proteins anywhere in the world, it's inexcusable, indeed unethical, for anyone to hunt, kill, or eat animal flesh. In this day and age, absolutely no one needs to eat meat!" Rarely have I heard a more culturally prejudiced, racially biased, environmentally naïve, and genetically-ignorant statement.

The Inuit have already been forced into permanent settlements against their will, had Christianity imposed upon them and our system of law shoved down their throats. Shall we also insist that they—and all indigenous hunters—consume *our* food, follow *our* lifestyle, and surrender their sacred animal culture and inherent right to full health?

Like human tribes everywhere, the genetic and dietary dictates of the Inuit have evolved alongside very explicit environmental conditions over tens of thousands of years. The result is a very high-fat diet that's essential in meeting the demands of the Arctic: up to 75% fat in the winter, with the remainder primarily protein—all from indigenous animals. Living among the Alaskan Inuit in the 1920s, Canadian anthropologist Dr. Vilhjalmur Stefansson was startled to observe the hearty good health that this exceedingly low-carbohydrate diet conferred on these people. Yes, the Inuit obtained all the necessary vitamins directly from their plant-free winter food, including vitamin C from the liver of ringed seals— findings greeted with great skepticism at the time but which subsequent studies have confirmed.

Stefansson himself lived almost exclusively on fish and other meat during nine years of Arctic exploration and easily maintained his robust health. The few times he got ill was when animal fat was unavailable. Upon his return, no one believed his claim. "The arguments ranged from metaphysics to chemistry [to] the Bible," Stefansson would later write. "He would get scurvy if he had no vegetables in [his] meat. The kidneys would be ruined by overwork. There would be protein poisoning and, in general, hell to pay." To convince the medical establishment and other doubters, Stefansson agreed to replicate his experience in a research trial that makes the paleo crowd look like wimps: 100% red meat and offal every day for an entire year. No fish, no plants, no supplements. Just 100-140 grams of daily animal protein (15-25%), 200-300 grams of fat (75-85%), and roughly 12 grams of carbs from the stored glycogen in organs. Radical.

The health results were published in *The Journal of Biological Chemistry* in 1930. They were as follows: no loss of physical or mental vigor; no deterioration of teeth (gingivitis disappeared); loss of only a few pounds (started at a healthy weight; daily calories: 2,000-3,000); same low blood pressure before and after; no digestive issues (except when protein was temporarily upped to 45%); no kidney problems; no calcium or vitamin deficiencies. Overall? Outstanding mental and physical health. Stefansson even had a healthier scalp and thicker hair at year's end. Can humans survive and even flourish on meat alone? The answer is yes, if the ancestors of those humans evolved in cold climate zones deficient in year-round plants and thick with animals. Stefansson was of Icelandic heritage.

Whatever our specific environment, nature provides and the human body adapts and evolves. In accord with this basic principle, humans from northern zones have precise, genetically-coded enzymes and morphological structures to break down large quantities of animal protein and fat. So envision if you dare, One World Vegans, the traditional Inuit, Inupiaq, and other indigenous tribes enjoying exceptional health and immunity while consuming several pounds of fatty meat a day. And chew on this—if fat-deprived brains allow for such focused consideration, mine certainly didn't during my final meatless years—humans who live in cold climes burn calories quickly, require high-fat animal foods to retain their health, and are not genetically equipped to survive as vegetarians, let alone skinny vegans.

I remember hearing vegan guru Dr. Gabriel Cousens express bafflement when a residential guest at his Tree of Life health center in southern Arizona declared that she absolutely could not function on 100% plants upon return to her native Canada, however hard she tried. Why are he and other plant eaters so surprised by this corporal reality? *Our smart human bodies evolved in synch with our natural environments, not our moral philosophies.*

REGRETTABLY, compulsory assimilation since the 1940s has taken a very heavy emotional and spiritual toll on the Inuit. Many feel lost and conflicted, drifting between two incongruent cultures. Enculturation has excised a toll on their physical health as well. As they stray from their traditional high-animal diet and eat ever more flown-in plant carbs (just as some vegans wished upon them), there's been a devastating increase in obesity, diabetes, heart disease and other conditions rarely seen even a generation ago. Along with the loss of an honorable and active lifestyle, inadequate nutrition for the Inuit's specific genetic makeup is a contributing factor to their alarming rates of infant mortality, depression, substance abuse and suicide.

Fighting to preserve their cultural identity through activism and art, the Inuit remain proud of their ancestral traditions, including their abiding relationship with the animals of *Nunatsiaq*, The Beautiful Land. Those who continue to hunt understand with great depth the ways of caribou, seal, whale, walrus and Arctic char—what the activist movement "Idle No More" rightly calls *Indigenous Ways of Knowing.* Similarly, the Plains Indians who once thrived in the grasslands of Colorado possessed precise, intimate knowledge of their living food sources—so astonishingly different from the obscure, disengaged relationship most of us now suffer with our daily food.

STREAK YOUR BODY WITH VERMILION AND MUD

That Colorado tribe was the Arapaho. Come late fall, these Algonquin-speaking people would split into smaller camps and move into the sheltering foothills of the Rockies, right where I live. Of course, "sheltering" is a relative term. Many a winter night plunges into the minus-zero digits around here, and just this week 70 mph winds ripped apart 100-foot tall cottonwoods. But compared to the icy blasts on the open plains where wind chills sink to 50 below? Where blizzards barrel through at 120 mph with nothing to hinder their way? This is a sanctuary.

With the welcome arrival of spring, the Arapaho people transformed into bison chasers, edging onto the gaping flatlands in search of sustenance. Like all Plains tribes, they depended on this majestic, lumbering herbivore for their existence. Even if green plants had been available year round, no amount of plant food alone could have supported their arduous lifestyle, sustained their health, and pulled them through the extreme winters. Acutely aware of their vulnerability, these people prayed to a higher power before each and every hunt. "Take pity on us," anthropologist George Bird Grinnell heard the Pawnee men and women cry out. "Send us plenty of buffalo….help the people—send us plenty of meat so that we may be strong and our bodies may increase and our flesh grow hard."

Were the bison also dependent on the Plains Indians? Absolutely. For 5,000 years, before white men arrived with their big firearms and profiteering mindset, Native Americans and *Bison bison* lived in mutually beneficial symbiosis. All the prescribed fires by natives helped to create these bison-nurturing grasslands, and regular hunting selected for herding behavior versus solitary wandering. Large herds meant added protection for the animals and a stable supply of protein-dense calories for the tribes, who grew brave and smart in their hunting tactics.

Despite weighing up to one ton each, these enormous, cumbersome-looking mammals can be frighteningly swift, agile, and hot tempered—capable of running up to 40 mph, pivoting abruptly, and jumping six feet vertical. When agitated, they don't hesitate to gore or break bones. (That's why Yellowstone visitors who try to get close are fools.) With few predators beyond wolves and the occasional grizzly, the plains bison thrived precisely *because* tribes like the Arapaho hunted and ate them, culling the herds, balancing their numbers, and preventing over-grazing of the grasses these animals depended upon.

This was no blood sport. These natives did not take the killing of their animal kin lightly, nor their responsibility to feed families who would otherwise starve, to provide them with thick robes and shelter against the killing cold. These people were deeply conflicted about their need to kill bison to survive. For in the sacred ecology of the Plains Indians, animals were not viewed as mere resources to be exploited; they were complex, autonomous, and sentient beings with families of their own. With each hunt, the Arapaho faced the elemental dilemma of killing their kin—animals they revered, even worshipped—or going hungry. As Howard Harrod explains in *The Animals Came Dancing*: "On the face of it the tensions were severe: one was eating the flesh of a being like oneself, a person with a kin-ship network, perhaps a wife and children, a being for whom relatives would grieve. Beliefs that individual animals possessed souls that were not destroyed when their bodies were taken for food helped to soften the conflicts embodied in this dilemma."

For sensitive moderns, there too is conflict. And that conflict is often intensely felt. Yet there are those among us who require some amount of animal flesh to be healthy and productive, including many former vegans, including the Dalai Lama, including myself. Do we wish it were different? Of course! We don't want to eat animals, no way. When I asked 45-year-old Diana—a small-boned sprite, barely 5'2" and 105 pounds—why she had given up her earnestly executed vegan diet, she didn't hold back for one second: "I NEED MY MEAT!" In truth, my own life would be so much easier without having to meet this fundamental need. Yet this is the genetic reality we've been handed and to argue with nature, we've learned the hard and debilitating way, is folly.

Instead of fighting our bodily needs, we need to embrace them, meet them full-on as the bison-slaying Arapaho did, even as we ponder why this has to be, this feeding of life for life, this need for death in order to continue our existence. And in the midst of our ponderings of this earthly mystery, we would be well served by exploring Plains Indian cosmology on a deeper level, for everything is reversed from the way we moderns think. The flesh that sustains life is no mere commodity or shameful necessity, but a timely and reverent bequest from nature. Listen to the words from a Cheyenne tale before the bison appeared, as recounted by Harrod and Grinnell:

379

> It was a hard time and the people were very hungry....Facing the pro-
> spect of starvation, the chiefs called two young men and instructed
> them to go ahead of the people in search of food....The chiefs' instruc-
> tions to the young men indicated the desperate condition of the people:
> "You must try hard. You hear the old people and the children crying for
> food. Be sure to find something. Do not come back until you do."

Yet even after the herds began to miraculously appear, the bison were never a given—some easily acquired, swipe-your-plastic, corporate-food provided 24/7 just around the urban corner. Nor were they a manipulated commodity, part of some Managed Futures portfolio. No, the bison were a profound and uncertain gift that had to be earned again and again by the Arapaho people. Theirs was no utilitarian ethic, but one of interdependence, grounded in mutual respect. In Plains Indian cosmology, it was the animals who offered themselves as food—but only to the honorable and deserving.

And how does one connect with a hulking, stomping, wild woolly beast of an animal to gain its respect? Intricate rituals are how the Plains Indians attempted to do this, taking on the appearance and persona, the very soul of the bison. Imagine if your own life depended on finding and slaying this 2,000 pound, unpredictable, bone-crushing creature—and the lives of your starving children and parents. You too would seek out extraordinary power, streak your body with vermilion and mud, don masks and horns in an attempt to access the consciousness of an animal. You too would dance out its movements and bellow its rough sounds into the dark night, trying in every way possible to comprehend its being. You might even experience what the Arapaho did in these elaborate and timeless ceremonies: a shattering of your limited consciousness as humans shape-shift into animals and animals into humans, signifying our transcendent oneness.

These people weren't simply acting out a dramatic role, fingers crossed. Aided by the shamans' relentless drums and wailing prayers, they entered into a parallel reality, connecting with the spirit of bison to attain its blessings. Praying in sweat lodges, smoking sweetgrass, ingesting sacred medicine and engaging in ritual sex, the Arapaho experienced visions and potent dreams to help them locate the herds and acquire the power needed to bring home the gift of food.

For many tribes, wild animals represented the feminine erotic principle and to have a sexual encounter in dreams was by far the most desirable omen. It not only symbolized the spiritual ties between humans and animals, with all our shared obligations, but an erotic rendezvous with a Buffalo Woman all but guaranteed supernatural powers and a successful hunt.

HIGH IN COLORADO'S Sangre de Cristo Mountains, two naked wood nymphs splash and cavort in a natural hot spring, thigh tattoos and rainbow scarves their only attire. They're in love with their own bodies as every twenty-year-old should be, wet dark hair clinging to unbearably smooth skin. Well-nourished beauties, euphoric. Their bright cries and laughter diminish as dusk settles in, and dozens of plump little wrens and chickadees prepare to roost among the pinyon pines and juniper. Here at 9,000 feet, I'm ready to do some roosting myself after a long hike to some higher-altitude hot springs that ooze into this mountain canyon: a pocket of lush, soggy green amidst the dry rocky terrain.

But the music of a droning human song pulls me back to the smallest spring-fed pool of this clothing-optional Shangri La. So I slide my naked self in and join the circle of beings gathered here: a tall Native American and his 30ish son, two motherly white women, and a pregnant young daughter whose long legs dangle into the warm water. Her swollen belly and radiant face rise serenely above, like a fertility goddess emerging out of the vaporous mist. A single crow flies back and forth, checking out the watery scene below. A deer peeks out of the thicket.

Chanting a song without words, plaintive and piercing, the bronzed son with black-seeming eyes accompanies his silver-haired father. Everything out here is getting blacker by the minute as their voices blend and ascend, punctuating the cool night air with quick yelps and sharp cries. Mesmerized, I gaze upward at the eternally exploding stars, tranquil in the velvety night sky. Oh, who would choose to live in a noisy closed-in city, cut off from the celestial source? It's like always wearing a too-tight hat instead of having the top of your head zipped open by the night wind, like brain surgery, like everything stupid and contradictory being sucked out, and the intelligent, elegant cosmos pouring in.

The singing climaxes, winds down. An easy peace envelops our little human group. Anyone who speaks, speaks softly. "Our tribe is small now," the father is saying, "and our sun dance almost upon us. I invite all of you to attend." Deeply honored, I accept at once, knowing this is a religious rite from which many tribes exclude non-members. In the Lakota, the Keeper of the Sacred White Buffalo Calf Pipe explicitly asked non-natives to stop attending their annual sun dance.

For generations, Plains tribes have been holding these sacred ritual dances, usually right before the summer's critical hunt. Preparation is intense: a year of meditation, sweat lodges, prayers and vision quests. The bravest of the brave then test their strength of will by taking vows of unsparing suffering. Some call it self-torture—whatever it takes to assist transcendent powers in renewing the earth's bounties: animals, plants, water, soil and seeds.

The tribe's holy man is there to assist and pray for them. Cutting each dancer's chest with ceremonial incisions, he pushes wooden pegs in and out of the torn and bleeding skin, pegs that attach to rawhide thongs dangling from a tall cottonwood pole. For four excruciating days, the men (and sometimes women) fast and dance and pray non-stop. "After you take that last drink of water, you are a ghost," a Saskatchewan elder testifies in *Nature's Laws*. "You are there with the spirits and they will cleanse you. You've got to prepare yourself and have faith to make it through." Pulling and pulling against the thongs for seemingly endless, tortuous hours, the dancer's flesh finally rips open and his anguished cries fill the air.

The ragged, bloody flesh is then buried in the soil, a symbolic sacrifice offered as a prayer. *Oh Great Spirit, help our families, our community, and the entire circle of life!* Depleted, utterly exhausted, the dancers lie on beds of fragrant sage and continue to fast and pray for a vision. In centuries past they prayed for prophecy: the location of the herds. Because the bison gave so much to the people, the sun dancers gave of themselves in return. Sacrifice, they realized, is required of all beings who are part of Nature. Those who partake must give back.

At this moment I can't help but think of amply fed Americans sitting in our cushy, air-conditioned, GPS-guided cars, pulling up to one of 160,000 drive-up windows across the country, annoyed or even angry if our fast food takes more than five minutes to arrive. *Five minutes.* If we're honest, we've all been there, if not at McDonald's then in some comfy café, edgy and impatient for our meal to be promptly served—whether braised beef or grilled tempeh—and scarfed down without a thought or prayer. Is it time for a reassessment of the gratitude principle in our own food culture? Time to bring out the wooden pegs and thongs?

The Plains people took nothing for granted when it came to nourishment. They bestowed enormous respect and moral standing on animals, greatly admiring their fortitude, intelligence, and swift intuitive actions. One widespread story motif even involved marriage between humans and bison in order to establish kinship connections and reciprocal responsibilities. Honoring these commitments meant the people would not only survive but thrive. Ethical violations—including over-hunting, wasting part of the animal, or an absence of appreciation—could bring disaster: ongoing hunger, suffering, or starvation of the entire tribe.

CONSIDERING MODERN HUMANS' extreme violations against animals on both land and sea—overharvesting, overeating, cruel disrespect, animals as commodities—is it any wonder we face our own disastrous consequences of dying species, depleted oceans, compromised health and moral apathy?

The Plains Indians show us how profoundly different human-animal relations can be. Envision a Cree hunter welcoming his buffalo kin as they enter the corral, as described by John S. Milloy: "My Grandfather, we are glad to see you, and happy that you have not come in a shameful manner, for you have brought plenty of your young men with you. Be not angry with us; we are obliged to destroy you to make ourselves live." Now picture modern city dwellers camped in front of our latest electronic toy, mindlessly masticating our easily acquired corporate food— animal or plant it doesn't matter—to which we have no sense of its unique spirit, no connection to its original form or source, no part in the gathering or slaying, and no clue as to how, where, or by whom it was grown or raised. And when is the last meal for which you danced an honor dance? Or belted out that song of gratitude to the life forms which sustain you?

Such complex rituals were never mere rationalizations for killing animals. They were spiritual practices that addressed head-on the mystical interpenetration of all life on this earth, the essential need to feed each other for food and power. No people ever understood these existential meanings with more depth or passion than the Plains Indians. Without killing and eating animals, they would perish.

After offering prayers of thanksgiving for the gift of its life, hunters quickly butchered a slain bison and every part of the animal was saved and put to good use, from sinews to gristle, heart to brain. The nutritional prize of the hunt, the still-hot, iron-rich liver, was mixed with gall fluid and immediately consumed. Shoulder blades emerged as digging hoes; scrotums transformed into a baby's rattle; the skin of a hind leg became soft moccasins for a child.

Think now of the immense, reckless waste and disrespect in today's planetary food culture. Think of the by-products of industrial production, both plant and animal, thrown into careless heaps without the slightest consideration or respect. Much of what gets wasted is "imperfect" produce, left to decay in the fields in favor of those flawless-looking red peppers and tomatoes we all insist upon. And consider the mega-tons of uneaten food indifferently pitched into garbage bins in all the grocery stores and all the households in just one city in just one night. We Americans throw out an outrageous 40% of our food, 31 million tons of it ending up in landfills each year where it releases methane, further roasting the planet.

New research puts the figure at up to *half of all food worldwide squandered or lost* along the supply chain, never reaching a human stomach—two billion tons—a scandalous waste not only of animals and plants, but of land, water, energy and human labor. In this context, veggie or omnie may be a moot point regarding the environment and reducing animal deaths. Changing the world's wasteful food habits might make considerably more difference.

In the Arapaho culture, by contrast, not one part of the animal was wasted, not a single connective tissue was tossed—from bladders for holding water, to tallow for healing wounds, to muscular hearts for nutritional richness. Everything was put to good use to energize and revitalize human beings, a practical philosophy echoed by today's "nose to tail" culinary crowd.

It is at this point we really must ask ourselves: who is the more ethical and conscious eater? The bison-consuming Arapaho who prayed, fasted and toiled for his precious meat, or the modern meatless vegan who buys commercial food from some far-flung, soil-dishonoring, wild animal-annihilating, monocrop corporate venture? Who is more aware of and more connected to his or her food source? Who understands the sacred interdependencies of sentient life more fully and with more gratitude? (For surely gratitude is the principal virtue.) So complete was the incorporation of this animal's body and spirit into their lives, the Arapaho nearly transformed into bison themselves. They celebrated them, honored them, danced with them, prayed to them, and became one with them in flesh and soul. Along with all Plains Indians, including their neighbors to the north, the Lakota, there was never a people whose lives were more physically and spiritually intertwined with one animal than the Arapaho.

Here in the West we cannot go back to being bison chasers, satisfying some primal urge to partake of a similarly rich and authentic food culture. Even though bison are again thriving, they contain cattle genes from hybridization and many roam behind padlocked gates. The last continuously wild bison herd, a few thousand individuals, still struggles to survive in Yellowstone, their ancestors having endured wanton slaughter by the tens of millions in the 1800s, their bodies left to rot on the ground by white men. Covertly sanctioned by a US government that favored white expansion, this annihilation amounted to attempted genocide of our nation's native people. Take away their food source and the tribes will starve. Give them modern food but take away their animal kin and sacred land, and they will simply die a slower death.

41.

YOUR ANCIENT ANIMAL SELF

HUNDRED YEAR FLOODS ASIDE, the Front Range of the Rocky Mountains is dry, appallingly dry by any Midwesterner's standards. Gathering a paltry 12-15 inches of annual rain, this is the geological zone where hundreds of miles of wide open plains—Arapaho country—abruptly rear up into heroic 14,000-foot snowy peaks. Arriving at this dramatic juncture, you'll find plenty of swirling dust, prickly yucca, and drought-tolerant ponderosa pine, their taproots reaching deep beneath the rocky surface to guzzle whatever water they can find. Out on the nearby plains, barely tolerable conditions can turn severe. You just have to breathe the brittle 100-degree air and watch all the creeks dry up by the 4th of July to understand what the Plains tribes were up against.

Water's limiting factor across the West is something that modern Americans, incredibly, don't seem to notice as we move into the territory in ever increasing numbers, pump rivers and aquifers dry, then cast an opportunistic eye elsewhere for yet more water to sustain our vast irrigated crop fields, plush green lawns, and $13 billion-dollar bottled water addiction. Talk about an ecological and spiritual disconnect!

Native hunter-gatherers didn't try to convert these dry plains and deserts into a counterfeit oasis. They lived within the natural constraints of their environment. They ate within the rhythms and limits of the seasons, whatever the earth was producing right then, right there. Wild plums and fresh greens in the springtime; lowbush blueberries and currants in summer; elk or duck during the autumn; and smoked bison, pemmican and wild roots through the long, punishing winter. They understood that sound ecological practices were essential, that over-indulgence meant a depleted landscape and hungry families.

I am not here to romanticize ancestral hunting societies. They existed in far fewer numbers; thus, their impacts were far less. Nor were they perfect humans. More stampeding bison could be killed in cliff jumps than intended. Camps could get messy. There was inter-tribal warring, most often to demonstrate honor and not to kill—at other times brutal. Their lives could turn horrible, starvation but one long, killing winter away.

But they were authentic. They were present. They were conscious of their place in the powerfully intricate web of life. They walked upon dirt and stones, honored the plants, lived respectfully among the animals, transformed creaturely muscle, blood and bones, as needed, into human muscle, blood and bones. They understood in a profound way that we are totally dependent upon and inseparable from other animals, inseparable from all-giving, all-consuming wild nature, and they chose to work with this truth, not against it.

LIKE MOST VEGANS, I used to loathe hunters. I found the hunt despicable and voiced my opinion to all who cared to listen. "How could anyone kill an animal as graceful as a deer? As vulnerable as a wild turkey? What's wrong with these crass humans? Shame on them!" Today I question who is the more principled: the vegan or the hunter? Indeed, the argument can be made that ethical hunters, deliberate and conscious in their actions to secure nourishment for their families, are acting in a more morally courageous manner than those who gain their grains and veggies easily and unconsciously from killing fields of incidental deaths.

Unlike our nationwide ritual of gobbling industrial food arriving from all over the globe, there's no detached non-presence when hunters gain their food directly. There is no killing by proxy. No invisible animals chewed up in fields of rice or kale, for which no one—plant eater or reaper—claims the least responsibility. No expatriated or endangered species from the blanket destruction of habitat. These men and women are wholly present, wholly responsible for their actions.

Nor is there unconscious waste in ethical hunting. As much as possible, all parts of the animal are used. This isn't food flown in from Chile, over-packaged and carbon-disgorging. It's local food, sometimes right outside the hunter's door, an integral part of his environment, an integral part of his awareness. Obtaining food from your own locality or bioregion uses up to 17 times less CO_2 than food distributed nationally (Pirog). So where did *your* last night's dinner come from?

And like those rare people in America who actually grow their own chow, hunters don't depend on strangers to do their difficult food labor for them. And in case you didn't know, the sowing, tending, weeding, and hand-harvesting of plant food is unbelievably arduous work. Latin American children as young as eight sweat and toil in hazardous conditions for our creamy banana smoothies (Pier). Poorly-paid illegal immigrants in California's Central Valley inhale a daily toxic soup of chemicals while gathering our juicy honeydews, living their lives in fear of deportation for doing the hard labor no one else wants to do.

Hand-picking commercial apples near Chelan, Washington in my 20s, I lasted but two miserable weeks, endlessly climbing up/down, up/down awkward, tippy ladders, clambering from tree to tree for up to ten hours a day—heavy cotton bag hanging from my raw, throbbing neck. I dragged myself back to Seattle like a sick animal, but all the migrant men and women I worked with continued to labor in those pesticide-soaked orchards seven days a week for very little money and zero respect—before moving on to the next punishing harvest. Do you know the grove your last apple came from? The species that pollinated it? The name of the human who carefully picked it for you?

Without defensiveness, ethical hunters will gladly talk to you about their solid connection to the land and its native beasts. Have you spoken to one lately? I'm not talking about slob hunters or trophy chasers, people pursuing not animals but their own egos, insensible to our obligations to nature. They are an embarrassment, an outrage to the men and women who feel something overpowering and yes, primeval when they're out in the homeland woods or prairie, whose contours, textures, and hidden features they know as well as their own weathered hands.

Responsible for bringing in essential protein for their families, these are the hunters who honor the fierce/raw/skittish otherness of animals and wish to explore their own wild being, an inner wildness out of which we've been badly cheated by our facile, disconnected suburban existence. "Our observation and detection abilities do not need to be so keen and alert anymore," writes Hans Kruuk in *Hunter and Hunted.* "Nor do we need to be able to sprint—and with all such faculties, it is known that if you don't use it, you lose it. One can afford to be an obese coach-potato." Or, for that matter, a too-skinny vegan.

Purposefully moving into untamed nature to seek sustenance is an inquiry, a passionate, visceral inquiry into that mystical connection between you and your food source, between consumer and consumed, flesh into flesh. Try doing it alone, head-deep in wilderness, and seriously protein-hungry if you want to truly understand the scary, sacred predator-prey connection. And for anyone who hunts out West in cougar or grizzly territory, there's opportunity to explore the fiercely

387

concentrated, zapped-in awareness of being possibly picked off at any moment, of tables turned, of predator swiftly turning into prey. As every hunter knows, the animals are already there, silently watching as you pass by. This is the kind of pure presence that Buddhists exalt. This is walking on thin ice meditation. "One sets out after one's quarry with senses fully engaged, wildly alert: entranced, nearly hypnotized," affirms author Rick Bass. "The tiniest of factors can possess the largest significance—the crack of a twig, the shift of a breeze, a single stray hair caught on a piece of bark, a fresh-bent blade of grass."

Females too are taking up ethical hunting, fired up by the sustainable food movement and, no doubt, admiration for skilled archer and spunky survivalist Katniss in *The Hunger Games*. Males still comprise the majority of the US and Canada's estimated 20 million hunters, but it's females who make most of the family food decisions and their hunting numbers are surging. In British Columbia, nearly 40 per cent of those attending EatWild hunter trainings are women.

One of them is Kesia, 25, a recovering vegetarian who refuses to support industrial meat. "I want my meat to be grass-finished and killed as ethically as possible," she disclosed to *The Vancouver Sun*. "Much as I firmly believe in the necessity of animal protein and saturated fats, the commercial stuff is all toxic." Kesia expressed amazement at the depth of knowledge required for skillful, principled hunting and the newly perceptive mind and body that arrived with her first experiences. "I realized this is how I want to be outside. It was like something had been missing."

Like the Inuit and Arapaho, today's ethical hunters are as conscious of the animal's world and highly sensitive body/mind as their own. They understand that strict rules and taboos comprise a strong hunting code: respect all living beings; express heartfelt thanks; take only what is needed and share the rest. In honoring this social contract, these hunters often distribute fresh, protein-rich food not only to their own families but to the frail, elderly, and less fortunate.

"Generous" is not a quality I would have credited to hunters in my past life as an outraged, self-righteous vegetarian—more like vile and contemptible. Bloody, heartless murderers! One of the grace notes of growing older is that we lose our irrational judgments based on incomplete experience and gain, let us hope, some measure of wisdom. The wisest, most gracious hunter I have ever encountered is Rick Bass. Living with his family in the animal-rich Yaak Valley of northwestern Montana, he writes of his love for this mountainous landscape, magically alive with human-animal symbiosis.

There is something mysterious happening here between the landscape and the people, a thing that stimulates our imagination, and causes many of us to set off deep into the woods in search of the unknown and sustenance—not just metaphorical or spiritual sustenance, but the real thing.....Nearly everyone who has lived here for any length of time has ended up—sometimes against one's conscious wishes—becoming a hunter. This wild and powerful landscape sculpts us like clay. I don't find such sculpting an affront to the human spirit, but instead, wonderful testimony to our pliability, our ability to adapt to a place.

Bass lives what he writes. A modern hunter-gatherer, he pursues nourishment for his family in the giving/unforgiving woods. Chopping firewood, gathering mushrooms, growing vegetables and later, come autumn, helping to dry, can, and freeze food for the long insular winter ahead, this man is, like many hunters, a dedicated environmentalist, working hard to preserve wild nature in the Yaak Valley and beyond.

Unlike modern agriculture, which scrapes away native flora and fauna by the millions of square acres, hunting demands protection of our remaining wild areas. In the US alone, hunters contribute over $1.6 billion annually to the conservation of land and wildlife. So they can go out and shoot an animal? Yes indeed. Besides saving dwindling habitat, this is part of the game plan. Tracking non-threatened species with healthy or unsustainably high populations, these people hunt for real food for their families—and for the deep-rooted pleasure of participating in wild nature on somewhat equal footing with other animals who possess advantages of speed, intuition, and sensory perception—against advantages of weaponry. Many a hunter has been left empty-handed by an animal far smarter than he. I'm talking about the solitary hunter who rises before dawn and quietly slips into his ancient animal self in order to confront, respectfully, the other.

HAVE HUNTERS ACTED in contemptible ways in the past and do some continue on this path today? Of course. After all, it was hunters, with our government's blessing, who killed off most of our large predators, those key carnivores that keep entire ecosystems balanced and healthy. Completely out of whack without them, our remaining natural areas now desperately need these predators back. Just 25 miles up the highway from our mountain cabin, you can find stark evidence of this missing-carnivore quandary at Rocky Mountain National Park.

Absent their historic predator—the critically important grey wolf—scrawny, overpopulated elk have devoured the native vegetation, denuding large areas of this rugged high-altitude park and damaging fragile streams. *No wolves allowed* might keep ranchers and other wolf-haters happy, but it's a perverse philosophy because *all* of our parks should be promoting healthy, intact ecosystems. At least Yellowstone saw the light, bringing back wolves a full seven decades after their extermination triggered missing species and a seriously degraded landscape. Today the world's first national park is experiencing ecosystem recovery. Inflated elk numbers are down, and in many areas the long-absent aspen, willow, native fish and song birds are once again thriving.

Ranchers who scream "Kill all Wolves!" and sometimes try to, seem ignorant of the fact that without this keystone carnivore, coyote and other mid-predator populations are exploding. And guess who loves to feast on calves and lambs? Wily coyote has been called the most intelligent, adaptable predator on earth (he knows what time you leave for work and what time you will return). Absent the wolf, he's now able to kill livestock in greater numbers than ever. Mess with nature and, ultimately, your own life gets messed with too.

Minus our top predators, rapid ecological decline is happening everywhere on the planet. Called a *trophic cascade,* missing or declining hunters like wolves, lions, great white sharks, and killer whales translates into unchecked populations of mid-size predators and grazers, denuded landscapes, and impoverished oceans. Take away these keystone carnivores, the foundation of all ecosystems, and the whole edifice starts to fall apart.

Thus, it is the natural hunter that ensures ecosystem health across the planet, including ethical human hunters who keep deer and other mid-tier wildlife from overpopulation and starvation. Acting on evolutionary instincts, both animal and human hunters seek the nourishment that sustains their lives and the lives of their families. And in that seeking and in that killing, a dynamic balancing act of taker/giver, the biodiversity of our luxuriant earth can flourish. Vegans, can you handle this? Without the animals-hunting-animals dynamic, there would be no earth as we know it. "There is neither cruelty nor compassion in a lion's quest for food," maintains the acclaimed biologist George Schaller, "and this impersonal endeavor strikes a responsive chord in man the hunter...as struggles of life and death at their most elemental. It is a time when each animal uses to its utmost those attributes with which evolution has endowed it."

PHILOSOPHERS HAVE LONG contemplated the amorality of animals that kill for food without any apparent pity for the killed. We cannot know the mind of a wild and hungry animal, yet we can come close. Who can even think of another's needs, let alone empathize, when your own body and brain are shutting down from lack of sustenance? Compassion, after all, is the province of the well-nourished. Wouldn't the most ardent vegan spear a deer if he found himself alone and starving in a winter wilderness? Hmm, maybe not. I momentarily forgot that martyr-vegan types claim to gladly put an animal's well-being before their own.

Yet how many have been put to the test on their principles? What if a refusal to eat animal food slowly delivered a puny, low-energy existence—as hundreds of thousands of former vegans suffered? Let us not forget the ailing Jenna who succumbed to eating wild game and experienced an astonishing recovery in her energy and brain health. Nor Alex, Jessica, Gabrielle and all the other ex-vegans who finally started popping eggs like crazy in order to feel fully alive. Nor the always tired and hungry vegan, Sylvie, who snatched fish from the barbeque and went home to dance away the night.

"So alright, our ancestors ate animals!" some vegans now reluctantly admit, "but it's not natural. They only did it out of necessity, to survive." Excuse me? What exactly is "not natural" about the urge to survive, to be healthy, to thrive? To secure the nutrition that allows this for the individual and the tribe? This kind of simplistic argument strips humans from our earthly environment, as if we are separate, free-floating entities. We are not separate from the environment that shaped our genetics and physiology, our exacting dietary needs. *We are not separate from nature.* Today's humans pretend to be and the results are disastrous.

We affluent moderns have it ridiculously easy. We are ruinously unaware. Strolling into Safeway to purchase pre-washed produce flown in from two continents, we know only that our food is already there, waiting for us. But what if you woke up ravishingly hungry every morning—like wild animals do, like poverty-stricken people do, like unhealthy individuals who need animal food do, as they try to survive on mere plants? And how would you behave if you had to venture into cold, raw nature to find your every morsel of food, exactly like your distant ancestors kicked out of those warm, nurturing, profusely-providing trees?

Well, if you cherished your own life, you would eat whatever non-poisonous food you could find. In other words, you'd be gathering and you'd be hunting and you'd be gathering some more. You would be a human omnivore. And that's who we are. But hold on, these same vegans will argue: "That was then; this is now.

Animal food is no longer necessary for optimal human health." Of which humans do they speak? Is it the long-living Japanese, with the planet's lowest incidence of heart disease and one of its highest consumption of fish? They couldn't possibly be referring to traditional Far North people who thrive on a 90% animal diet. Nor to the Swiss, the healthiest population in the western hemisphere, who suck down plentiful grass-fed dairy—their high-mountain ancestors having consumed warm frothy milk every morning, straight from the goat. It's time for vegan activists to grasp that when proto-humans clambered out of the trees and began to slowly fan across the face of the earth, these groups encountered and genetically adapted to extraordinarily varied climates and food availability.

I will concede this: if we humans persist in heating up the planet, engendering monster storms and heavy rainfall; if we continue to have our food virtually handed to us while sitting on our collectively-spreading bottoms for endless hours before the altar of our computers; then perhaps over the millennia we will indeed devolve into quasi-vegetarians, much like our non-hunting, low-IQ, hominoid ancestors—engulfed by opulent heat, copious fruit, and similar easy pickings.

WHAT DIFFERENCE DOES it make, really, what our ape ancestors were eating in the African rainforest 20 million years ago? Fruit or insects, their primitive needs don't dictate what seven billion, genetically diverse humans "should" be eating today. And with 88 million possible variations in human DNA, what does any of this have to do with *you*, a 21st century *Homo sapien* with precise biochemical requirements? Obviously, human physiology has evolved and will continue to evolve. What's important are *your* individual needs at this time in your life. And for most of us, that means some optimal proportion of both plants and animals.

As ex-vegan Kent Schoberle perceptively concludes: "The decision is not so simple as eating meat or not eating meat. There are many variables to consider and we have the information now to be more specific with our unique dietary needs. Anyone who claims otherwise is ignoring the big picture."

We need animals in our lives. We need their company and their courage, their beauty, power, and grace. We need their intricate predator-prey relationships to keep the whole planetary system running. And yes, many of us *need* their protein-dense muscles and rich slippery fat to be healthy and strong. And we will partake of our essential nourishment with deep appreciation and no apology.

42.

THE FOOD CHAIN:
INCLUDING YOU, MY FRIEND

Death is the mother of beauty.

—Wallace Stevens

Upon witnessing the brutal reality of an open-air French butcher shop, I could no longer tolerate animals being slaughtered, sliced, and served up on fat deli sandwiches. But what I really could not bear at such a tender young age was the biological truth of our earthly existence. Every creature is food for others, including me, including you. Each of us will suffer and die, along with the ego and all individuality. It's called dissolution: breaking down into our original parts in order to merge with the universal and become mere stuff of life—the fertile soil, the fruitful field—edibles for other life forms. All flesh is grass: the poet never spoke more truly.

The vegan argument is, in fact, is a profound denial of nature. We are animals. And our living and dying and nourishing are utterly entangled with other animals. Genetically, it is well encoded for humans to consume animal food for full health. No need to feel guilty taking your fair share of sustenance along the way. Your own turn will come to offer up your body to the communal compost heap that feeds all living things. You too will be graciously paying back the debt all beings must pony up for having lived and dined on this dynamic planet. Maybe vegans think they can opt out of this sacred reciprocity by not eating other animals. So sorry. It doesn't work that way.

Youth can't get this because most haven't truly witnessed death, up close and personal. The man in white sharpening the butcher knife, nor the one in black who harvests souls, yielding the scythe. Most haven't spent days and nights in the closed room of the dying, desperate and gasping for her final breath. They haven't watched the light in a loved one's eyes extinguish and blow out forever. Nor helped to dig an earthly grave, lying down to grieve on the broken ground beside it, disbelief swept away by a cold hard wind. Nor gathered up the displaced soil, rich and teeming with new life, to help cover the remains of the one they adore. *"We are perishable, friends,"* poet Robert Bly quietly reminds us. *"We are salty, impermanent kingdoms."*

As youth we live in a cocoon of innocence. No animal should have to suffer and die to nourish a human being! Our own death, our own transformation into life-food is mere abstraction. It has no visceral reality. Many strict vegans, not yet ready to own up, live in this same sweet bubble, chanting their no-meat, no-suffering songs of innocence. I certainly did. All my young vegetarian friends did. Visionary poet William Blake's earliest verses were likewise painfully innocent: *Pipe a song about a Lamb! So I piped with merry cheer. Piper, pipe that song again! So I piped: he wept to hear.*

It's not just the madness of the method that ethical vegans abhor. Take away all factory farms, demolish all CAFEs, and offer them well-tended Priscilla the Pig from a caring, earth-wise family farm and it won't matter. It's the suffering and the killing that's intolerable, the feeding and the eating, animal into animal, tissue into tissue, bone into bone, nature's enduring gift exchange of life for life. This is frighteningly intimate stuff and they will tolerate none of it. The organic food chain itself appears to be their real issue, "using" other animals to sustain the human animal. But if we humans continue to remove ourselves from the natural food chain, consuming fake industrial concoctions and synthetic supplements, nature's cycles will eventually move on without us. "It is our choice to be a part of nature," writes Diane Schwarzbein. "Choosing to be part of the food chain again is one way we humans can restore our collective health."

Honorable plant-eaters: you too are part of this complex chain of beings. You too will die and be used as nutritious food for other organisms, possibly even sentient creatures. Humans suffer just like other animals, and often not only on their final day, but for weeks, months or even years before their death. It's totally understandable, even commendable, all this tender passion, all this longing for non-suffering. Untested by the hard lessons of time, removed from wild nature and the food chain's beautiful, terrifying truths—the endless impersonal cycles of life, death and regeneration—young vegans aren't yet ready to sing their own songs of experience. This book is my hymn to experience. And here is the mature Blake's:

Tyger! Tyger! burning bright/ In the forest of the night/ What immortal hand or eye/ Could frame thy fearful symmetry?

I know how easy it is to be an ethical vegetarian or vegan and condemn those who eat animals—even those whose failing bodies insist they must. *Easy* because all killing is unacceptable to the idealistic. *Easy* because many of these innocents live in cities, largely removed from nature's exquisite yet lethal net of beings, its complex field of interrelationships. *Easy* because most haven't been on their diet long enough to comprehend the long-term health consequences. Some may continue to thrive and that is a good thing. Others will suffer and eventually turn to animals for their deliverance, as humans have for millions of years.

NOW THAT I'M OLDER and somewhat wiser, I live in the natural world and can look a coiled rattlesnake in its cold reptilian eyes, even as its muscular throat still undulates with a hapless mouse. This late-arriving acceptance of the food chain, including the hunting human, shatters the Edenic idealism of my youth to cause no animal suffering, to do no harm, and to certainly never suffer, die, and turn into animal fodder myself. My participation in this natural cycle is now a conscious and reverent one. It has to be. Once you fully grasp the ultra-personal significance of food interchange, you can no longer mindlessly eat and run and feel good about it. You sit down to the table in awe and gratitude. Eating becomes a deeply moral act. With every mouthful, animal or plant, you are eating death, transforming it into pulsating new life.

This "sacred gift exchange" has existed since life began on this earth and has absolutely nothing to do with modern industrial agriculture and factory farms, which exist as an abomination, a cruel perversion of nature's truth. (Not to mention nonstop bad karma for humanity.) And nature's truth is interdependency. We are here to respect one another, to serve one another and yes, to feed one another with our very bodies: communion of the most crass and high order. Reciprocity is the reality of our organic world and like it or not, you will be both eater and eaten in this vast and intricate system.

"To acknowledge that each of us at the table will eventually be part of the meal is not just being realistic," writes Gary Snyder in *The Practice of the Wild*. "It is allowing the sacred to enter and accepting the sacramental aspect of our shaky, temporary personal being."

You can't love just the animals; you have to love the whole system! And the universal organic system isn't interested in your no-meat ethics. Truthfully, it's not that interested in you at all. It's interested in the persistence of soil and water and myriad life forms, the persistence of nature. Unfortunately, as karmically kind as plant eating appears, plant eaters are not exempt from the great cycles of life and death which pay no attention to individuals. Ecologically and spiritually, we are all here in service to one thing: the continuation of Life itself.

You can either abhor the set-up and try to opt out by engaging in abstention, fasting, and self-mortification like a Pythagorean monk, denying yourself proper sustenance. Or you can joyously embrace your integral role in the banquet of life. To answer the original question: How can I love animals and then eat them? Because they heal me, nourish me, serve me, and sustain me. And exactly as the laws of nature demand, my own body will one day nourish, serve, and sustain them. "The crawling of new life out of the old," Galway Kinnell has written, "is what we have for eternity on earth."

OUR CULTURE EXERCISES an entrenched resistance to the reality of death and the transformative food cycle. We erect barriers of metal and wood against the soil, enclosing our loved ones in ostensibly sturdy boxes lined with smooth blue satin. We pretend they'll last, separate and forever. In truth, the soil longs for us and we the soil: our home, our origin, our transfiguration.

Most gardeners have a real feel for this because we spend long, sweaty hours working and fingering the soil, crucible for the living and the dying. Late summer afternoons, when I can stand the insipid glare of my computer screen no longer—my entire being reduced to a yapping, analytical brain—I escape to my vegetable garden and fling myself nose-down in the soil, inhaling the divine fragrance of our 4.5 billion year-old earth: nitrogen-rich, alkaline, primeval. Today we have fancy kits, probes, and meters to measure PH but our grandpas used to just sniff and know: sweet or sour, alkaline or acidic.

Torrid sun beating on my back, I spread my limbs just like the elegant water striders suspended upon our pond's placid surface. So very delicate, are they not? In reality, these slender pond skaters are aggressive carnivores patiently waiting for tell-tale vibrations—picked up by their sensitive body hairs—whereupon they dart madly across the water and instantly devour their startled prey. Face-down in the soil, I too discern subtle vibrations as life and death mingle their vital energies beneath me. I haven't eaten dirt since I was a little kid but right now I am nearly sucking soil, soaking up its primordial scent, breathing in the bouquet of billions of micro-organisms which enhance our life and spur our dissolution.

Instead of trying to deny or slow down the body's alteration by these invisible beings, these hungry ghosts, Tibetan Buddhists consciously hasten the process, helping nature along. Carrying a deceased loved one to a Himalayan mountaintop for sky-burial, a family will intentionally leave the body exposed to the elements, as both generous gift to animals and swift instruction to humans on the transience of all life. While chanting monks burn incense of juniper, several "body-breakers" quickly disassemble the corpse, speeding the arrival of vultures: an auspicious omen in the Tibetan world. The bones are crushed, ground together with barley, tea and yak butter, then freely offered to the high-circling raptors and other living beings.

Sky-burial strikes most westerners as bizarre and grotesque, especially since we rarely reflect on our own demise, but it's actually a sound ecological practice that's been around since the 12th century. First recorded in *The Book of the Dead*, this devout ceremony serves Tibetans as both a practical interment method at high-altitude (hard stony dirt, little to no timber) and a spiritual celebration of release and transformation.

We Americans may be hush-hush and fearful about death but not so in other cultures. Day of the Dead in Mexico is an annual bank holiday, a three-day, high-jinks celebration! Originating as an Aztec ritual to honor all ancestors, this garish fiesta abounds with sugar skulls and homemade skeletons as families beckon the spirits of adults and especially children, *angelitos,* to return for a friendly visit. Similar glitzy celebrations take place throughout Brazil and Spain; and in African and Asian cultures, ancestor veneration is common. The dead continue to exist, they believe, but in wholly different form, invisible to the limited human eye.

Is this ancient belief really that different from new understandings in atomic biology that allow us to see earth's life forms in brilliant new light? At an atomic level, nothing is fixed; everything is in flux, constantly constructing and decon-structing. That's why your own genes' DNA is always busy creating new protein, rebuilding bones, replacing brain neurons, even replacing the DNA itself. The body you had as a child does not in any way exist today, maybe even the body you had last year. Their half-lives vary but almost all of your atoms are constantly being replaced by atoms from the food you eat and the air you breathe. And yet "you" are still here. *How is this possible?*

Think of that lovely blue-flowing river observed from a distance: always the same to your mind's eye, never the same in reality. In this same way, you are not your body, a fixed entity, but a vibrant process. A pattern drawn in the sand, not the sand itself. "You are not the stuff of which you are made," contends science writer Steve Grand. Who then are you? Your very cells die and slough off. Your molecules migrate into the soil, into the waterways, into the bodies of animals. Biologists call this sustained dynamic transience. Physicists call it energy in flux. The ancient Greeks named it transmigration of souls. And the Buddha called it impermanence.

Other cultures seem to get this on an intuitive level. So why in our culture do we hide from aging and death, especially our own? Because we are ego-driven, not soul-driven, and our ego clings to separation and superiority until its dying day. Yet at the moment of liberation, that final breath-sucking *zap! zap! zap!* of passing through the unseen veil, that razor-thin, diaphanous membrane separating life from beyond-life—your trickster ego will finally be outfoxed and you will have no choice but to join the great Kibbutz of Beings.

The joy is in the sharing of the feast! proclaimed a colorful springtime banner at Seattle's Pike Market and you better believe it. As we nourish one another and continuously transform into the other, the great cycle continues and Life goes on *within you and without you*, as the gentle poet sang. End of story (beginning of another).

43.

AUTOBIOGRAPHY OF A VEG'N

"YOU MUST NOT BEG, either for food or money," Ananta instructed his young brother Yogananda, as recounted in *Autobiography of a Yogi*. "You must not reveal your predicament to anyone; you must not go without your meals; and you must not be stranded in Brindaban." The divine faith of Yogananda was being put to the test. If he agreed to his brother's proposal, he and his friend Jitendra would be sent to this ancient Hindu city, knowing not one soul and possessed of nothing but simple dhoti-cloths wrapped around their waists. When the bold challenge was accepted, Ananta presented his brother and anxious friend one-way tickets to Brindaban, then left them penniless at the train station.

I'd never heard of Yogananda when I purchased my solitary, one-way ticket to Europe without a clue or a plan. I departed America with a few hard-earned dollars and little else: no credit cards, no cell phone, nobody waiting at the airport. All I knew at nineteen years of age was this: I urgently needed to shake things up, to transform myself and my insular life. And I had to start out alone, just me and my stubborn faith. Faith that somehow I would find my way, find shelter, food, and good people—a more bighearted existence. For wherever you travel in life, if you are possessed of a kind of wild enthusiasm, a trust in the open-ended journey, synchronicity will unfold.

This happened to the young Yogananda and Jitendra as they relinquished their fears, receiving abundant blessings and wholesome meals from strangers. And it happened to me. Even bumping into my French friend Lasserre was full-blown serendipity—I thought she was still teaching in the States. But she spotted my distinctive, toes-out amble as I wandered like a lost child through Luxembourg Gardens, clutching my few remaining francs and wondering where in all of Paris I would sleep that night.

This is a journey we must all take in one form or another, shedding our safe harbors and false selves to leap into the grand unknown. Where will your own courageous quest lead you? To beauty and freedom? To inner exploration? To veg'nism? Decades later, the bigger trip that is my unfolding life pushed me out of that dietary side canyon and back into the valley of complete nourishment and individual truth.

Most ethical vegetarians and vegans who end up needing meat will embark on a difficult path of self-inquiry. The sage Yogananda, who introduced millions of westerners to yoga and meditation, put it well: "Meat eating and vegetarianism is a very complicated and controversial subject…and I believe that no absolute view can be given which would be good for all times and all people." Absolutism, Yogananda well understood, is neither a lofty nor intelligent principle to live by.

So what did my own journey teach a comically naïve if earnest youth who thirsted for carnal knowledge and hungered to abolish all animal suffering? Its hard truth was this: the very real dangers of a rigid ideology, born of the mind and the emotions, which does not line up with the biological realities of the body. For as much as I longed to honor and respect my animal brethren by not eating them, the earthly reality is that I need to do exactly that.

Compassion is a primary tenant of all religions, but it must be offered first to oneself. If we are to honor our own life and health, we must participate in nature's community feast and this includes, for many of us, feasting on other animals. Yes indeed, we are *eating animals*—and with great appreciation. Conscious living is not about following fixed, albeit lovely concepts. It is about being fearlessly present to the truth of your own experience as it unfolds, however unwelcome or unexpected. Finding your dharma means staying with the inquiry, being willing to break old beliefs about who you think you are and graciously accepting each new metamorphosis.

Could I have done a better job being a vegetarian? Could my daughter have been a better vegan? Ingested even more supplements? Moved to a more conducive climate like India or Hawaii, meditating throughout the day in the manner of traditional plant-eating ascetics who avoid physical activity? Spent my time in quiet, undemanding repose instead of working hard and raising a family? These are valid questions but the answer is no. This is not who I am. For this is my individual truth: I'm of Scotch-Irish and German stock. My ancestors were fish, meat, and dairy eaters, one reason my health soars when I eat heartily of these same foods. "Forbidden" for some, very nourishing for me. Furthermore, I am a high-oxidizer, burn through food at hyper speed, thrive on outdoor physical labor and prosper in colder climes. Bottom line: I require a high-fat, high-purine diet. A good amount of this nutrition, my body has made relentlessly clear, must derive from animals if I am to sustain my health and have any energy to give back. This is my genetic and biochemical reality. What's yours?

I am aware that guard-dog, one-world vegans will attempt to trash everything presented in this book, from bountiful personal testimony to peer-reviewed scientific studies. They will then offer their own opposing testimony and research. Perfect! I welcome them. Yet more evidence of the splendid bio-individuality of humanity. There's really nothing to contest. Those of us who faithfully followed a veg'n diet for years, and now eat meat, realize in a deeply intimate way—no outside verification necessary—that there is something fundamentally different about the way our body utilizes animal food. And we are grateful for that difference for it bestows upon us the good health we could not find with plants alone, despite supplementation. Even the Dalai Lama was forced to end his sincere veganism in order to regain his energy and health. ("A loathsome spiritual crime!" clueless absolutists continue to shriek.) He became frail eating all-plants, a diet his ancestors never came close to consuming in their rock-strewn, high-altitude landscape of meager vegetables and many grazing beasts. Eating native yak meat again, small amounts every other day, His Holiness quickly returned to full health.

> *Take. Eat. This is my body,*
> *this real milk, thin, sweet, bluish,*
> *which I give for the life of the world.*
> —Robin Morgan

OUR FIRST FOOD was animal food, straight from our mother's beautiful swollen tits; that is, if you were fortunate enough to be nurtured in this superior manner. From our very first breaths on earth, humans are designed to eat animal food: tiny mouths instinctively sucking, straight away seeking real milk.

All the carninutrients, critical to human growth and health but found nowhere in plants, are further testimony to this truth. High-purine, amino-acid-complete protein, essential cholesterol, conjugated linoleic acid, abundant DHA and EPA fatty acids, vitamins A, B12, D3, and K2 add profound weight to the argument. Millions of years of evolution must be respected. We are supposed to eat animals.

401

If you are able to live long and well on an animal-free diet, go for it. Truly, I mean this. But never assume that your friend, your brother, or the person running next to you on the hardrock trail can do the same. Those of you who are pushing your agenda on the young and naïve, or simply insisting it's the healthiest diet for all: *stop it.* You may be contributing to the long-term harm of others. And I am speaking to all the "veganism can work well for everybody in all stages of life" official promoters, as well as the pushy PETA crowd, plus all the skinny bitches who write their look-like-me missives, i.e., anyone indiscriminately encouraging "come one, come all" to this nonhistorical diet. As you make all your fantastic, unfounded health claims, I assume you are listening closely to your own wise body as the years unfold. So leave us be to listen to ours.

Three resources should guide your nutritional choices. First, highly respected research, preferably peer-reviewed large cohort studies or double-blind controlled clinical trials. Just as important: study the traditional diet of your ancestors, both sides of your lineage, for valuable clues about the kinds of food your body is best suited to metabolize. Most valuable of all is your own private and irrefutable experience—every food choice, every meal—as you carefully monitor any changes in your health over time. If you decide to embark on the journey of restrictive eating, be a skeptic like the Mahayana Buddhists and rely on inquiry and investigation, not blind faith. And ask yourself one all important question before starting out: "How extensive is my knowledge of human nutrition?"

I don't pretend that my own experience—nor that of Linda, Sylvie, Annie, Rhys, Jade, Jessica, on and on, my daughter, my yoga students, and all the former vegans interviewed and the doctors who healed them—constitute any kind of conclusive evidence. But something is up—the Internet is exploding with tales of ex-veggies lamenting their compromised health. What *is* conclusive is the hearty good health bestowed by traditional, whole-food diets over the centuries, patterns of eating that deliver the full spectrum of nutrients found in animals and plants. Based on real biochemistry and actual outcomes, not an idealist's philosophy, these are nutritional truths you can depend on.

Meanwhile, the verdict on long-term veganism is still out and will be for many generations. So what exactly are we doing here, blindly experimenting with ourselves and our children? Even Pythagoras didn't ask his outer circle of devotees, working men and women leading normal lives, to give up meat. And the third century Buddha, spiritual boss for millions? As the young, wandering Siddhartha he was probably a lacto-veg'n, but scholars believe he renounced his vegetarianism and occasionally ate meat after emerging from the forest to become a revered teacher. What we know for certain is the Buddha never prohibited meat for his followers and asked them to eat any animal food offered them, respecting both the generosity of the giver and the sacrifice of the animal.

Spiritually inclined people have never been dependent upon any prescribed diet regime. My own post-veg'n mysticism is alive and well, just as it was as a meat-eating child, awakening to rapture in the deepest hours of the night while my three sisters slept peacefully nearby. Lips parted, eyes flown open, I never knew when or why these ecstatic states would happen, never telling my family, never forgetting these spontaneous hours with the divine. It was the early Syrian philosopher Iamblichus who believed in our capacity for rapturous union with the source, once we let go of our reductionist minds, our ego's hardened resistance.

In my local *sangha* we share a monthly feast of "finger food" and everyone contributes something of benefit, including modest amounts of meat. Sitting cross-legged in a big circle, we are waited on by all the children in attendance: barefoot, scrappy, happy, eager to serve. Texts are sung, Buddhist prayers are offered, and all Beings are invited to join us at the table, to participate as One in the divine Yum. Then right before eating as a grateful community, we chant with great gusto and delight from The Sublime Green Tara: *Smell Taste Touch/ All things offered with respect in oneness/ Nectar Torma Blood Eat!*

Throughout the ages, ethical men and women have eaten meat. Today we are mindful of its source, eschewing factory farms and eating the minimum required to secure our health. Your own spiritual life will not suffer if you return to being an omnivore. Indeed, it will flourish as you come to a more mature understanding of the interpenetration of all life, right down to our holy comingling as eater and eaten. It doesn't get any more intimate than this. With each conscious, reverential mouthful, we are eating the divine.

I PUT OFF WRITING this book for years. Why? Because I wanted to be certain my omnivorous diet returned me to excellent health that continues over time. It has— and then some. I have more energy and stamina in my 50s than I did in my 20s. But as the legions of young vegans began to burgeon—taking on this novel diet with overnight zealousness—I could not remain silent any longer. So heartfelt and committed they are, but with little to no knowledge of this diet's non-history. And some are taking on veganism for all the wrong reasons: to be skinny, to be accepted, to be cool.

And I felt compelled to reply to the sanctimonious, finger-pointing vegans that remind me so much of my young self, smugly presuming to know the "right" diet, the "superior" diet for all, calling the omnivore's diet—the natural diet of human-kind and our pre-human ancestors—aberrant and unethical, a sin and a vice. The Venerable Shravasti Dhammika addresses this kind of nonsense:

> In the Buddha's teachings, the important thing is the quality of your heart, not the contents of your diet. Many Buddhists take great care never to eat meat, but they are not concerned about being selfish, dis-honest, cruel or jealous. They change their diet which is easy to do, while neglecting to change their hearts which is a difficult thing to do. So whether you are a vegetarian or not, remember that the purifica-tion of the mind is the most important thing....

Conscious omnivores, you are on a noble path, the path of your hunting and foraging ancestors. Grow as much of your own food as possible, honoring the carbon cycle and the soil, respecting the rotations of the seasons. Choose local, organic, pastured and sustainable. If you hunt for your own meat, that too is a righteous path if your ethics stay strong. Eat with sublime awareness. Express genuine gratitude. Consume the minimum animal-based nourishment that you require for good health, no more.

Vegans, you're beautiful. You are on the path of spiritual seekers and sadhus. This too is a noble journey, but only if you divest yourself of any sense of superi-ority you may be harboring. Do not allow your original act of compassion to dete-riorate into a tribute to your own self-image. Respect the dietary needs of others. If you grow your own food, this is especially righteous; honoring the seasons and the fertility of the soil; expressing thankfulness. Be discriminating in the food sources you support. Ecologically and health-wise, eating nutrient-dense whole food is a far better rock to stand on than processed, industrial fare.

Take in enough protein and good fat for exceptional health, not too little. For many individuals, veganism will be best utilized as a short-term diet for cleansing and healing. If you are determined to go the long haul, all best wishes. You are bravely testing a new path that translates into fewer choices, missing nutrients, and constant supplementation. If your body thrives as a vegan over the years, be grateful. If not, be truthful. Pay attention and the food that best serves your unique body will become very clear. And its language is *radiant energy*. If you are suffering and choose to continue to do so for the animals, electing to be a martyr and practice reverse speciesism, be aware that over time you will have less and less to give to your own family, your own species.

And may we all begin to free ourselves from our former adolescent gross-out issues and denials regarding the visceral body, suffering and death, including, inevitability, our own. This is your scared-shitless ego digging in. But your spirit relishes transformations, delights in them! As my friend Anne's elderly hospice patient called out in her final hours, as she moved back and forth between the two worlds: *Wonderful! Wonderful!*

The act of eating is a biological process, evolutionary based. It is not a theory about animal sentience versus plants. It is not a beguiling belief system based on the way we would like our living earth to be, free of all suffering. The underlying workings of the natural world are not for us to change, much as idealists would like to, much as profit-driven corporations blindly, foolishly attempt to. We are part of nature and just like breathing, sleeping, and engaging in fabulous ego-liberating sex, eating other life forms is a most natural act of our embodied souls.

Welcome to our elegant, interdependent, all nurturing world. Even as animals and plants feed the bodies of you and your kin, so shall you one day feed the plants and animals that live through you and beyond you. Vegetarian, omnivore, and carnivore: we are on this earth to celebrate and nourish one another.

SOURCES

Primary resources referenced in this book are listed below, along with texts that contributed to my analysis or perspective. Notes and recommended readings are included.

PREFACE: Failure to Thrive

Asher, Kathyrn, et al. *Study of Current and Former Vegetarians and Vegans*. Humane Research Council. Dec 2014, p. 4. This pro-vegan research council concludes: "70% of vegans abandon their diet."

Dyall, Simon. "Long-chain omega-3 fatty acids and the brain: a review of the independent and shared effects of EPA, DPA, and DHA." *Frontiers in Aging Neuroscience* 7 (2015): 52.

Fabelo, N., et al. "Severe alterations in lipid composition of frontal cortex lipid rafts from Parkinson's disease." *Molecular Medicine* 17 (2011): 1107-18.

Fuhrman, Joel, MD. "Leaders of Vegan Movement Develop Parkinson's: Case Studies." *Drfuhrman*.com. n.d. Web. 9 Jun 2014.

Hall, Harriet. "The China Study Revisited: New Analysis of Raw Data Doesn't Support Vegetarian Ideology." *Science-Based Medicine*. 20 July 2010. Web. 9 Feb 2012.

Klaper, Michael, MD, and J.A. Mollenhauer, "Failure to Thrive: Speculations on the Nutritional Adequacy of 100% Plant-Based Diets." *Nutrientrich*. 12 Nov 2012. Web. 3 Mar 2013.

Masterjohn, Chris. "The Truth About the China Study." *Cholesterol and Health*. 2005. Web. 14 Jan 2012.

McCarty, Mark F. "Failure to Thrive as a Vegan—Could Supplemental Carninutrients Help?" *Catalytic Longevity*. n.d. Web. 25 Feb 2014.

Stover, P.J. "Influence of human genetic variation on nutritional requirements." *Am Journal of Clinical Nutrition* 83.2 (2006): 436S-42S.

1: At First Bite

This scene took place after years of delay tactics and self-searching. Eating small amounts of bison and other local meat after her vegan health crash, my daughter had encouraged me to do the same—and witness if healing followed, as it had for her.

3: Vegan Health

Asher, Kathyrn, et al. *Study of Current and Former Vegetarians and Vegans*. Humane Research Council. Dec 2014, p. 4. The study also concludes: "84% of vegetarians/vegans abandon their diet."

Craig, Winston J., and Ann R. Mangels. "Position of the American Dietetic Association: Vegetarian Diets. *Journal of the American Dietetic Association* 109.7 (2009): 1266-82. Of the 204 studies cited, only 19 are specific to vegans, revealing the dearth of data on plants-only eating and vegan health outcomes.

Esselstyn, C.B., Jr. "Updating a 12-year experience with arrest and reversal therapy for coronary heart disease." *Am J of Cardiology* 84.3 (1999): 339-41, A8. These studies pertain to heart patients only.

-----. "Resolving the Coronary Artery Disease Epidemic Through Plant-Based Nutrition." *Preventive Cardiology* 4.4 (2001): 171-77. Note: a plant-based diet is very different from a plants-only diet.

-----. *Prevent and Reverse Heart Disease*. New York: Penguin, 2008. Esselstyn recommends zero animal products and these "supplements": statin drugs, a multivitamin, vitamins D and B12, plus flax seeds.

Ferrieres, Jean. "French paradox: lessons for other countries." *Heart* 90.1 (2004): 107-11.

Herzog, Hal, PhD. "Why Do Most Vegetarians Go Back To Eating Meat?" *Psych Today*. 20 Jun 2011. Web. 5 Dec 2012. In this survey of ex-veg'ns, "declining health" was cited as the primary reason for quitting.

Key, T.J., et al. "Health effects of vegetarian and vegan diets." *Proceedings of the Nutrition Society* 65.1 (2006): 35-41. (Refer to chapter 7 for more studies on vegetarian and vegan diets.)

Messina, G., RD. "How the Health Argument Fails Veganism." *theveganrd.* 30 Nov 2010. Web. 9 Oct 2013.

Newport, Frank. "In US, 5% Consider Themselves Vegetarians." *Gallup.* 26 July 2012. Web. 30 Jan 2013. This works out to 12 million vegetarians and 5 million vegans (aged 18+). The pro-vegan Asher study cited far less: just 2% of the US population (aged 17+) "is considered to be a current vegetarian/vegan."

Ornish, Dean, et al. "Intensive lifestyle changes re reversal of heart disease." *JAMA* 280.23 (1998): 2001-7.

Sofi, F., et al. "Accruing evidence on benefits of adherence to the Mediterranean diet on health: updated systematic review and meta-analysis." *American Journal of Clinical Nutrition* 92.5 (2010): 1189-96.

United States. Depts. of Agriculture and Health and Human Services. *Dietary Guidelines for Americans.* Washington DC: GPO, 2010, p. 45.

"Vegetarian Statistics." Vegetarian Resource Group. Harris Service Bureau. May 2015. Web. 3 Dec 2015. This survey also found smaller numbers of veg'ns than the Gallup survey (where respondents self-defined categories; see Newport, F.): approximately 4.3 million vegetarians and 3.7 million vegans.

5: The Ethical Vegetarian

Bourette, Susan. *Meat: A Love Story.* New York: G. P. Putnam's Sons, 2008. Bourette's remarks about her slaughterhouse experience appear on pages 9, 10, and 24.

"Go Vegetarian, Go Vegan! Starter Kit." *People for the Ethical Treatment of Animals.* Norfolk, VA, 2010.

Imhoff, Daniel, ed. *CAFO: The Tragedy of Industrial Animal Factories.* San Rafael, CA: Earth Aware, 2010.

"Vegetarian Starter Guide." *Compassion Over Killing.* Washington DC: n.d.

West, Brittany. "Human Rights Situation of Workers in the Meatpacking and Poultry Industry in the United States." *Human Rights Brief.* 27 March 2014. Web. 19 May 2014.

7: Young Bitchin' Females: Get Skinny!

Aloufy, A., and Y. Latzer. "The linkage between vegetarianism and anorexia nervosa." *Harefuah* 45.7 (2006): 526-31, 549.

Ambroszkiewicz, J., et al. "The influence of vegan diet on bone mineral density and biochemical bone turnover markers." *Pediatric Endocrinology Diabetes and Metabolism* 16.3 (2010): 201-04.

Appleby, P., et al. "Mortality in vegetarians and comparable nonvegetarians in the UK." *Am J of Clinical Nutrition* 103.1 (2016): 218-230. "Similar all-cause mortality" is the conclusion from this study of pooled data from > 60,000 UK–based vegetarians/vegans and comparable meat eaters.

-----. "Comparative fracture risk in vegetarians and nonvegetarians in EPIC-Oxford." *Eur Journal of Clinical Nutrition* 61.12 (2007): 1400-06. Vegans had 30% higher fracture rates than meat eaters.

-----, et al. "Mortality in British Vegetarians." *Public Health Nutrition* 5.1 (2002): 29-36.

-----, et al. "Oxford vegetarian study: an overview." *Am Journal of Clinical Nutrition* 70 (1999): 525S–31S.

Bardone-Cone, Anna, PhD, et al. "The Inter-relationships between Vegetarianism and Eating Disorders among Females." *Journal of Academy of Nutrition and Diet* 112.8 (2012): 1247–1252.

Bouckenooghe, T., et al. "Is taurine a functional nutrient?" *Cur Opin Clin Nutr Met Care* 9.6 (2006): 728-33.

Bousquet, M., et al. "Beneficial effects of dietary omega-3 polyunsaturated fatty acid on toxin-induced neuronal degeneration in an animal model of Parkinson's disease." *FASEB Journal* 22 (2008): 1213-25.

Chang-Claude, J., et al. "Lifestyle determinants and mortality in German vegetarians and health-conscious persons: results of a 21-year follow-up." *Cancer Epidemio Biomarkers & Prevention* 14.4 (2005): 963-68.

Craig, Winston J. "Health effects of vegan diets." *Am Journal of Clinical Nutrition* 89.5 (2009): 1627S-33S.

Crowe, F.L., et al. "Risk of hospitalization or death from ischemic heart disease among British vegetarians and nonvegetarians: results from the EPIC-Oxford cohort study." *Am Journal of Clinical Nutrition* 30 Jan 2013. Web. 28 May 2013.

Daniel, Kaayla, PhD. "The High Fructose Diet of Steve Jobs." *Psych Today* 19 Jan 2012. Web. 18 Nov 2016.

Davis, Brenda, RD, and Vesanto Melina, RD. *Becoming Vegan.* Summertown, TN: Book Publishing Co., 2000, pp. 21, 24, 35, 94-95. For an excellent discussion of vegan diets & chronic disease, see pp. 19-37.

Dyall, Simon. "Long-chain omega-3 fatty acids and the brain: a review of the independent and shared effects of EPA, DPA, and DHA." *Frontiers in Aging Neuroscience* 7 (2015): 52.

Elmadfa, I., and I. Singer. "Vitamin B-12 and homocysteine status among vegetarians: global perspective." *Am Journal of Clinical Nutrition* 89 (2009): 1693S–98S.

EPIC-Oxford Study. Refer to Appleby, P.; Crowe, F.; Gilsing, A.; Key, T.J.; and Romieu, I. in this chapter.

Fabelo, N., et al. "Severe alterations in lipid composition of frontal cortex lipid rafts from Parkinson's disease." *Molecular Medicine* 17 (2011): 1107-18.

Fraser, G.E. "Vegetarian Diets: What do we know of their effect on common chronic diseases." *Am Journal of Clinical Nutrition* 89.5 (2009): S1607-12.

-----. *Diet, Life Expectancy, and Chronic Disease: Studies of Seventh-Day Adventists and Other Vegetarians.* Oxford University Press, 2003, pp. 231-39.

Freedman, Rory, and Kim Barnouin. *Skinny Bitch.* Philadelphia: Running Press, 2005.

Fuhrman, Joel, MD. "Leaders of Vegan Movement Develop Parkinson's: Case Studies." *Drfuhrman*.com. n.d. Web. 9 Jun 2014.

Gaull, G.E. "Taurine in pediatric nutrition: review and update." *Pediatrics* 83.3 (1989): 433-42. "Absence from the diet of a conditionally essential nutrient does not produce immediate deficiency disease but, in the long term, can cause problems." Taurine is added to infant formulas for improved nourishment.

Gilsing, Anne, et al. "Serum concentrations of B12 and folate in British male omnivores, vegetarians, and vegans: the EPIC-Oxford cohort study." *Eur Journal of Clinical Nutrition* 64.9 (2010): 933-39.

Heidelberg Study. Refer to Chang-Claude, J., et al. Conclusion from 21-years of follow-up: "Being a vegan was associated with a higher mortality risk than being a lacto-ovo vegetarian."

Huang, T., et al. "Cardiovascular Disease Mortality & Cancer Incidence in Vegetarians: A Meta-Analysis and Review." *Annals Nutrition and Metabolism* 60.4 (2012): 233-240.

Key, T.J., et al. "Mortality in vegetarians and nonvegetarians." *Am J Clinical Nutrition* 70.3S (1999): 516-24. No statistically significant differences found between vegans and meat-eaters for any causes of death.

Kies, Constance. "Effect of Dietary Fat & Fiber on Calcium Bioavailability." *ACS Symposium* (1985): 175-87.

Liu, Haibo, et al. "Fructose Induces Transketolase Flux to Promote Pancreatic Cancer Growth." *Cancer Research* 70.15 (2010): 6368-76.

Mangels, Reed, PhD, RD, and Davida Breier. *Vegan & Vegetarian FAQ: Answers to Your Frequently Asked Questions.* Baltimore: Vegetarian Resource Group, 2001.

McCoy, Krisha, MS. "The Dangers of Hidden Abdominal Fat." *NYU Langone Medical Center.* Jun 2014. Web. 9 July 2014.

Michalak, Johannes, et al. "Vegetarian diet & mental disorders: results from representative community survey." *Int Journal of Behav Nutri and Phys Activity* 9:67 (2012): Web 9 Feb 2014.

Mozes, A. "Underweight Even Deadlier Than Overweight." *HealthDay.* 28 March 2014. Web. 4 July 2014.

Obersby, D., et al. "Plasma total homocysteine status of vegetarians compared with omnivores: a systematic review." *British Journal of Nutrition* 109.5 (2013): 785-94.

O'Neill, Brighid. "Scientific review of the reported effects of vegan nutrition on occurrence and prevalence of cancer and cardiovascular disease." *Bio Horizons* 3.2 (2010): 197-212.

Orlich, M.J., et al. "Vegetarian dietary patterns and mortality in Adventist Health Study 2." *JAMA Internal Med* 173.13 (2013): 1230-38. A total of 73,308 Adventists participated.

Paradis, Sébastien, et al. "Emotional and instrumental aggressiveness and body weight loss." *Europe's Journal of Psychology* 3.4 (2007) n.p. Web. 18 Feb 2014.

Pedersen, A.B., et al. "Menstrual differences due to vegetarian and nonvegetarian diets." *Am Journal of Clinical Nutrition* 53.4 (1991): 879-85.

Ray, Joel , and Sissi Cao, et al. "J-shapedness: an often missed, often miscalculated relation: the example of weight and mortality." *J of Epidemiology and Community Health* 28 Mar 2014. Web. 19 May 2014.

Reimer, S. "More girls & women take up vegan banner." *Baltimore Sun.* 26 March 2008. Web. 2 July 2012.

Romieu, Isabelle, et al. "Dietary glycemic index & glycemic load and breast cancer risk in the EPIC Study." *Am Journal of Clinical Nutrition* 96.2 (2012): 345-55.

Seventh-Day Adventist Studies. Refer to Fraser, G.E., et al; Key, T.J., et al; and Orlich, M.J., et al.

Thomas, E.L., et al. "Excess body fat in obese and normal-weight subjects." *Nutrition Research Reviews* 25.1 (2012): 150-61. Explores disease risk factors in lean individuals with hidden abdominal fat.

Wachob, J. "Q & A with Skinny Bitch Author Rory Freedman." *MindBodyGr.* 3 Aug 2010. Web. 1 Nov 2012.

8: Liberation Road

Cromwell, Bob. "What do French schoolchildren eat for lunch?" *Cromwell-intl.* 2014. Web. 15 Jun 2014.

David, Marc, Director. Institute for the Psychology of Eating. Interview. 8 Mar 2014.

-----. *The Slow Down Diet.* Rochester, VT: Healing Arts Press, 2005.

Dominé, André, ed. *Culinaria: FRANCE.* Konigswinter: Konemann, 2004.

Ferrieres, Jean. "French paradox: lessons for other countries." *Heart* 90.1 (2004): 107–11. The French have low coronary heart disease death rates, despite high intakes of cholesterol and saturated fat.

Gide, André. *La Porte Étroite.* Cambridge, MA: Schoenhofs Foreign Books, 1972.

Guiliano, Mireille. *French Women Don't Get Fat.* New York: Vintage Books, 2007.

Haurant, Sandra. "French government 'banning vegetarianism' in school canteens." *Guardian.* 26 Oct 2011. Web. 18 Aug 2013.

Keroac, Jack. *On the Road.* New York: Signet Books, 1958.

Le Billon, Karen. *French Kids Eat Everything.* New York: HarperCollins, 2012.

Lorgeril, M. de, et al. "Mediterranean diet and the French paradox." *Cardio Research* 54.3 (2002): 503-15.

Organization for Economic Co-operation Development. *Obesity Update.* 2014. Web. 30 May 2015.

Pereira, M., et al. "Fast-food habits, weight gain, and insulin resistance." *Lancet* 365.9453 (2005): 36-42.

Rozin, P., et al. "Attitudes to food and the role of food in life in the USA, Japan, Flemish Belgium, and France." *Appetite* 33 (1999): 163-180.

Schama, Simon. *Citizens: A Chronicle of the French Revolution.* New York: Knopf. 1989.

Whitman, Walt. "Passage to India." *Complete Poetry & Collected Prose.* New York: Literary Classics, 1982.

9: Vegetarian Class Wars

Alao, B., et al. "The Potential of Animal By-Products in Food Systems." *Sustainability* 9 (2017): 1089.

"Classifications of Vegetarians: Comments." *The Veg Blog.* 2006-07. Web. 8 Dec 2012.

Dominé, André, ed. *Culinaria: FRANCE.* Konigswinter: Konemann, 2004, p. 46.

Hall, Donald. "O Cheese." *White Apples and the Taste of Stone.* New York: Houghton Mifflin, 2006.

"Pescatarian—A vegetarian who eats….what?" *Hubpages.* 2009. Web. 28 Dec 2012.

Richter, Allan. "Alanis Morissette Sings a Song of Wellness." *Energy Times.* July 2013, pp. 21-24.

10: The Vegetarian's Dilemma

Bailey, N. W., et al. "Testing acoustic communication in plants." *Behavioral Ecology* 24.4 (2013): 797.

Baluška, F., D. Volkmann, and S. Mancuso, eds. *Communication in Plants: Neuronal Aspects of Plant Life.* Berlin: Springer-Verlag, 2006.

Baluška, F., and S. Mancuso. "Plant Neurobiology as a Paradigm Shift Not Only in the Plant Sciences." *Plant Signaling & Behavior* 2:4 (2007): 205-07.

-----, et al. "The 'root-brain' hypothesis of Charles and Francis Darwin: Revival after more than 125 years." *Plant Signaling & Behavior* 4.12 (2009): 1121-27.

Bentham, Jeremy. *Introduction to the Principles of Morals and Legislation.* 1823. Oxford: Clarendon, 1907.

Borrelli, Luca, et al. "Insect-based diet, a promising nutritional source, modulates gut microbiota composition in laying hens." *Scientific Reports* 7:16269 (2017). Web. 10 Mar 2018.

Brahic, Catherine. "Solar-powered sea slug harnesses stolen plant genes." *New Scientist* 17 (2008): 24.

Braithwaite, Victoria. *Do Fish Feel Pain?* New York: Oxford University Press, 2010.

Chow, B., and P. McCourt. "Plant hormone receptors: perception is everything." *Genes and Development* 20.15 (2006): 1998-2008.

Cox, Peter. *You Don't Need Meat.* New York: St. Martin's Press, 2002, p. 322.

Crowley, Pat. "The World's First Cricket Bar." *Kickstarter.* 3 July 2012. Web. 20 Dec. 2013.

Darwin, Charles. *The Power of Movement in Plants.* Whitefish, MT: Kessinger, 2004.

Durst, Patrick B., et al. *Forest Insects as Food: Humans Bite Back.* UN Food and Agriculture Organization. 2010. Web. 3 Nov. 2013.

Frick-Wright, Peter. "Eat Your Bugs!" *Sierra.* July/Aug 2013, 32-33.

Garzon, F.C. "The Quest for Cognition in Plant Neurobiology." *Plant Signaling Behavior* 2.4 (2007): 208-11.

Goh, C.H., et al. "Stress memory in plants." *The Plant Journal* 36.2 (2003): 240-55.

Goldin, Ryan. "Eat Insects and Benefit Your Gut Biome." *Entomo Farms.* 12 Jan 2016. Web. 9 Mar 2017.

Gordon, David George. *The Eat-a-Bug Cookbook.* 1998. New York: Ten Speed Press, 2013.

Grandin, Temple, and Mark Deesing. "Distress in Animals: Is it Fear, Pain, or Physical Stress?" Dept. of Animal Sciences, Colorado State University. Sept 2003. Web 2 Oct. 2013.

Kandel, Eric R., and Robert D. Hawkins. "The Biological Basis of Learning and Individuality." *Scientific American.* Sept 1992, pp. 79-86.

Looijer-van Langen, M., and L. Dieleman, "Prebiotics in Chronic Intestinal Inflammation." *Inflammatory Bowel Disease* 15.3 (2009): 454-62.

Lovejoy, Arthur. *The Great Chain of Being: A Study of the History of an Idea.* 1936. Harvard U Press, 2001.

Madsen, David B. "A Grasshopper in Every Pot." *Natural History* 2.2 (1989): 22-5. Dried cakes of layered grasshoppers were called "desert fruitcake" by early white travelers to Utah.

Marder, Michael. "Plant intentionality and the phenomenological framework of plant intelligence." *Plant Signaling and Behavior* 7.11 (2012): 1365-72.

Martinelli, Nicole. "Smarty Plants: Inside the World's Only Plant-Intelligence Lab." *Wired.* 30 Oct 2007. Web. 3 Mar 2012.

Naik, Gautam. "Switzerland's Green Power Revolution: Ethicists Ponder Plants' Rights." *Wall St Journal.* 10 Oct. 2008. Web. 29 Mar 2012. Ecuador has gone bravely further, granting rights to entire ecosystems to "exist, flourish, and evolve," supported by 2/3 of voters.

Nichiren Daishonin. "The Oral Tradition Regarding the Enlightenment of Plants." *The Writings of Nichiren Daishomnin.* Nichiren Buddhism Library. n.d. Web. 17 Oct 2013.

Peak, D.A., et al. "Evidence for complex, collective dynamics and emergent, distributed computation in plants." *Proceedings of the Natl Academy of Sciences* 101.4 (2004): 918-22.

Rose, J.D., "The Neurobehavioral Nature of Fishes and the Question of Awareness of Pain." *Reviews in Fisheries Sciences* 10.1 (2002): 1-38.

Sanabria, Natasha, et al. "Self/non-self perception in plants in innate immunity and defense." *Immune Recognition and Signaling* 1.1 (2010): 40-54.

Schmidt, Charles. "Mental Health May Depend on the Creatures in the Gut." *Scientific American.* March 2015. Web. 9 Mar 2018.

Sneddon, L., V. Braithwaite, and M. Gentle. "Do fish have nociceptors? Evidence for the evolution of a vertebrate sensory system." *Proc of the Royal Society* 270.1520 (2003): 1115-21.

Spencer, Colin. *Vegetarianism, A History.* New York: Eight Walls Four Windows, 2000, pp. 2-3.

Stone, C. *Should Trees Have Standing? Law, Morality, and the Environment.* 1972. Oxford U Press, 2010.

Theophrastus. *Enquiry Into Plants, Vol. 1: 1-5.* Trans. Arthur F. Hort. Harvard Press, 1916.

Thomas, Elizabeth Marshall. *The Hidden Life of Deer.* New York: Harper Collins, 2009.

Tompkins, Peter, and Christopher Bird. *The Secret Life of Plants.* New York: Harper & Row, 1973. In its Dec. 30, 1973 review, *The New York Times* called the book "whimsical" and "very interesting, if true."

Trewavas, A. "Green plants as intelligent organisms." *Trends in Plant Science* 10.9 (2005): 413-9.

-----. "How Plants Learn." *Proceedings of the National Academy of Sciences* 96.8 (1999): 4216–18.

United States. Food and Drug Administration. "Levels of natural or unavoidable defects in foods that present no health hazards for humans." *Defect Levels Handbook.* 20 Jun 2014.

Van Huis, Arnold, et al. *Edible insects: future prospects for food and feed security.* United Nations Food and Agricultural Organization. Rome, 2013.

Watt, Simon. "Ugly Animal of the Week." *Ugly Animals Preservation Society.* 2014. Web. 15 Oct 2014.

"You Can Fool Climate Deniers but You Can't Fool Mother Nature: Plants Pack Up and Move North."
   Climate News Network. 10 Mar 2013. Web. 20 Apr 2013.
Zimmermann, M.R., et al. "System Potentials, a Novel Electrical Long-Distance Apoplastic Signal in Plants,
   Induced by Wounding." *Plant Physiology* 149.3 (2009): 1593–1600.

11: The Meaning of Meat

Agapakis, C. "Steak of the Art: The Fatal Flaws of In Vitro Meat." *Discover.* 24 Apr 2012. Web. 19 Feb 2013.
Arens, William. *The Man Eating Myth: Anthropology and Anthropophagy.* Oxford University Press, 1979.
Barnes, Jonathan. *The Presocratic Philosophers, 2 vols.* London: Routledge, Kegan Paul: 1979. A respected
   historian, Barnes claims no evidence exists that Pythagoras was a vegetarian.
Bloom, Harold, ed. *Stephen Crane.* InfoBase, 2009, p. 54. Web. 9 Jan 2015.
"Classifications of Vegetarians: Comments." *The Veg Blog.* 19 Jun 2007. Web. 3 Apr 2012.
Cranston, Maurice. *The Solitary Self: Jean-Jacques Rousseau in Exile and Adversity.* University of Chicago
   Press, 1999. The venison and wine quote appears on pages 89-90.
Einstein, Albert. *The New Quotable Einstein.* Ed. Alice Calaprice. Princeton University Press, 2005.
Guthrie, Kenneth. *The Pythagorean Sourcebook and Library.* Grand Rapids: Phanes, 1988.
Harmon, Leon, "The Meat of Argentina Would Make a San Francisco Vegetarian's Head Explode." *Huff-
   ington Post.* 17 Jun 2010. Web. 5 May 2012.
Jochems, Carlo, et al. "The use of fetal bovine serum: ethical or scientific problem?" *Alternatives to Lab
   Animals* 30 (2002): 219-227.
Porphyry. *On Abstinence from Animal Food.* Ed. E. Wynne-Tyson. Whitefish, MT: Kessinger, 2006.
-----. *Vie de Pythagore.* Ed. Edouard Des Places. Paris: Société d'édition les Belles Lettres, 1982.
Preece, Rod. *Sins of the Flesh: A History of Ethical Vegetarian Thought.* Vancouver: UBC Press, 2008, pp. 7,
   8, 11, 15, 21, 336. Read chapter 9 for a fascinating historical account of "Preaching Without Practicing."
Rousseau, Jean-Jacques. *Emile: or On Education.* Allan Bloom, Trans. New York: Basic Books, 1979. Refer
   to page 154 for Rousseau's quote.
Rumble, Victoria. "The Laird's Table: Scottish Fare for the Upper Class." *The Historic Foodie.* 8 Jan 2013.
   Web. 29 Apr 2013.
Schwartz, John. "PETA's Latest Tactic: $1 Million for Fake Meat." *NY Times.* 21 Apr 2008. Web. 3 Aug 2012.
Sears, William, Dr. "Soy Formula." *Ask Dr. Sears.* 2014 Web. 30 Nov 2013.
Spencer, Colin. *Vegetarianism: A History.* 1993. New York: Four Walls Eight Windows, 2000.
Stuebe, Alison, MD. "The Risks of Not Breastfeeding for Mothers and Infants." *Reviews in Obstetrics and
   Gynecology* 2.4 (2009): 222–31.
"Use of Fetal Calf Serum." *Humane Research Australia.* 2016. Web. 9 May 2016.
Williams, Howard. *The Ethics of Diet: A Catena of Authorities Deprecatory of the Practice of Flesh-Eating.*
   Ed. Carol J. Adams. 1883. Reprint. University of Illinois Press, 2003. Porphyry's statement on the per-
   sonal diet of Pythagoras appears on page 7. Voltaire's "frightful inconsistency" quote is on page 145.

13: Brains, Bliss, and Pythagoras

Arthen, Inanna. "The Eightfold Path: Fasting." *Fireheart* 4. n.d. Web. 22 Dec 2012.
Bardone-Cone, Anna, PhD, et al. "The Inter-relationships between Vegetarianism and Eating Disorders
   among Females." *J of Academy of Nutrition and Diet* 112.8 (2012): 1247–1252.
Bell, Rudolph M. *Holy Anorexia.* Chicago: University of Chicago Press, 1985.
Buettner, Dan. *The Blue Zones: Lessons for Living Longer.* Washington, DC: Nat. Geographic Society, 2010.
Chisholm, Kate. *My Hungry Hell.* London: Short Books, 2002.
Cohen, Marc, et al. *Readings in Ancient Greek Philosophy: Thales to Aristotle.* Indianapolis: Hackett, 2001.
Darby, William, et al. *Food: The Gift of Osiris.* San Diego: Academic Press, 1977.
Deary, Ian. Refer to Gale, Catherine, 1970 British cohort study.
Estruch, Ramón, MD, et al. "Primary Prevention of Cardio Disease with Mediterranean Diet." *New England
   Journal of Medicine* 368 (2013): 1279-90.

Franklin, Benjamin. *The Autobiography & Other Writings.* Ed. K. Silverman. London: Penguin, 1986, p. 98.

Fraser, Gary E. *Diet, Life Expectancy, and Chronic Disease: Studies of Seventh-Day Adventists and Other Vegetarians.* Oxford University Press, 2003, pp. 231-39.

-----, et al. "Possible protective effect of nut consumption on risk of coronary heart disease; The Adventist Health Study." *Archives of Internal Medicine* 152 (1992): 1416-24.

Gale, Catharine, et al. "Childhood and vegetarianism in adulthood." *British Medical* 334.7587 (2007): 245.

Mantel, Hilary. "Holy Disorders." *The Guardian.* 3 March 2004. Web. 12 Dec. 2012.

Mazess, R., and S. Forman. "Longevity and age exaggeration in Vilcabamba, Ecuador." *J of Gerontology* 34.1 (1979): 94-98.

McEvoy, C.T., et al. "Vegetarian diets, low-meat diets and health." *Pub Health Nutri* 15.12(2012): 2287-94.

Micha, R. PhD, et al. "Red vs Processed Meat Consumption and Risk." *Circulation* 121.21 (2010): 2271-83.

Mills, P.K. "Cancer Incidence Among California Seventh-Day Adventists, 1976-1982." *Am Journal of Clinical Nutrition* 59.5S (1994): 1136S-42S.

Norris, Jack, RD. "Disease Rates of Vegetarians & Vegans." *VeganHealth.org.* Dec 2013. Web. 29 Jan 2014.

Orlich, M.J., et al. "Vegetarian dietary patterns and mortality in Adventist Health Study 2." *JAMA Internal Med* 173.13 (2013): 1230-38. A total of 73,308 Adventists participated.

Perry, Susan. "Study on vegetarianism: interesting but not definitive," *Minn Post.* 6 Jun 2013.

Riedweg, Christoph. *Pythagoras: His Life, Teaching, and Influence.* Trans. S. Rendall. Cornell U Press, 2008.

Shaw, George Bernard. *The Star.* London. 5 Apr 1890. Digital. 2013.

Spencer, Colin. *Vegetarianism, A History.* New York: Four Walls Eight Windows, 2000, pp. 45, 48, 52.

"Vegetarians Live Longer Than Meat-Eaters, Loma Linda Study Finds." *Science Times.* 4 Jun 2013.

Verducci, Tino. "Vegetarians are More Intelligent." *The Future is Vegan.* 20 Jun 2010. Web. 5 Oct 2012.

Yokoyama, Y., et al. "Vegetarian diets and blood pressure." *JAMA Internal Med* 174.4 (2014): 577-87.

14: *Martine on the Rocks*

Cannavan, Tom. "Pouilly-Fuissé with Audrey Braccini." *wine-pages.* 2013. Web. 5 Oct 2013.

Chelminkski, Rudolph. *I'll Drink to That: Beaujolais and the French Peasant Who Made It the World's Most Popular Wine.* New York: Penguin Group, 2007.

Counihan, Carole. Quoted in "Food Taboos." *National Geographic News.* 28 Oct 2010. Web. 5 Nov 2012.

Dominé, André, ed. *Culinaria: FRANCE.* Konigswinter: Konemann, 2004, p. 81.

15: *The Kinship of Cuisine*

Blaisdell, Aaron, et al. "From heart beats to health recipes: The role of fractal physiology in the Ancestral Health movement." *Journal of Evol and Health* 1.1 (2013): n.p. Web. 30 Dec 2013.

Chan, Laurie, and Harriet Kuhnlein. "Traditional food and participatory research: a Canadian experience." *GRID Arendal.* n.d. Web. 8 Sept 2012.

Crandall, Russ, PhD. *The Ancestral Table.* Las Vegas: Victory Belt Publishing, 2013.

Humane Research Council. (Asher et al.) *Study of Current and Former Vegetarians and Vegans.* Dec 2014, p. 7. Nearly 60% of veg'ns who quit did not view the diet as part of their identity.

Pope, Sarah. "Determining Best Traditional Diet for You." *Healthy Home Eco* 7 Jun 2012. Web. 9 July 2012.

Schmid, Ron. *Native Nutrition: Eating According to Ancestral Wisdom.* Rochester, VT: Healing Arts, 1994.

Scruton, Roger. "The Conscientious Carnivore." *Food for Thought: The Debate Over Eating Meat.* Ed. Steve Sapontzis. Amherst, NY: Prometheus, 2004, pp. 81-91.

16: *Renegades: A Brief History of Veg'nism in the West*

Antiphanes. Quoted in "The Deipnosophistae of Athenaeus." Vol. II. Loeb Classical, 1928. Digital. 2013.

Aristophanes. *The Frogs.* Jeffrey Henderson, Trans. Newburyport, MA: Focus/Pullins, 2008.

Bramley, S. *Leonardo: The Artist and the Man.* London: Penguin, 1994. See page 240 for da Vinci quote re keeping his body from becoming "a container of corruption."

Detienne, Marcel. *Dionysos Slain.* John Hopkins University Press, 1979, p. 70.

Edmonds, John M., ed. *The Fragments of Attic Comedy.* Leiden, Netherlands: E.J. Brill, 1959. Digital. 2013.

Forward, Charles W. *Fifty Years of Food Reform: History of the Vegetarian Movement in England.* London: Ideal Publishing, 1898. Digital 2013. *Manchester City News* quote re Simpson appears on page 44.

Godwin, Joscelyn. *Mystery Religions in the Ancient World.* New York: Harper Row, 1981, p. 28.

Haran, Dan. "Why I'm giving up vegetarianism." *K5 Tech and Culture.* 14 Oct 2003. Web. 18 July 2012.

Herzog, H. "Why Do Vegetarians Go Back To Eating Meat?" *Psych Today.* 20 Jun 2011. Web. 19 Oct 2013.

Holroyd, Michael. *Bernard Shaw, Vol 1: 1856-1898.* New York: Vintage Books, p. 88.

-----. *Bernard Shaw: The One-Volume Definitive Edition.* Random House, 1990.

Homer. *The Odyssey.* Trans. Rodney Merrill. University of Michigan Press, 2002, Books 12, 14.

Joyce, James. *Ulysses.* New York: Modern Library, 1992. The mutton kidney espisode appears in chapter 4.

LaMartine, Alphonse de. Quoted in Williams, H. *The Ethics of Diet,* London, Pitman: 1883, p. 251. Digital.

Manchester City News. Quoted in *Fifty Years of Food Reform: History of the Vegetarian Movement in England.* Refer to Forward, Charles (above).

Porphyry. *On Abstinence from Animal Food.* Ed. E.W. Tyson. Trans. T. Taylor. Fontwell, UK: Centaur, 1965.

Preece, Rod. *Sins of the Flesh: A History of Ethical Vegetarian Thought.* Vancouver: UBC Press, 2008, pp. 252-260. Preece delivers a fascinating account of Shelley's vegetarianism. The "renewed enjoyment in life" quote re Shelley's partaking of mutton chops appears on page 257.

Ritson, Joseph. *An Essay on Abstinence from Animal Food as a Moral Duty.* London: Richard Phillips, 1802.

Rousseau, Jean-Jacques. *Emile et Julie: Selections.* Great Neck, NY: Barrons, 1964, p. 89.

Saint Augustine. *The City of God Against the Pagans.* Ed. and Trans. R.W. Dyson. Cambridge U Press, 1998. Refer to Book 19, chapter 16.

Sax, Boria. *Animals in the Third Reich.* Providence, RI: Poet's Press, 2013.

Shaw, George Bernard. Refer to Holroyd, Michael (above).

Shelley, Percy Bysshe. *The Complete Works of Percy Bysshe Shelley,* V. 6. Eds. Roger Ingpen and Walter Peck. New York: Gordian, 1965, pp. 6, 8, 11, 17, 18.

-----. A *Vindication of Natural Diet.* Pamphlet, 1813. Nabu Press, 2010.

Spencer, Colin. *Vegetarianism, A History.* New York: Four Walls Eight Windows, 2000.

Voltaire. *Elements de la Philosphie de Newton,* 1738, V. Refer also to Williams, H. in chapter 11 sources.

Wilkins, John. "Public and Private Eating in Greece, 450-300 BC." Oxford Symposium of Food, 1991.

Wright, John. *The Vegetarian Messenger.* August 1850. "Archives of the Vegetarian Society." Altrincham, Cheshire, England. Digital. 2013.

17: To Kill or Not to Kill

Gandhi, M.K. *How to Serve the Cow.* Ahmedabad: Navajivan Publishing, 1954. Gandhi's quote on "Mother Cow" appears in Jha's *The Myth of the Holy Cow,* p. 17.

Jha, Dwijendra. *The Myth of the Holy Cow.* London: Verso, 2002, p. 17. The cow is valued in India, Jha writes, "because of its resource value in an agrarian society whose members derive a substantial part of their sustenance from its milk and other dairy products." Refer to Gandhi also (above).

Thomas of Celano. "First Life of St. Francis." *St. Francis of Assisi: Writings and Early Biographies.* Ed. M.A. Habig. Chicago: Franciscan Herald Press, 1983, Book I.

18: What Are Veg'ns Eating, Really?

Cherbuin, N., PhD, et al. "Higher normal fasting plasma glucose is associated with hippo-campal atrophy: The PATH Study." *Neurology* 4.79 (2012): 1019-26.

Crane, P.K., et al. "Glucose levels and risk of dementia." *New England J of Medicine.* 369.6 (2013) 540-548.

Davis, William, MD. "Wheat is an Opiate." *Wheat Belly.* 17 Apr 2012. Web. 12 Sept 2012.

Emond, J.A., et al. "Risk of Breast Cancer Recurrence Associated with Carbohydrate Intake and Tissue Expression of IGF-1 Receptor. *Cancer Epidem Biomarkers Prev* 23.7 (2014): 1273-79.

Franz, M.J. "Carbohydrate and diabetes: Is the source or the amount of more importance?" *Cur Diabetes Report* 1.2 (2012): 177-86. Findings: total amount of carbs in a meal is more important than the source.

Fung, T.T., et al. "Low carbohydrate diets, dietary approaches to stop hypertension-style diets, and the risk of postmenopausal breast cancer. *Am Journal of Epidem* 174.6 (2011): 652-60.

Graham, Douglas. *The 80/10/10 Diet.* Key Largo, FL: FoodnSport Press, 2006, p. 171.

Havel, P.J., et al. "Adverse metabolic effects of dietary fructose." *Current Op Lipidol* 24.3 (2013): 198-206.

Henderson, S.T. "High carbohydrate diets and Alzheimer's disease." *Medical Hypoth* 62.5 (2004): 689-700.

Hu, J., et al. "Glycemic index, glycemic load and cancer risk." *Oncology* 24.1 (2013): 245-51. Glycemic load is calculated by multiplying the glycemic index of a food by its grams of carbohydrates, divided by 100.

Jeppesen, J., et al. "Effects of low-fat, high-carb diets on risk factors for ischemic heart disease in post-menopausal women." *Am Journal of Clinical Nutrition* 65.4 (1997): 1027-33.

Josefsen, Deborah. "High carbohydrate diet implicated in pancreatic cancer." *Brit Med J* 325 (2002): 566.

Lennerz, Belinda S., et al. "Effects of dietary glycemic index on brain regions related to reward and craving in men." *Am Journal of Clinical Nutrition* 064113 (2013) n.p. Web. 15 Oct 2013.

Liu, Simin, et al. "Dietary glycemic load, carbohydrate intake, and risk of coronary heart disease in US women." *Am Journal of Clinical Nutrition* 71.6 (2000): 1455-61.

Michaud, D.S., et al. "Dietary glycemic load, carbohydrate, sugar, and colorectal cancer risk in men and women." *Cancer Epidemiology Biomarkers and Prevention* 14.1 (2005): 138–47.

Muti, Paola, et al. "Fasting Glucose is a Risk Factor for Breast Cancer, A Prospective Study." *Cancer Epidemiology, Biomarkers and Prevention* 11 (2002): 1361.

Nordmann, A.J., et al. "Effects of low-carb vs. low-fat diets on weight loss and cardiovascular risk factors: a meta-analysis." *Archive of Internal Medicine* 166.3 (2006): 285-93.

Parks, Elizabeth , et al. "Effects of a low-fat, high-carbohydrate diet on VLDL-trigylceride clearance." *Journal of Clinical Investigation* 104.8 (1999): 1087-96.

-----, and Marc Hellerstein. "Carbohydrate-induced hypertriacylglycerolemia: a historical perspective and review of biological mechanisms." *Am Journal of Clinical Nutrition* 71.2 (2000): 412-33.

Perlmutter, David, MD. *Grain Brain.* New York: Little, Brown and Company. 2013.

Petrova, Nadia. "The biggest mistakes people make on a vegan diet." *Nature Insider.* 20 Nov 2012. Web. 27 Sept 2013.

Roberts, R.O., et al. "Relative intake of macronutrients impacts risk of mild cognitive impairment or dementia." *Journal of Alzheimer's Disease* 32.2 (2012): 329-39.

Romieu, Isabelle, et al. "Dietary glycemic index and glycemic load & breast cancer risk in the EPIC Study." *Am Journal of Clinical Nutrition* 96.2 (2012): 345-55.

Schwarzbein, Diane, MD, and Nancy Deville. *The Schwarzbein Principle.* Deerfield Beach, FL: Health Communications, 1999, pp. 110-126.

Seneff, S., et al. "Nutrition and Alzheimer's disease: the detrimental role of a high carbohydrate rate diet." *European Journal of Internal Medicine* 22.2 (2011): 134-40.

Sieri, S., et al. "Dietary glycemic index, glycemic load, and the risk of breast cancer in an Italian prospective cohort study." *Am Journal of Clinical Nutrition* 86.4 (2007): 1160-66.

Spencer, Colin. *Vegetarianism: A History.* New York: Four Walls Eight Windows, 2000. Tolstoy's high-carb porridge diet is described on page 270.

"Thoughts on Raw Vegan, 80/10/10 & Paleo Diets." *Open Mind Required.* 28 Jun 2009. Web. 5 Nov 2013.

Twigg, Julia. *Prospectus of Concordium.The Vegetarian Movement in England 1847-1981.* U of London PhD thesis. 1981. Web. 20 Nov 2013.

Weil, Andrew, MD. "Anti-Inflammatory Diet and Pyramid." *Dr Weil.* Web. 3 Jan 2014.

19: Liebig and 15 Cups of Rice

Brock, William H. *Justus von Liebig: The Chemical Gatekeeper.* 1997. Cambridge U Press, 2002.

Campbell, T. Colin, PhD. "Animal versus Plant Protein." T. Colin Campbell Center for Nutrition Studies. *Nutritionstudies.* 2014. Web. 20 May 2014.

Enig, Mary, PhD, and Sally Fallon. *Nourishing Traditions.* Washington DC: New Trends, 2001, p. 26.

Illinois Dept. of Agriculture. "Crop Production, 1950-1997: Soybeans." 2001. Web. 9 July 2013.

Lappé, Francis M. *Diet for a Small Planet.* 1971. New York: Ballantine, 1991.

Liebig, Justus, MD, PhD. *Chemistry in Its Application to Agriculture and Physiology.* Ed. Lyon Playfair. Philadelphia: T.B. Peterson, 1847. Digital. 30 Oct 2013.

Mangels, Reed, PhD. "Protein in the Vegan Diet." *The Vegetarian Resource Group.* 2014. Web. 1 Oct 2013.

Norris, Jack, RD. "Lysine: Limiting Amino Acid in Vegan Diets." *veganhealth.* Dec 2010. Web. 10 Oct 2013.

"Reviews for Diet for a Small Planet." *Goodreads.* 21 July 2013 Web. 12 Oct 2013.

Wasserman, D., and R. Mangels, PhD. *Simply Vegan.* Baltimore: Vegetarian Resource Group, 2006, p. 140.

20: Hunger, Caffeine, and Seattle's Naked Beauty

Bourette, Susan. *Meat: A Love Story.* New York: G. P. Putnam's Sons, 2008, p. 35.

Carpenter, M. *Caffeinated: How Our Daily Habit Helps, Hurts and Hooks Us.* New York: Hudson St, 2014.

Johnson, Steven. *Where Good Ideas Come From.* New York: Riverhead Books, 2011.

Pendergrast, Mark. *Uncommon Grounds: The History of Coffee.* New York: Basic Books. 2010.

22: Annoying Attitudes/Dubious Research

Campbell, T. Colin, PhD, and Thomas M. Campbell II. *The China Study: Startling Implications for Diet, Weight Loss, and Long-term Health.* Dallas: BenBella Books, 2005, Introduction and pp. 4, 132, 242.

Chen, Junshi, et al. *Diet, Lifestyle and Mortality in China: A Study of the Characteristics of 65 Chinese Counties.* Oxford University Press. 1990.

"Classifications of Vegetarians: Comments." *The Veg Blog.* 2007. Web. 25 Jan 2011.

"Confessions of an Ex-Vegetarian." *FoodVibe.* 15 Oct 2008. Web. 15 Dec 2011.

Gannon, Sharon, and David Life. *Jivamukti Yoga.* New York: Ballantine, 2002, p. 65.

Hall, Harriet. "The China Study Revisited: New Analysis of Raw Data Doesn't Support Vegetarian Ideology." *Science-Based Medicine.* 20 July 2010. Web. 9 Feb 2012.

"Health and Wellness: Forum." *Above Top Secret.* n.d. Web. 4 Mar 2012.

Hu, F., and W. Willett. "Reply to TC Campbell." *Am Journ of Clin Nutrition* 71.3 (2000): 850-51.

"Imogen." Should Vegans Hate Meat Eaters? *Let Them Eat Meat.* 12 July 2010. Web. 30 Jan 2011.

King, Barbara J. "Do Vegetarians and Vegans Think They Are Better Than Everyone Else?" *Culture: npr.org.* 30 Aug 2012. Web. 10 Jan 2013.

Masterjohn, Chris. "The Truth About the China Study." *Cholesterol and Health.* 2005. Web. 14 Jan 2012.

Messina, Virginia, RD. "Dr. Lanou Responds to Jack's Post about Calcium: Comments." *JackNorrisRD.* 31 Dec 2009. Web. 12 Aug 2012.

Minger, Denise. *Death by Food Pyramid: How Shoddy Science, Sketchy Politics and Shady Special Interests Have Ruined Our Health.* Malibu: Primal Blueprint, 2013.

-----. "The China Study: Fact or Fallacy?" *Raw Foods SOS.* 7 July 2010. Web. 13 Feb 2012.

Morley, Dan. "Vegans." *The Human Guide to North America.* n.d. Web. 29 Jan 2012.

Naughton, Tom. "Outstanding Critique of the China Study." *Goodscience.* 13 July 2010. Web. 19 Nov 2012.

Norris, Jack, RD, and Virginia Messina, RD. *Vegan for Life.* Boston: Da Capo Press, 2011, pp. 11, 12. 177.

"People Eating Tasty Animals." *doughney.net.* n.d. Web. 30 Nov 2012.

Preece, Rod. *Sins of the Flesh.* Vancouver: UBC Press, 2008, p. 8.

Shaw, George Bernard. *Man and Superman.* Preface. Digireads Publishing: Stilwell, KS, 2007.

Southan, Rhys. "Interview with Ex-Vegan Heather Mamety." *Let Them Eat Meat.* 2012. Web. 21 Mar 2013.

Turner, Lisa. "Vegetarianism for Dummies: Everything You Need to Know." *Nexus.* Nov/Dec 2006.

23: Into the Wilds

Corral, Roy. *Alaska Native Ways: What the Elders Have Taught Us.* Graphic Arts Books, 2002.

Rosen, Y. "Keevan Dinkel, Alaska Boy, Wins Cabbage Contest." *Reuters.* 31 Aug 2013. Web. 30 Jan 2014.

State of Alaska. Department of Fish and Game. "Historical Commerical Salmon Catches and Values, 1873-2013." Web. 7 Feb 2014.

24: Protein 101: Don't Get Wasted

Albert, Paul, and Chawki Benkelfat. "The neurobiology of depression: revisiting the serotonin hypothesis." *Philos Trans of the Royal Society* 368:1615 (2013): n.p. Web. 2 Oct 2012.

Ambroszkiewicz, J., et al. "The influence of vegan diet on bone mineral density and biochemical bone turnover markers." *Pediatr Endocrinol Diabetes Metab* 16.3 (2010): 201-04.

Armas, L.A., et al. "Vitamin D2 is much less effective than vitamin D3 in humans." *Journal of Clinical Endocrinology & Metabolism* 89 (2004): 5387-91.

Campbell, W.W. "Dietary Protein Requirements of Older People: Is the RDA Adequate?" *Nutrition Today* 31.5 (1996): 192-97.

Cordain, Loren, PhD. "Cereal grains: humanity's double-edged sword." *World Rev Nutri* 84 (1999): 19-73.

-----. "The late role of grains and legumes in human diet, and biochemical evidence of their evolutionary discordance." *Beyond Veg.* 1999. Web. 28 Aug 2012.

-----, and Campbell, T. Colin, PhD. "The Protein Debate." *Catalyst Athletics: J of Nutrition and Athletic Excellence* (2006) n.p. Web. 14 Sept 2012.

-----, et al. "Origins and evolution of the Western diet: health implications for the 21st century." *American J of Clinical Nutrition* 81.2 (2005): 341-54.

Davis, B., RD, and V. Melina, RD. *Becoming Vegan.* Summertown, TN: Book Publishing Co., 2000. "Vegan Food Guide" appears on page 154.

Eades, Michael, MD, and Mary D. Eades, MD. *Protein Power.* New York: Bantam Books, 1996.

Edwards, Pamela. "Haiku." *Vital Choices.* Newsletter. 19 Jun 2006.

Elango, R., et al. "Evidence Protein Requirements Have Been Significantly Underestimated." *Current Op in Clinical Nutrition and Metabolic Care* 13.1 (2010): 52-57.

Feng, R., et al. "High carb intake from starchy foods is positively associated with metabolic disorders." *Scientific Reports* 5 (2015): 16919.

Floersheim, G.L. "Treatment of brittle fingernails with biotin." *Z Hautkr* 64.1 (1989): 41-48.

Fulgoni, Victor. "Current protein intake in America; analysis of National Health and Nutrition Examination Survey, 2003-2004." *Am Journal of Clinical Nutrition* 87.5 (2008): 15545-75.

Gilani, G.S., et al. "Effects of antinutritional factors on protein digestibility and amino acid availability in foods." *Journal of AOAC International* 88.3 (2005): 967-87.

Institute of Medicine. *Dietary Reference Intakes for Energy, Carbohydrate, Fiber, Fat, Fatty Acids, Cholesterol, Protein & Amino Acids.* Washington, DC: National Academy Press, 2005.

Int'l Society of Sports Nutrition. "Position stand: protein and exercise." 4.8 (2007): n.p. Web. 3 Sept 2012.

Kasarda, Donald. "Can an Increase in Celiac Disease Be Attributed to an Increase in the Gluten Content of Wheat?" *Journal of Ag and Food Chemistry* 61.6 (2013): 1155-59.

Kerti, L., et al. "Higher glucose levels associated with lower memory and reduced hippocampal microstructure." *Neurology* 81.20 (2013): 1746-52.

Klaper, Michael, MD, and John Mollenhauer. "Failure to Thrive: Speculations on the Nutritional Adequacy of 100% Plant-Based Diets." *Nutrient Rich.* 12 Nov 2012. Web. 3 Mar 2013.

Klement, Rainer, and U. Kämmerer. "Is There a Role for Carbohydrate Restriction in the Treatment and Prevention of Cancer?" *Nutrition Metabolism* 8.75 (2011): 75.

Lees, S.J., and F.W. Booth. "Sedentary death syndrome." *Can Journal Appl Physiology.* 29.4 (2004): 444-60.

Liener, I.E., "Implications of antinutritional components in soybean foods." *Critical Reviews: Food Science and Nutrition* 34.1 (1994): 31-67.

Liu, Simin, et al."Dietary glycemic load, carbohydrate intake, and risk of coronary heart disease in US women." *Am Journal of Clinical Nutrition* 71.6 (2000): 1455-61.

Ludvigsson, J.F., et al. "Increasing incidence of celiac disease in a North American population." *Am Journal of Gastroenterology* 108.5 (2013): 818-24.

Mathieson, I., et al. "Genome-wide patterns of selection in 230 ancient Eurasians." *Nature* 528:7583 (2015): 499-503.

Michaud, D.S., et al. "Dietary glycemic load, carbohydrate, sugar, and colorectal cancer risk in men and women." *Cancer Epidemiology Biomarkers and Prevention* 14.1 (2005): 138–47.

Mollenhauer, John A. Refer to Klaper, Michael, MD, "Failure to Thrive," in this chapter.

Nagle, C., et al. "Glycemic index, load, and endometrial cancer risk." *Euro J Nutrition* 52.2 (2013): 705-15.

Norris, Jack, RD. "Protein." *Vegan Health.* 2014. Web. 30 Jan 2014.

-----, and Virginia Messina, RD. *Vegan for Life.* Boston: Da Capo Press, 2011, pp. 23, 173 (low HDL levels).

Paddon-Jones, D., and B.B. Rasmussen. "Dietary protein recommendations and prevention of sarcopenia." *Current Op in Clinical Nutrition and Metabolic Care.* 12.1 (2009): 86-90.

Pencharz, Paul, et al. "Recent developments in understanding protein needs—How much and what kind should we eat?" *Applied Physiology, Nutrition and Metabolism* 41.5 (2016): 577-80.

Pfeiffer, Carl, MD. *Mental and Elemental Nutrients.* New Canaan: Keats, 1975, p. 103.

Pullen, Kate. "Dangers of Veganism." *vegetarian.lovetoknow.com.* 2012. Web. 5 May 2012.

"Reader Comments." *Primal Living in the Modern World.* 2013. Web. 8 Jan 2014.

Robbins, John. "Ask John." *Foodrevolution.com.* n.d. Web. 12 Nov 2013.

Rodriguez, N.R., et al. "Position of the ADA, Dietitians of Canada, and the American College of Sports Medicine: Nutrition and Athletic Performance." *Journal of Am Dietetic Association* 109 (2009): 509-27.

Romieu, Isabelle, et al. "Dietary glycemic index, glycemic load, and breast cancer risk in the EPIC Study." *Am Journal of Clinical Nutrition* 96.2 (2012): 345-55.

-----, et al. "Carbohydrates and Risk of Breast Cancer among Mexican Women." *Cancer Epidem Biomarkers* 13.8 (2004): 1283-89. Carbohydrate intake was positively associated with breast cancer risk. Strongest associations were observed for sucrose and fructose.

Rubio-Tapia, Alberto, MD. "The Prevalence of Celiac Disease in the United States." *American Journal of Gastroenterology* 107 (2012): 1538–1544.

Schwarzbein, Diane, MD, and Nancy Deville. *The Schwarzbein Principle,* Deerfield Beach, FL: Health Communications, 1999, pp. 17-27.

Sebastian, Anthony. "Isoflavones, protein, and bone." *Am Journal of Clinical Nutrition* 81.4 (2005): 733-35.

Sieri, S., et al. "Dietary glycemic index, glycemic load, and the risk of breast cancer in an Italian prospective cohort study." *Am Journal of Clinical Nutrition* 86.4 (2007): 1160-66.

-----, and V. Krogh. "Dietary glycemic index, glycemic load, and cancer." *Nutri, Metab, and Cardio Diseases* 27.1 (2017): 18-31. High glycemic load is associated w/increased risk of breast and endometrial cancer.

Stead, I.M., and John Bourke. *Lindow Man: The Body in the Bog.* Ed. Don Brothwell. Cornell U Press, 1986.

Tieman, Jill, Dr. "Your Brain on Fake Food." *Real Food Forager.* 7 Apr 2011. Web. 23 Jan 2014.

United States. Depts. of Agriculture and Health and Human Services. *Dietary Guidelines for Americans.* Washington, DC: 2010. Revised every five years. The 2015 Guidelines finally call for less sugar.

Waldmann, A., et al. "Dietary iron intake and iron status of German female vegans: results of the German vegan study. " *Annals Nutrition Metab* 48.2 (2004): 103-08.

Wolfe, Robert R., PhD, and Sharon L. Miller, PhD. "The Recommended Dietary Allowance of Protein: A Misunderstood Concept." *JAMA* 299.24 (2008): 2891-93.

Wong, E. "Pollution Rising, Chinese Fear for Soil & Food." *New York Times.* 30 Dec 2013. Web. 5 Jan 2014.

Yu, D., et al. "Dietary glycemic index, glycemic load, and refined carbohydrates are associated with risk of stroke." *Am Journal Clinical Nutrition* 104.5 (2016): 1345-51.

25: Soy Stories

Adgent, M., et al. "Early-life soy exposure and age at menarche." *Perinatal Epidemiol* 26.2 (2012): 163-75.

Adlercreutz, Herman. Refer to Sandbeck, E. for this scientist's quote re soy isolates.

American Academy of Environmental Medicine. "Genetically Modified Foods Position Paper." Presented by Amy Dean, DO, and Jennifer Armstrong, MD. 8 May 2009. Web. 3 Aug 2013.

Antoniou, Michael, et al. "Roundup and birth defects: Is the public being kept in the dark?" *Earth Open Source.* Jun 2011. Web. 18 Oct 2014.

Badger, T.M., et al. "The health implications of soy infant formula." *Am Journal of Clinical Nutrition* 89S (2009): 1668S–72S.

Balk, Ethan, MD., et al. U.S. Dept. of Health and Human Services. "Effects of Soy on Health Outcomes." Aug 2005. Web. 28 Nov 2013.

Barrett, J. "The Science of Soy: What do we really know?" *Enviro Health Perspect* 114.6 (2006): A352–58.

Bhatia, Jatinder, et al." Use of Soy Protein-Based Formulas in Infant Feeding." *Pediatrics* 121.5 (2008). Refer to Welch, Claudia, p. 228, for source of Bhatia's quotation.

Carrasco, Andres. "Glyphosate-Based Herbicides Produce Teratogenic Effects on Vertebrates by Impairing Retinoic Acid Signaling." *Chem Res Toxicology* 23.10 (2010): 1586–95.

Cassidy, A., et al. "Biological effects of diet of soy protein rich in isoflavones on the menstrual cycle of pre-menopausal women. *Am Journal for Clinical Nutrition* 60.3 (1994): 333-40.

Clark, J.D., et al. *Food processing operations and scale-up*. New York: CRC Press, 1991.

"Classifications of Vegetarians: Responses." *The Veg Blog*. 10 Sept 2007. Web. 30 Dec 2011.

Condor, Bob. "The Milk Debate: Soy vs. Cow." *Chicago Tribune*. 20 May 2001. Web. 5 Dec 2013.

Cornucopia Institute. *Behind the Bean: The Heroes and Charlatans of the Natural and Organic Soy Foods Industry*. 2009. Web. 28 May 2014.

-----. *Dirty Little Secret in Natural Foods Industry: Toxic Chemical Use*. 28 Nov 2010. Web. 14 May 2014.

Daniel, Kaayla, PhD. *The Whole Soy Story*. Washington DC: Newtrends Publishing, 2005, p. 331.

Davis, B., RD, and V. Melina, RD. *Becoming Vegan*. Summertown, TN: Book Publishing, 2000, p. 154.

Dean, Amy, DO, and Jennifer Armstrong, MD. "Genetically Modified Foods Position Paper." *Am Academy of Environmental Medicine*. 8 May 2009. Web. 30 Jan 2014.

Doerge, Daniel R., and Daniel M. Sheehan. "Goitrogenic and estrogenic activity of soy isoflavones." *Enviromental Health Perspectives* 110.S3 (2002): 349–53.

Druker, S.M. *Altered Genes, Twisted Truth*. Clear River Press, 2015. Exposé of the GM food industry.

Enig, M.G., and S. Fallon. "Food in China: Variety and Monotony." *Traditional Diets*. Jan 1 2000: Web. 10 Mar 2014. Average daily soy consumption in China cited: a mere 9 grams.

Ewen, Stanley, PhD, et al. "The Case for a GM-Free Sustainable World." *The Independent Science Panel on GM Final Report*. 15 Jun 2003. Web. 8 Feb 2014.

Guyton, Kathryn, et al. "Carcinogenicity of tetrachlorvinphos, parathion, malathion, diazinon, and glyphosate." *The Lancet Oncology*. 20 March 2015. Web. 28 Apr 2015.

Kent, George, PhD. "Skewed Soy Studies." *Pediatrics*. Published Letters. 14 Jun 2012. Web. 30 Mar 2014.

Krajcovicova-Kudlackova, M., et al. "Iodine defiency in vegetarians and vegans." *Annals of Nutrition and Metabolism* 47.5 (2003): 183-85.

Krüger, Monika, et al. "Detection of Glyphosate Residues in Animals and Humans." *Journal of Enviro and Analytical Toxicology* 4.2 (2014): n.p. Web. 9 Dec 2014.

Levis, S., et al." Soy isoflavones in the prevention of menopausal bone loss and menopausal symptoms: a randomized, double-blind trial." *Archives Internal Med* 171.15 (2011): 1363-69. "A significantly larger proportion of participants in the soy group experienced hot flashes compared with the control group."

Liener, I.E. "Implications of antinutritional components in soybean foods." *Critical Reviews in Food Science and Nutrition* 34 (1994): 31–67.

Mesnage, Robin, et al. "Potential toxic effects of glyphosate." *Food Chem Toxicology* 84 (2015): 133-53.

Myers, J.P., et al. "Concerns over use of glyphosate-based herbicides and risks associated with exposures: a consensus statement." *Enviro Health* 15 (2016): 19.

Nguyen, Andrea. "Is Tofu Healthy or Harmful?" *Viet World Kitchen*. Apr 2012. Web. 2 Dec 2013.

Palmer, Brian. "The risks of hexane in soy products." *Slate*. 26 Apr 2012. Web. 14 May 2014.

Pope, Sarah. "170 Scientific Studies Confirm the Dangers of Soy." *Healthy Home Economist*. 27 Apr 2014. Web. 17 May 2014.

Roccisano, D., et al. "A possible cause of Alzheimer's dementia—industrial soy foods." *Medical Hypotheses* 82.3 (2014) 250-4.

Sacks, F.M., et al. "Soy Protein, Isoflavones, and Cardiovascular Health." *Circulation* 113 (2006): 1034-44.

Samsel, Anthony, and Stephanie Seneff. "Glyphosate's Suppression of Cytochrome P450 Enzymes, Amino Acid Biosynthesis by Gut Microbiome: Pathways to Modern Diseases" *Entropy* 15.4 (2013): 1416-63.

Sandbeck, Ellen. *Green Barbarians: Live Bravely on Your Home Planet.* New York: Scribner, 2009. Scientist Adlercreutz's quote about his fear of soy isolates appears on page 77. Dr. White's quote about phytoestrogens as drugs appears on pages 76-77.

Sebastian, Anthony. "Isoflavones, protein and bone." *Am Journal of Clinical Nutrition.* 81.4 (2005): 733-35.

Sheehan, D.M., and D.R. Doerge. "Goitrogenic and estrogenic activity of soy isoflavones." *Environmental Health Perspectives* 110.S3 (2002): 349–53. Refer also to Condor, B. for Sheehan's soy formula quote.

Siepmann, T., et al. "Hypogonadism and erectile dysfunction associated with soy product consumption." *Nutrition* 27.7-8 (2011): 859-62.

Smith, Jeffrey. *Seeds of Deception: Exposing Industry and Government Lies About the Safety of the Genetically Engineered Food You're Eating.* Fairfield, IA: Yes! Books. 2003.

"Straight Talk About Soy." *The Nutrition Source.* Harvard School of Public Health. 2014. Web. 5 Apr 2014.

Terrain, Mary Vance. "The Dark Side of Soy." *Utne Reader.* July/Aug 2007. Web 25 Aug 2012.

Thongprakaisang, S., et al. "Glyphosate induces human breast cancer cells growth via estrogen receptors." *Food Chem Toxicol.* 59 (2013): 129-36.

Union of Concerned Scientists. *Heads They Win, Tails We Lose: How Corporations Corrupt Science at the Public's Expense.* Cambridge: UCS Publications, 2012.

United Nations. Food and Agricultural Organization, Statistics, 2003. Average daily intake of soy protein in China is just 3.4 grams; 8.7 grams in Japan. Refer to Barrett, 2006.

United States. Dept. of Health and Human Services. "New Report on Soy Finds Limited Evidence for Health Outcomes." 24 Aug 2005. Web. 28 Oct 2013.

Warner, Melanie. *Pandora's Lunchbox: How Processed Food Took Over.* New York: Scribner, 2013.

Welch, Claudia. *Balance Your Hormones, Balance Your Life.* Cambridge, MA: DaCapo Press, 2011, p. 208.

White, Lon. "Association of High Midlife Tofu Consumption with Accelerated Brain Aging." *Third Int'l Soy Symposium.* Nov 1999, p. 26. Web. 3 Oct 2013. Refer to Sandbeck for White's quote re phytoestrogens.

26: The Nervous Vegetarian

Ames, Bruce, PhD, and Joyce C. McCann. "Vitamin K, an example of triage theory." *Am Journal of Clinical Nutrition* 90.4 (2009): 889-907.

Armas, L.A., et al. "Vitamin D2 is much less effective than vitamin D3 in humans." *J of Clinic Endocrinology and Metabolism* 89 (2004): 5387-91.

Aro, A., et al. "Inverse relation between CLA in adipose breast tissue and risk of breast cancer. A case-control study in France." *Inform* 10.5 (1999): S43.

Blesso, Christopher, et al. "Whole egg consumption improves lipoprotein profiles and insulin sensitivity to greater extent than yolk-free egg substitute." *Metabolism* 62.3 (2013): 400-10.

Boldyrev, A., et al. "Biochemical and physiological evidence that carnosine is endogenous neuroprotector against free radicals." *Cell & Mol Neurobiology* 17.2 (1997): 259- 71.

-----, et al. "Carnosine Protects Against Excitotoxic Cell Death Independently of Effects on Reactive Oxygen Species." *Neuroscience* 94:2 (1999): 571—77.

Burke, D.G., et al. "Effect of creatine and weight training on muscle creatine and performance in vegetarians." *Medicine and Science in Sports and Exercise* 35.11 (2003): 1946-55.

Chan, J., et al. "Vitamin D status of vegetarians, partial vegetarians, and nonvegetarians: Adventist Health Study 2." *Am Journal of Clinical Nutrition* 89 (2009): 1686S–92S.

Cordain, L., et al. "Detailed fatty acid analysis of selected tissues in elk, mule deer, and antelope." *FASEBJ* 13 (1999): A887.

Costa da, K.A., et al. "Choline deficiency increases lymphocyte apoptosis and DNA damage in humans." *Am Journal of Clinical Nutrition* 84.1 (2006): 88-94.

Davis, B., RD, and V. Melina, RD. *Becoming Vegan.* Summertown, TN: Book Publishing Co., 2000, p. 104.

Deans, Emily, MD. "Your Brain on Creatine." *Evolutionary Psychiatry.* 10 Feb. 2012.

Etzioni, A., et al. "Systemic carnitine deficiency exacerbated by strict vegetarian diet." *Archives of Disease in Childhood* 59 (1984): 177-79.

Gast, G.C.M., et al. "A high menaquinone (K2) intake reduces the incidence of coronary heart disease." *Nutrition, Metabolism & Cardiovascular Disease* 19 (2009): 504-10.

Geleijnse, J.M., et al. "Dietary intake of vitamin K-2 reduces the risk of cardiac events and aortic athero-sclerosis: The Rotterdam Study." *Journal of Nutrition* 134 (2004): 3100-105.

Goodman, Gary, et al. "Beta-Carotene and Retinol Efficacy Trial." *J Nat Cancer Inst* 96.23 (2004): 1743-50.

Higdon, Jane, PhD, et al. "Choline." *Linus Pauling Institute.* 18 Aug 2009. Web. 30 Mar 2014.

Hipkiss, A.R. "Glycation, aging and carnosine: Are carnivorous diets beneficial?" *Mechanisms of Aging & Development* 126.10 (2005): 1034-39.

-----. "Could carnosine or related structures suppress Alzheimer's disease?" *Journal of Alzheimer's Disease* 11.2 (2007): 229-40.

Hu, Frank, et al. "A prospective study of egg consumption and risk of cardiovascular disease in men and women." *JAMA* 281.15 (1999): 1387-94.

Hunt, Janet R. "Bioavailability of iron, zinc, and other trace minerals from vegetarian diets." *Am Journal of Clinical Nutrition* 78.3 (2003): 6335-95.

Jamieson, A. "I'm Not Vegan Anymore." *Alexandra Jamieson.* 27 Feb 2013. Web. 5 Mar 2013.

Jones, Peter J.H. "Dietary cholesterol and the risk of cardiovascular disease in patients: a review of the Harvard Egg Study and other data." *Int Journal Clinical Pract Suppl* 163.1-8 (2009): 28-36.

Kim, K.J., et al. "ATF3 Mediates Anti-Cancer Activity of Trans-10, cis-12-Conjugated Linoleic Acid in Human Colon Cancer Cells." *Biomolecules and Therapeutics* 23.2 (2015): 134-40.

Koba, K., and T. Yanagita. "Health benefits of conjugated linoleic acid (CLA)." *Obesity Res Clinical Practice* 8.6 (2014): 525-32.

Krajcovicova-Kudlackova, M., et al. "Correlation of carnitine levels to methionine and lysine intake." *Physiological Research* 49.3 (2000): 399-402.

Laidlaw, S., et al. "Plasma and urine taurine levels in vegans." *Am J of Clinic Nutrition* 47.4 (1988): 660-63.

Lee, K.W., et al. "Role of CLA in the Prevention of Cancer." *Crit Rev Food Sci Nutrition* 45.2 (2005): 135-44.

Lin, Y., et al. "Variability of conversion of beta-carotene to vitamin A in women measured using a double-tracer study design." *Am J of Clinical Nutrition* 71.6 (2000): 1545-54.

Littlejohns, T., et al. "Vitamin D and the risk of dementia and Alzheimer disease." *Neurology* 10.1212 (2014): n.p. Web. 10 Aug 2014.

Masterjohn, Christopher. "On the Trail of the Elusive X-Factor: 62-Year-Old Mystery Finally Solved." *Wise Traditions in Food, Farming & Healing Arts.* Spring 2007. Details Dr. Weston Price's discovery of Vit K2.

McCarty, Mark F. "Failure to Thrive as a Vegan—Could Supplemental Carninutrients Help?" *Catalytic Longevity.* n.d. Web. 25 Feb 2014.

Murphy S.P., and L.H. Allen. "Nutritional Importance of Animal Sourced Foods." *Journal of Nutrition* 133S (2003): 3932S-35S.

"Natto: Steve, Don't Eat It! Vol. 6." *TheSneeze.* 24 Jun 2004. Web. 5 Jan 2014.

Nierenberg D.W., et al. "Effects of 4 yrs of oral supplementation with beta-carotene on serum concentrations of retinol." *Am Journal of Clinical Nutrition* 66.2 (1997):315-19.

Nimptsch, K., et al. "Dietary Vitamin K intake: relation to cancer incidence & mortality: EPIC-Heidelberg." *Am Journal of Clinical Nutrition* 91 (2010): 1348-58.

Norris, Jack, RD. "Choline." *VeganHealth*.org. Apr 2013. Web. 20 Dec 2013.

Obersby, D., et al. "Plasma total homocysteine status of vegetarians compared with omnivores: a systematic review." *British Journal of Nutrition* 109.5 (2013): 785-94.

Pasantes-Morales, H., et al. "Taurine enhances proliferation, promotes neuronal specification of murine and human neural stem/progenitor cells. *Adv Exp Med Biology* 803 (2015): 457-72.

Poliquin, C. "Vegetarians Beware: Nutrient Deficiencies." *Poliquin Group.* 29 Mar 2012. Web. 2 Dec 2013.

Pope, Sarah. "The Benefits of Emu Oil." *The Healthy Home Economist.* 28 Jan 2014. Web. 17 Feb 2015.

Preston, J.E., et al. "Toxic Effects of Beta-amyloid on Immortalised Rat Brain Endothelial Cell: Protection by Carnosine, Homocarno and Beta-alanine." *Neuroscience Letters* 242:2 (1998): 105-108.

Price, Weston, DDS. *Nutrition and Physical Degeneration: A Comparison of Primitive and Modern Diets and Their Effects.* 1939. Price-Pottenger Nutrition Foundation, 2009, p. 282. See also Masterjohn, C.

Rae, Caroline, et al. "Oral creatine monohydrate supplementation improves brain performance: a double-blind, placebo-controlled, cross-over trial." *Proc Biol Science* 270: 1529 (2003): 2147–50.

Rheaume-Bleue, Kate. *Vitamin K2 and the Calcium Paradox.* Ontario: John Wiley and Sons, 2012.

Scott, Jenna. "From Vegan to Paleo" with Comments. *Robb Wolf: Revolutionary Solutions to Modern Life.* 15 Oct 2012. Web. 8 Jan 2013.

Shao, L., et al. "L-carnosine reduces telomere damage and shortening rate in cultured normal fibroblasts." *Biochem and Biophys Research Comm* 324 (2004): 931–36.

Stephens, Francis B., et al. "Vegetarians have a reduced skeletal muscle carnitine transport capacity. *Am J of Clinical Nutrition* 94.3 (2011): 938-44.

Stewart, Desmond. "The Limits of Trooghaft." *Encounter* 38.2 (1972): 3-7.

Wylie, C. "New Studies Validate Age-Delaying Effects of Carnosine." *Life Ext.* Dec 2016. Web. 7 May 2017.

Yamano, E., et al. "Effects of chicken essence." *Med Science Monit* 19 (2013): 540-47.

Yamori, Y., et al. "Taurine as the nutritional factor for the longevity of the Japanese." *Adv Exp Med Biol* 643 (2009): 13-25.

Xiao, Y., et al. "Creatine for Parkinson's disease." *Co Database Syst Rev* 17 (2014): n.p. Web. 28 Feb 2015.

Zeisel, S. "Choline: Needed for normal development of memory." *JACN* 19.5 (2000): 528S-31S.

27: Into The Light

Andreasen, Nancy. *The Creating Brain: The Neuroscience of Genius.* Dana Press: New York, 2011. Examines "extraordinary creativity" in science, including that of German chemist Friedrich Kekulé.

Bucky, Peter A. *The Private Albert Einstein.* Kansas City: Andrews & McMeel, 1992, p. 86. This is but one of many statements Einstein made about mysticism and science.

Dunn, Stephen. "Tiger Face." *What Goes On: Selected and New Poems.* New York: W.W. Norton, 2009.

Einstein, Albert. Refer to Bucky, Peter (above).

Ernst, Edzard, MD. "Public's enthusiasm for complementary/alternative medicine amounts to a critique of mainstream medicine." *Int Journ Clinical Practice* 64. 11 (2010): 1472-74.

Jain, S., et al. "Healing Touch with Guided Imagery for PTSD in returning active duty military: a randomized controlled trial." *Military Medicine* 177.9 (2012): 1015-21.

Leape, L., et al. "Counting deaths from medical errors." *JAMA* 288 (2002): 2405.

Messina, G., RD. "How the Health Argument Fails Veganism." *theveganrd.* 30 Nov 2010. Web. 9 Oct 2013.

Naparstek, Belleruth. "What Is Guided Imagery?" *Health Journeys.* 2014. Web. 20 Apr 2014.

Nelson, Jeff. "How the Ethical Argument Fails Veganism." *Vegsource.* 8 Aug 2012. Web. 3 Feb 2014.

O'Brien, Chris. "Medical Intuition: More Than A Hunch. *Nexus.* July/Aug 2006, pp. 27-28.

Schwarzbein, Diane, MD, and Nancy Deville. *The Schwarzbein Principle.* Deerfield Beach, FL: Health Communications, 1999, pp. 3-27, 61-65. Quote appears on page 22.

Shealy, C. Norman, MD. *Medical Intuition: Your Awakening to Wholeness.* Virginia Beach: ARE Press, 2010.

Trakhtenberg, E.C. "The effects of guided imagery on the immune system: a critical review." *Int Journal of Neuroscience* 118 (2008): 839-55.

28: Praise the Lard and Pass the Butter

Agrawal, R., and F. Gomez-Pinilla. "Metabolic syndrome in the brain: deficiency in omega-3 fatty acid exacerbates dysfunctions in insulin receptor signaling & cognition." *J of Physiology* 590.10 (2012): 2485.

Allen, Mark. Personal Interview. 30 Jan 2013.

----- . "Nutrition and Endurance Training." *Mark Allen Online.* 10 July 2013. Web. 30 Jun 2014.

Bazzano, Lydia A., et al. "Effects of Low-Carbohydrate and Low-Fat Diets: A Randomized Trial." *Annals of Internal Medicine* 161.5 (2014): 309-18.

Blaylock, R., MD. "DHA Supports Brain Development, Protects Neurological Function." *Life Ext.* Jan 2008.

Bousquet, M. et al. "Beneficial effects of dietary omega-3 polyunsaturated fatty acid on toxin-induced neuronal degeneration in an animal model of Parkinson's disease." *FASEB Journal* 22 (2008): 1213-25.

Campbell, T. Colin, PhD, and Thomas Campbell II, MD. *The China Study: Startling Implications for Diet, Weight Loss, And Long-term Health.* Dallas: BenBella Books, 2005.

Campbell, Thomas, MD. "How Can I Lower My Triglycerides?" *T. Colin Campbell Center for Nutrition Studies.* 1 Aug 2013. Web. 19 Apr 2017.

Chowdhury, Rajiv, MD, et al. "Association of Dietary, Circulating, and Supplement Fatty Acids With Coronary Risk: A Systematic Review and Meta-analysis." *Annals of IntMedicine* 160.6 (2014): 398-406.

Datz, Todd. "Eating processed meats, but not unprocessed red meats, may raise risk of heart disease and diabetes." *Harvard School of Public Health.* 17 May 2010. Web. 30 Sept 2014.

Davis, B., RD, and V. Melino, RD. *Becoming Vegan.* Summertown: Book Pub Co., 2000, pp. 21, 58, 63, 64.

Dehghan, M., et al. "Association of nutrients with blood lipids in 19 countries and 5 continents: the PURE study." *Global Heart.* 11.2S (2016): e6.

Enig, Mary, PhD. *Know Your Fats: The Complete Primer for Understanding the Nutrition of Fats, Oils, and Cholesterol.* Bethesda, MD: Bethesda Press, 2000.

Fallon, Sally, and Mary Enig, PhD. *Nourishing Traditions.* Washington DC: New Trends, 2001, pp. 12, 26.

Ferrieres, Jean. "French paradox: lessons for other countries." *Heart* 90.1 (2004): 107-11.

Fuhrman, Joel, MD. "Leaders of Vegan Movement Develop Parkinson's: Case Studies." *Drfuhrman.com.* n.d. Web. 9 Jun 2014.

Gunnars, Kris. "23 Studies on Low-Fat/Low-Carb Diets." *Authority Nutrition: An Evidence-Based Approach.* Nov 2013. Web. 30 Mar 2014.

Hayek, T, et al. "Dietary fat increases high density lipoprotein (HDL) levels." *J of Clinical Investigation* 91.4 (1993): 1665-71. HDL is known as "the good cholesterol" and high levels reduce risk for heart disease.

Hudgins, L.C. "Effect of high-carbohydrate feeding on triglyceride and saturated fatty acid synthesis." *Proc of the Society for Exp Medicine* 225.3 (2000): 178-83.

Ingenbleek, Y., and K. McCully. "Vegetarianism produces subclinical malnutrition, hyperhomocysteinemia, and atherogenesis." *Nutrition* 28.2 (2012): 148-53.

Keith, Lierre. *The Vegetarian Myth: Food, Justice, and Sustainability.* Crescent City, CA: Flashpoint, 2009, pp. 9-10.

Knopp, R., and B. Retzlaff. "Saturated fat prevents coronary artery disease? An American paradox." *Am Journal of Clinical Nutrition* 80.5 (2004): 1102-03.

Kornsteiner, M., et al. "Very low n-3 long-chain polyunsaturated fatty acid status in Austrian vegetarians and vegans." *Annals of Nutrition Metabolism* 52.1 (2008): 37-47.

Lee, Robyn. "Why You Should Eat Animal Fat: An Interview with Jennifer McLagan: Comments." *Seriouseats.com.* 26 Sept 2008. Web. 18 July 2013.

Lin, Biing-Hwan, and Joanne Guthrie. "Nutritional Quality of Food Prepared at Home and Away From Home, 1977-2008." *USDA: ERS Report Summary.* Dec 2012. Web 27 Feb 2016.

Lorgeril, M. de, et al. "Mediterranean diet & the French paradox." *Cardio Research* 54.3 (2002): 503-515.

Malhotra, S. *Indian Journal of Industrial Medicine* 14 (1968): 219.

Millard, Elizabeth, Ed. " Want to eat healthier? Add more animal fat, butter, eggs and raw milk to your diet: Comments." *Simple, Good and Tasty.* 11 Oct 2009. Web. 8 Mar 2014.

Mozaffarian D., et al. "Dietary fats, carbohydrate, and progression of coronary atherosclerosis in post menopausal women." *Am Journal of Clinical Nutrition* 80 (2004): 1175-84.

Newport, Mary T., MD. *Alzheimer's Disease: What if There Was a Cure?* Laguna Beach, CA: Basic Health Publications, 2011. Newport investigates the role of saturated fat in brain health.

Nicholson, John. *The Meat Fix: How a Lifetime of Healthy Living Nearly Killed Me.* London: Biteback, 2012.

Norris, Jack, RD, and Virginia Messina, RD, *Vegan for Life*. Boston: Da Capo Press, 2011, p. 178.

Okuyama, H., et al. "Excess linoleic acid and relative n-3 deficiency syndrome seen in Japan." *Prog Lipid Res* 35 (1997): 409-57.

Parks, Elizabeth, and Marc Hellerstein. "Carbohydrate-induced hypertriacylglycerolemia: historical perspective and review of biological mechanisms." *Am Journal of Clinical Nutrition* 71.2 (2000): 412-33.

Pearce, K.L., et al. Egg consumption as part of an energy-restricted high-protein diet improves blood lipid and blood glucose profiles in individuals with type 2 diabetes. *Brit J of Nutrition* 105.4 (2011): 584-92.

Price, Weston. *Nutrition and Physical Degeneration: A Comparison of Primitive and Modern Diets and Their Effects*. 1939. Price-Pottenger Foundation, 2009, p. 282. Refer to Schmid, R. re "perfect babies."

Ravnskov, U. "Questionable role of saturated and polyunsaturated fatty acids in cardiovascular disease." *Journal of Clinical Epidemiology* 51.6 (1998): 443-60.

Roberts, R., et al. "Relative intake of macronutrients impacts risk of mild cognitive impairment or dementia." *Journal of Alzheimers Disease* 32.2 (2012): 329-39.

Sarter, B., et al. "Blood DHA and EPA in vegans: Associations with age and gender and effects of an algal-derived omega-3 supplement." *Clinical Nutrition* 13 Mar 2014. Web. 19 May 2014.

Schmid, Ron. *The Untold Story of Milk: Green Pastures, Contented Cows and Raw Dairy Foods*. Washington DC: New Trends, 2003. The fish eggs = perfect babies quote appears on page 136.

Schwartz, Robert S., et al. "Increased Coronary Artery Plaque Volume Among Male Marathon Runners." *Journal of the Missouri Med Assoc* 111.2 (2014): 85-90.

Schwarzbein, Diane, MD. Interview. 19 Dec 2014.

-----, and Nancy Deville. *The Schwarzbein Principle*. Deerfield Beach, FL: Health Communications, 1999, pp. 23-27, 61-71, 88, 144, 278.

Shin, J., et al. "Egg Consumption in Relation to Risk." *American J of Clinical Nutrition* 98.1 (2013): 146-59.

Simopoulos, A.P. "The importance of the omega-6/omega-3 fatty acid ratio in cardiovascular disease and other chronic diseases." *Experimental Bio & Med* 233.6 (2008): 674-88.

Siri-Tarino, Patty, et al. "Meta-analysis of cohort studies evaluating association of saturated fat w/cardiovascular disease." *Am Journal of Clinical Nutrition* 91.3 (2010): 535-46.

Taubes, Gary. "What If Fat Doesn't Make You Fat?" *New York Times Magazine,* July 7, 2002.

Weil, Andrew, MD. "Triglycerides too High?" *drweil.com.* 30 May 2007. Web. 25 Oct 2013.

Wells, A.S., et al. "Alternations in mood after changing to a low-fat diet." *Brit J of Nutri* 79.1 (1998): 22-30.

Wessen, Albert, ed. *Migration and Health in a Small Society: The Case of Tokelau*. Oxford U Press, 1992.

Willett, Walter C., MD, and Rudolph L. Leibel, MD. "Dietary fat is not a major determinant of body fat." *Am Journal of Medicine* 113.9 (2002): 47-59.

Yurko-Mauro, Karin, et al., "Beneficial effects of docosahexaenoic acid (DHA) on cognition in age-related cognitive decline." *Alzheimer's and Dementia* 6.6 (2010): 456-64.

29: BUSTED: The Cholesterol Myth

Abbott, C., et al. "Low cholesterol and noncardiovascular mortality." *Mil Medicine* 165.6 (2000): 466-69.

Anderson, J., et al. "Breast-feeding and cognitive development." *Am J of Clinical Nutri* 70.4 (1999): 525-35.

Beck, Melinda. "Can a Drug That Helps Hearts Be Harmful to the Brain?" *Wall Street Journal* 12 Feb 2008. Web. 1 Feb 2015. Source of Dr. Etingin's quote that "statins make women stupid."

Brescianini, S, et al. "Low total cholesterol & increased risk of dying." *J of Am Geriatric* 51.7 (2003): 991-96

Campbell, T. Colin, PhD. *The China Study*. Dallas: BenBella Books, 2005, p. 132.

Castelli, William, MD. "Response to the Adventist Health Study." *Arch of Int Medicine* 152 (1992): 1371-72.

Christie, Megan. "Why Dietary Cholesterol is Important." *Int Dietary Mgmt.* 18 Apr 2014.

Coburn, Brendan, RD. "Historical Context 3: Ancel Keys." *Thehealthycow.* 24 Mar 2011. Web. 19 Aug 2014.

Colpo, A. "LDL Cholesterol: Bad Cholesterol or Bad Science?" *J of Am Phys and Surg* 10.3 (2005): 83-89.

-----. *The Great Cholesterol Con*. Lulu Books, 2006. pp. 34, 49.

Couzens, C.K., refer to Taubes, Gary, "Big Sugar's Sweet Little Lies."

Diamond, D.M., and U. Ravnskov. "How statistical deception created the appearance that statins are safe and effective." *Expert Review of Clinical Pharmacology* 8.2 (2015): 201-10.

DuBroff, R., and M. de Lorgeril. "Cholesterol confusion and statin controversy." *World Journal of Cardio* 7.7 (2015): 404–09.

Enig, Mary, PhD. *Know Your Fats: The Complete Primer for Understanding the Nutrition of Fats, Oils, and Cholesterol*. Bethesda, MD: Bethesda Press, 2000.

Etingin, Orli, MD. Refer to "Beck, Melinda" re Dr. Etingin's quote about statin drugs.

Fallon, Sally, and Mary Enig, PhD. *Nourishing Traditions*. Washington DC: New Trends, 2001, pp. 12, 26.

Fernandez, M.L. "Dietary cholesterol provided by eggs and plasma lipoproteins in healthy populations." *Current Opinion in Clinical Nutrition and Metabolic Care* 9.1 (2006): 8-12.

Goldstein, Mark R., et al. "Do statins prevent or promote cancer?" *Current Oncology* 15.2 (2008): 76–77.

Golomb, B.A. "Impact of statin adverse events in the elderly." *Exp Op on Drug Safety* 4.3 (2005): 389-97.

Gunnars, Kris. "How many eggs can you safely eat?" *Healthline*. 18 Aug 2016. Web. 30 Oct 2016.

Jones, Peter J.H. "Dietary Cholesterol Feeding Suppresses Human Cholesterol Synthesis." *Arteriosclerosis, Thrombosis, and Vascular Biology* 16 (1996): 1222-28.

Keys, Ancel, et al. *Seven Countries: A multivariate analysis of death and coronary heart disease*. Harvard U Press, 1980.

-----. "Atherosclerosis: A problem in newer public health." *Journal of the Mt. Sinai Hospital* 20.2 (1953): 118-39. This is the source of Keys' Six Countries Graph.

Lustig, Robert, MD. *Sugar: The Bitter Truth*. University of California TV. 27 July 2009. Web. 5 Mar 2014.

-----. *Fat Chance: Beating the Odds Against Sugar, Processed Food, Obesity and Disease*. New York: Hudson Street Press, 2012.

Mann, George, MD, et al. "Atherosclerosis in the Masai." *Am Journal of Epidemiology* 95 (1972): 26-37.

-----, Ed. *Coronary Heart Disease: Dietary Sense and Nonsense*. London: Veritas Society, 1993.

Miller, Donald J., MD. "Enjoy Saturated Fats, They're Good for You!" 29th Annual Meeting of Doctors for Disaster Preparedness. *Lew Rockwell*. 2014. Web. 30 Mar 2014.

Minger, Denise. "The Truth About Ancel Keys." *Raw Food SOS*. 22 Dec 2011. Web. 8 July 2013.

Rosedale, R., MD. "Cholesterol is Not Cause of Heart Disease." *Loveforlife*. 28 Oct 2007. Web. 1 Aug 2014.

Sachdeva, Amit, MD, et al. "Lipid levels in patients hospitalized with coronary artery disease: An analysis of 136,905 hospitalizations." *American Heart Journal* 157.1 (2009): 111-17.

Schreurs, Bernard, PhD. "Effects of Cholesterol on Learning and Memory." *Neuroscience & Biobehavioral Review* 34.8 (2010): 1366-79.

Schwarzbein, Diane, MD, and Nancy Deville. *The Schwarzbein Principle*. Deerfield Beach, FL: Health Communications, 1999, pp. 61-71, 88, 144, 278.

Stuebe, Alison, MD. "The Risks of Not Breastfeeding for Mothers and Infants." *Reviews in Obstetrics and Gynecology* 2.4 (2009): 222–31.

Taubes, Gary, and Cristin Kearns Couzens. "Big Sugar's Sweet Little Lies." *Mother Jones*. Nov/Dec 2012.

Tedders, S.H., et al. "Low cholesterol is associated with depression among US household population." *Journal of Affective Disorders* 135 (2011): 115-21

Willett, Walter C., MD, and Rudolph L. Leibel, MD. "Dietary fat is not a major determinant of body fat." *Am Journal of Medicine* 113.9 (2002): 47-59.

Yudkin, John. *Pure, White and Deadly: How Sugar Is Killing Us*. New York: Penguin Books, 2012.

30: Rising Casualties

Douillard, John. *The Three Season Diet: Eat the Way Nature Intended*. New York: Three Rivers Press, 2000.

-----. Interviews. 30 Nov 2010 and 5 Oct 2014.

Gandhi, M.K. "Moral Basis of Vegetarianism." *Address to the London Vegetarian Society, 20th November 1931*. Reprint. International Vegetarian Union. 5 Mar 2011. Web. 28 May 2014.

Hesse, Hermann. *Siddhartha*. Trans. Hilda Rosner. New York: New Directions, 1951.

Klaper, Michael, MD. "Failure to Thrive: Speculations on the Nutritional Adequacy of 100% Plant-Based Diets." *Nutrientrich.com.* n.d. Web 30 Mar 2014.

Meredith. "Yoga Journal's Recipes: No Meat Allowed." *MeatYoga.com.* 16 Jan. 2010. Web. 29 Feb 2012.

Nanamoli, Bhikkhu. *Life of the Buddha: According to the Pali Canon.* Pariyatti Publishing, 2003.

Ninivaggi, Frank, MD. *Ayurveda: Comprehensive Guide to Traditional Indian Medicine for the West.* Lanham, MD: Rowman and Littlefield, 2010.

Shaw, George Bernard. *The Diaries, 1885-1897.* Ed. Stanley Weintraub. Pennsylvania State U Press, 1986.

Svoboda, Robert, Dr. *Prakriti: Your Ayurvedic Constitution.* Bellingham, WA: Sadhana, 1998.

Walters, Kerry, and Lisa Portmess. *Ethical Vegetarianism: From Pythagoras to Peter Singer.* Albany: State U of New York, 1999. See page 143 for Gandhi's quote.

Witte, A.V., et al. "Long-chain omega-3 fatty acids improve brain function and structure in older adults." *Cereb Cortex.* 24 Jun 2013. Web. 3 Aug. 2013.

31: Young and Vegan: Get Worried

Contie, Vicki. "Choline Deficiency May Hinder Fetal Brain Development." *National Institutes of Health.* 26 July 2010. Web. 30 Nov 2013.

Cousens, Gabriel. "Problems with Vegan Diets." *GreenMedInfo.* 14 Sept 2012. Web. 2 May 2014.

Dasarathy, Jaividhya, et al. "Methionine metabolism in human pregnancy." *Am J of Clinical Nutrition* 91.2 (2010) 357-65. Methionine is implicated in neural tube defects, preeclampsia, and premature delivery.

Davis, Brenda, RD, and Vesanto Melina, RD. *Becoming Vegan.* Summertown: Book Pub Co., 2000, p. 35.

Diogena. "Vegetarian Brains: Comments." *Brainwaving.* 8 Jan 2011. Web. 19 Dec 2011.

Edison, R.J., et al. "Adverse birth outcome among mothers with low serum cholesterol." *Pediatrics* 120.4 (2007): 723-33.

Imbard, Apolline, et al. "Neural Tube Defects, Folic Acid and Methylation." *Int J Enviro Res Public Health* 10.9 (2013): 4352-89. Examines low B12 and high homocysteine as risk factors for neural tube defects.

Kovacs, C.S. "Vitamin D in pregnancy and lactation: maternal, fetal, and neonatal outcomes from human and animal studies." *Am Journal of Clinical Nutrition* 88S (2008): 520S-8S.

Lambrinoudaki, I., and D. Papadimitriou. "Pathophysiology of bone loss in the female athlete." *Annals of the NY Academy of Sciences* 1205 (2010):45-50.

Lu, Henry C. "Traditional Chinese Medicine: An Authoritative and Comprehensive Guide." Basic Health Publications, 2005.

Master-Hunter, T., and D.L. Heiman. "Amenorrhea." *Am Family Physician* 73.8 (2006): 1374-82.

Mehedint, M.G., et al. "Choline deficiency alters angiogenesis in the fetal brain." *FASEB* 22 (2008): 1122.

Novakovich, J. "Female Athletes and Amenorrhea." *Sunwarrior* 2 Apr 2013. Web. 1 Dec 2013.

Sears, William, Dr. "Soy Formula." *Ask Dr. Sears.* 2014 Web. 30 Nov 2013.

Shaw, G., et al. "Periconceptional dietary intake of choline & betaine re neural tube defects in offspring." *Am Journal of Epidemiology* 160 (2004): 102-09.

Southan, Rhys. "Interview with Ex-Vegan: Tasha." *Let Them Eat Meat.* 6 Feb 2011.

-----. "Interview with Ex-Vegan: Erim." *Let Them Eat Meat.* 24 Feb 2011.

-----. "Interview with Ex-Vegan: Devon." *Let Them Eat Meat.* 2 Jun 2010.

Tochitani, S. "Functions of Maternally-Derived Taurine in Fetal and Neonatal Brain Development." *Adv Exp Med Biology* 975 (2017) 17-25.

Turner, L. "A meta-analysis of fat intake, reproduction, and breast cancer risk." *Am J of Human Biology* 23.5 (2011): 601-08. Dietary fat's preventative effect in pre-menopausal women.

Vyver, E., et al. "Eating disorders and menstrual dysfunction in adolescents." *Annals of the NY Academy of Sciences* 64:135 (2011): 253-64.

Yan, Y., et al. "Pregnancy alters choline dynamics." *Am Journal of Clinical Nutition* 98 (2013): 459-67.

Zeisel, S. "Choline: Needed for normal development of memory." *JACN* 19.5 (2000): 528S-31S.

-----. "Choline: Critical role during fetal development." *Annual Rev Nutrition* 26 (2006): 229-50.

32: Skinny Vegan Bitches Over 35: Beware

Bauer, J., et al. "Evidence-based recommendations for optimal dietary protein intake in older people." *J of the American Medical Directors Assoc* 14.8 (2013): 542–59.

Cantley, Lewis, MD. Refer to Taubes, Gary (below).

Chernoff, R. "Protein and Older Adults." *J of the American College of Nutrition* 23.6S (2004): 627S-30S.

Douillard, John, Dr. Interview. 30 Nov 2010.

Goldin, B.R., et al. "Estrogen excretion patterns and plasma levels in vegetarian and omnivorous women." *New England Journal of Medicine* 307 (1982): 1542-47.

Graham, Nicholas A., et al. "Glucose deprivation activates a metabolic and signaling amplification loop leading to cell death." *Mol Systems Bio* 26 Jun 2012. Web. 1 Aug 2013.

Halpern, Marc, AD. "The Journey into Ayurveda." *AyurvedaCollege.* n.d. Web. 17 Feb 2012.

Holmes, Marcy, NP. "Perimenopause." *Women to Women.* 2012. Web. 27 Dec 2012.

Liu, Haibo, et al. "Fructose Induces Transketolase Flux to Promote Pancreatic Cancer Growth." *Cancer Research* 70.15 (2010): 6368-76.

Martinez-Lapiscina, E., et al. "Mediterranean diet improves cognition: PREDIMED-NAVARRA randomised trial." *Journal of Neurology, Neurosurgery, and Psych.* 13 May 2013. Web. 2 July 2013.

Muti, Paola, et al. "Fasting Glucose is a Risk Factor for Breast Cancer, A Prospective Study." *Cancer Epidemiology, Biomarkers, and Prevention* 11 (2002): 1361.

Ninivaggi, Frank, MD. *Ayurveda: A Comprehensive Guide.* Lanham, MD: Rowman and Littlefield, 2010.

Schwarzbein, Diane, MD, and Nancy Deville. *The Schwarzbein Principle.* Deerfield Beach, FL: Health Communications, 1999, pp. 61-65.

Shuster, Lynne, et al. "Premature menopause or early menopause: long-term health consequences." *Maturitas* 65.2 (2010): 161.

Sircus, Mark. "Cancer and Sugar: Strategy for Selective Starvation of Cancer." *GreenMedInfo.* 27 Feb 2013. Web. 5 Apr 2013.

Southan, Rhys. "Bad News for Vegans in the ADA's Position Paper on Vegetarian Diets." *Let Them Eat Meat.* 21 Feb 2010. Web. 30 Jan 2012.

Spangenburg, Espen, et al. "Metabolic Dysfunction Under Reduced Estrogen Levels." *Exercise and Sport Sciences Reviews* 40.4 (2012): 195-203.

Suba, Zau." Circulatory estrogen level protects against breast cancer in obese women." *Recent Patents in Anticancer Drug Discovery* 8.2 (2013): 154-67.

Svoboda, Robert, Dr. *Prakriti: Your Ayurvedic Constitution.* Bellingham, WA: Sadhana, 1998. The description of a Vata "constitution" is a concise blend from three Ayurvedic authorities cited for this chapter.

Taubes, Gary. "Is Sugar Toxic?" *The New York Times.* 13 Apr 2011. Web. 3 Nov 2012. This article is the source of Dr. Lewis Cantley's quote, "Sugar scares me."

Turgeon, J.L., et al. "Complex actions of sex steroids in adipose tissue, the cardiovascular system, and brain." *Endocrinology Review* 27.6 (2006): 575–605.

Valls-Pedret, C., et al. "Mediterranean Diet and Age-Related Cognitive Decline, A Randomized Clinical Trial." *JAMA Intern Med* 175.7 (2015): 1094-103.

Vance, Mary. "Deep Nutrition." *Mary Vance NC.* 22 Jun 2012. Web. 25 Aug 2012.

Waterhouse, Debra, RD. *Outsmarting the Mid-Life Fat Cell.* New York: Hyperion, 1998.

-----. Personal Correspondence. 31 Mar 2015.

Wolf, R. et al. "Factors associated w/calcium absorption efficiency in pre- & peri-menopausal women." *Am Journal of Clinical Nutrition* 72.2 (2000): 466-471.

33: Raw and Exposed

Aluli, N.E. "Prevalence of obesity in a Native Hawaiian population." *Am Journal of Clinical Nutrition* 53 (1991): 1556S-60S.

Boutenko, Victoria. *Raw Family Newsletter.* Jan 2010. Web. 8 Sept 2012. Queen of Raw does a U-Turn.

Bratman, Steven, MD. *Health Food Junkies: Orthorexia Nervosa: Overcoming the Obsession with Healthful Eating.* New York: Broadway Books, 2001.

-----. "Fatal Orthorexia." *orthorexia.* 3 Jun 2010. Web. 22 Sept 2012.

Dewanto, Veronica, et al. "Thermal Processing Enhances the Nutritional Value of Tomatoes by Increasing Total Antioxidant Activity." *Journal of Agr and Food Chem* 50.10 (2002): 3010-14.

Douillard, John. *The Three Season Diet: Eat the Way Nature Intended.* New York: Three Rivers Press, 2000.

-----. Interview. 5 Oct 2014.

Finn, Kate. "Finding balance between the extremes of denial and indulgence." *Beyondveg.* 2003. Web. 14 Sept 2014.

Garcia, Ada L., et al. "Long-term strict raw food diet is associated with favourable plasma b-carotene and low plasma lycopene concentrations in Germans." *British Journal of Nutrition* 99 (2008): 1293–1300.

Miglio, Cristiana, et al. "Effects of different cooking methods on nutritional and physiochemical characteristics of selected vegetables." *J of Agr and Food Chem* 56.1 (2008): 139-47.

Reinfeld, Mark, Bo Rinaldi, and Jennifer Murray. *Eating Raw.* New York: Alpha Books, 2008.

Robbins, John. *Diet for a New America: How Your Food Choices Affect Your Health, Happiness and the Future of Life on Earth.* Stillpoint Publishing, 1987.

Shintani, T.T., et al. "Obesity and cardiovascular risk intervention through the ad libitum feeding of traditional Hawaiian diet." *Am J of Clinical Nutrition* 53 (1991): 1647S-51S.

Southan, Rhys. "Interview: Ex-Vegan Kaleigh Mason." *Let Them Eat Meat.* 19 Mar 2010. Web. 5 Jan 2012.

Spencer, Colin. *Vegetarianism: A History.* 1993. New York: Four Walls, Eight Windows, 2000, p. 88. See pages 87-92 for a revealing look at Greek food in the Hellenic age.

Subramanian, Sushma. "Fact or Fiction: Raw veggies are healthier than cooked ones?" *Scientific American.* 31 Mar 2009. Web. 4 Jun 2013.

Wolfe, David. *Eating for Beauty.* San Diego: Maul Brothers, 2003, pp. 3, 9. Admantius quote is on page 3.

34: Body of Evidence: The One and Only You

Abuissa, Hussam, et al. "Realigning our 21st Century Diet and Lifestyle With Our Hunter-gatherer Genetic Identity." *Directions in Psychiatry* 25 (2005): SR1-10.

Appelby, P.N., et al. "The Oxford vegetarian study: an overview." *Am J of Clin Nutri* 70 (1999): 525S–31S.

Bieler, Henry, MD. *Food Is Your Best Medicine.* New York: Random House, 1966.

Camp, Kathyrn, and Elaine Trujillo. "Position Paper: Nutritional Genomics." *Academy of Nutrition and Dietetics* 114.2 (2014): 299-312.

Choi, H., et al. "Intake of purine-rich foods, protein, and dairy products." *Arthritis Rhe* 52.1 (2005): 283-89. Purines are found not only in molecules of DNA and RNA, but in ATP, NADH, GTP, and co-enzyme A.

Cronin, Cornelius, and Fergus Shanahan. "Why is Celiac Disease So Common in Ireland?" *Perspectives in Biology and Medicine* 44.3 (2001): 342-52.

Dagnelie, P., et al. "Vit B-12 from algae appears not bioavailable." *Am J of Clin Nutri* 53 (1991): 695-97.

Dauncey, M. "Recent advances in nutrition, genes and brain health." *Proc of Nutri Soc* 71.4 (2012): 581-91.

Dunn, Robb. "Human Ancestors Were Nearly All Vegetarians." *Scientific American.* 23 July 2012. Web. 3 Mar 2013. This thesis has been discredited by abundant anthropological findings.

Elliott, Ruan, and Teng Jin Ong. "Nutritional Genomics." *British Medical Journal* 324.7351 (2002): 1438-42.

Eriksson, P., et al. "Neurogenesis in the adult human hippocampus." *Nature Medicine* 4 (1998): 1313–17.

Grand, Steve. *Creation: Life and How to Make It.* Harvard University Press, 2003.

Halpern, Marc, Dr. "The Journey into Ayurveda." *AyurvedaCollege.* n.d. Web. 17 Feb 2012.

James, Gary D. ""Biomedical Anthropology and Climate: Exploring Physiological Adaptations as Causes of Ethnic Variation in Metabolic Diseases." *Anthropology* 1 (2013): e115

Leach, Jeff, PhD. *Honor Thy Symbionts.* Jeff D. Leach and Human Food Project, 2012.

Mangels, Reed, PhD. "Dr. Lanou Responds to Jack's Post about Calcium: Comments." *JackNorrisRD.* 31 Dec 2009. Web. 12 Aug 2012.

"Metabolic Typing Diet: A Review." *American Nutrition Association*. 1 Jun 2007. Web. 2 Apr 2012.

Miloslavich, Edward L. "Racial studies on the large intestine." *Am Journal of Physical Anthropology* 8.1 (1925): 11-22. Web. 5 Mar 2013.

Moore, E., et al. "Cognitive impairment and vitamin B12." *Int Psychogeriatrics* 24.4 (2012): 541-56.

Myss, Carolyn, PhD. *Energy Anatomy*. Audio. Sounds True, 2001.

Noë, Alva. *Out of Our Heads: Why You Are Not Your Brain, and Other Lessons from the Biology of Consciousness*. New York: Hill and Wang, 2009.

Preece, Rod. *Sins of the Flesh*. Vancouver: UBC Press, 2008.

Rumi, Jelaluddin. "Special Plates." *The Essential Rumi*. Trans. C. Barks. New York: HarperCollins, 1995.

Santillo, Humbart. *Intuitive Eating: Everybody's Guide to Vibrant Health & Lifelong Vitality Through Food*. Prescott, AZ: Hohm Press, 1993.

Schueller, Gretel. "The Wild World Within." *Eating Well*. July/Aug 2014, pp. 82-91.

Stover, P.J. "Influence of human genetic variation on nutritional requirements." *Am J of Clinical Nutrition* 83.2 (2006): 436S-442S.

Triche, Tim, Jr. "Protein Debate: Cordain vs. Campbell: Response." *Crossfit*. 13 Dec 2006. Web. 2 Dec 2012.

Vakili, S., and M.A. Caudill. "Personalized nutrition: nutritional genomics as a potential tool for targeted medical nutrition therapy." *Nutrition Reviews* 65.7 (2007): 301-15.

Van Buren, C.T., et al. "Role of Dietary Nucleotides in Adult Nutrition." *J of Nutrition* 124 (1994): 124S-60S.

Watson, George. *Nutrition and Your Mind: The Psychochemical Response*. HarperCollins. 1972.

Wiley, Carol. "Six Steps to a Balanced Diet." *Vegetarian Times*. Aug 1991. Reed Mangel's quote on lower protein and calcium intake in vegans appears on p. 40.

Williams, Roger. *Biochemical Individuality*. 1956. New Canaan, CT: Keats Publishing, 1998.

-----. *Nutrition and Disease*. London: Pitman Publishing, 1971.

Wolcott, William, and Trish Fahey. *The Metabolic Typing Diet*. New York, Broadway Books, 2000, pp. 6, 8, 173. Refer to pages 129-158 for metabolic typing tests.

Van Zile, Jon. "Eat for Your Genes: Interview with S. Moalem." *Life Extension*. Dec 2016. Web. 7 Apr 2017.

35. Sniffing Like a Black Bear
Grand, Steve. "Where do those damn atoms go?" *Artificial Life in Real Life*. 12 Jan 2009. Web. 9 Apr 2014.

-----. *Creation: Life and How to Make It*. Harvard University Press, 2003.

His Holiness the Dalai Lama. *The Middle Way: Faith Grounded in Reason*. Somerville, MA: Wisdom, 2014.

Rumi, Jelaluddin. "A Great Wagon." *The Essential Rumi*. Trans. C. Barks. New York: HarperCollins, 1995.

Watts, Alan. *The Way of Zen*. New York: Vintage Books, 1989, E-Book: 2016, chapter 2, pp. 1-2.

Wolcott, W., and T. Fahey. *The Metabolic Typing Diet*. New York, Broadway Books, 2000, pp. 6, 8, 173.

36: The Buddha Ate Meat

Early Buddhist tradition and practice did not include vegetarianism, as confirmed in the Pali Canon, the earliest recording of the historical Buddha's teachings. Scholars believe the Buddha ate meat on occasion and did not forbid his followers from doing so. He explicitly refused a suggestion to include vegetarianism in the monastic code, believing it was not a requisite for enlightenment. Today's followers of Theravada Buddhism, the oldest branch of Buddhism and closest to its origins, generally continue to eat meat. The other main branch, Mahayana Buddhism, teaches abstention. Even these teachings are not strictly followed: Chinese and Vietnamese monks and nuns are vegetarians (not vegans), while vegetarianism among Japanese and Tibetan Buddhists is rare. The Buddha would no doubt be pleased. Freedom of thought was one his primary teachings.

Adams, Carol. *Neither Man nor Beast: Feminism and the Defense of Animals*, New York: Continuum, 1995, p. 177.

-----. *The Sexual Politics of Meat: A Feminist-Vegetarian Critical Theory*. New York: Continuum, 2010. p. 13.

Audrey. "Facing Failing Health as a Vegan: Comments." *Bonzai Aphrodite*. 20 Jan 2013. Web. 20 May 2014.

Bodhi, Bhikkhu. *In the Buddha's Words: Discourses from the Pali Canon*. Somerville, MA: Wisdom, 2005.

Brester, Gary W., PhD. "Corn." *Agricultural Marketing Resource Center.* 2015. Web. 9 Mar 2015. Statistics continue to change as human consumption of corn for ethanol now outstrips livestock feed usage.

"Collateral included deaths in organic rice production." *googleforum: animal.ethics.vegetarian* 1 Jan 2000. Web. 30 Oct 2013.

Davis, Steven. "The Least Harm Principle May Require that Humans Consume a Diet Containing Large Herbivores, Not a Vegan Diet." *Journal of Agricultural and Enviro Ethics* 16.4 (2003): 387-94.

Dhammika, Shravasti. *Good Question, Good Answer.* Buddhist Association of USA, 2000. Web. 1 Oct 2013.

-----. "The Buddha and His Disciples." Buddha Dharma Mandala Society. n.d. Web. 3 Oct 2013.

Dingwall, Dawna. "Alexandra Jamieson: I'm not vegan anymore." *The Current Review: CBC Radio."* 15 May 2013. Web. 10 Oct 2013.

Dubay, Eric. "Judgmental Vegan Nazis." *Atlantean Conspiracy.* 8 Dec 2011. Web. 2 Sept 2013.

Edge, W.D. "Wildlife of Agriculture, Pastures, and Mixed Environs," *Wildlife-Habitat Relationships in Oregon and Washington.* Corvallis: Oregon State Press, 2000, pp. 342-60.

Farrer-Halls, Gill. *Buddhist Wisdom.* Wheaton, IL: Quest Books, 2000, pp. 46-7, 110, 121-2.

Francione, Gary. *Animals as Persons: Essays on the Abolition of Animal Exploitation.* Columbia Press, 2008.

-----. *Introduction to Animal Rights: Your Child or the Dog?* Philadelphia: Temple University Press, 2000.

Gandhi, M.K. Refer to Yogananda, P. (below) re Gandhi's refusing eggs for his dying daughter.

Johnson, N. "Can meat actally be eco-friendly?" Grist.org. 15 July 2015. This fact-rich article says "yes."

Joy, Melanie. *Why We Love Dogs, Eat Pigs, and Wear Cows: An Introduction to Carnism.* San Francisco: Conari Press, 2010, p. 29.

Keith, Lierre. *The Vegetarian Myth: Food, Justice, and Sustainability.* Crescent City, CA: Flashpoint Press, 2009, pp. 37, 40-41.

Kerasote, T., *Bloodties: Nature, Culture, and the Hunt.* New York: Random House, 1993, pp. 232-3, 254-55.

Kingsolver, Barbara, *Prodigal Summer.* New York: HarperCollins, 2001, pp. 322-23.

Lamey, Andy. "Food Fight! Davis vs. Regan on the Ethics of Eating Beef." *Journal of Social Philosophy* 38.2 (2007): 331-48.

"Massive Bird Kills from Building Collisions." *American Bird Conservancy.* 15 Nov 2010. Web. 29 Apr 2013.

Matheny, Gaverick. "Least harm: a defense of vegetarianism." *J of Ag and Enviro Ethics* 16 (2003): 505-11.

Nanamoli, Bhikkhu. *Life of the Buddha: According to the Pali Canon.* Pariyatti Publishing, 2003.

Nass, R.D., et al. "Fate of Polynesian Rats in Hawaiian Sugar Cane Fields During Harvest." *Journal of Wild-Life Management* 35 (1971): 353-56.

Pollard, E., and T. Relton, "A Study of Small Mammals in Hedges and Cultivated Fields." *Journal of Applied Ecology* 7 (1970): 549-57.

Rahula, W. *What the Buddha Taught: Texts from Suttas and Dhammapada.* New York: Grove Press, 1974.

Reid, Anna. *Leningrad: The Epic Siege of World War II, 1941-1944.* London: Walker Books, 2012.

Robertson, Ken. "The Tallgrass Prairie in Illinois." *Illinois Natural History Survey.* 2012. Web. 3 Dec 2012.

Saddhatissa, H. *The Sutta-Nipata: A New Translation from the Pali Canon.* London: Routledge, 1995.

Schoberle, Kent. "Schobiz Says." *brainwaving.* 21 July 2010. Web. 17 Oct 2012.

Slobodchikoff, C.N., et al. "Prairie Dogs: Communication & Community." Harvard University Press, 2009.

Southan, Rhys. "Veganism is Not the Lifestyle of Least Harm, and 'Intent' Does Nothing For Animals." *Let Them Eat Meat.* 23 Jun 2011. Web. 30 Mar 2015.

-----. "Interview with an Ex-Vegan: Jessica Pelkey." *Let Them Eat Meat.* Web. 12 May 2010.

-----. "Interview with an Ex-Vegan: Jade Vanacore." *Let Them Eat Meat.* Web. 9 Mar 2012.

Suzanne. "Vegan life is not bloodless: Comments." *fleshisgrass.* 7 Aug 2010. Web. 3 Apr 2015.

Tew, T.E., and D.W. Macdonald. "The Effects of Harvest on Arable Wood Mice." *Biological Conservation* 65 (1993): 279-283.

-----, et al. "Herbicide Application Affects Microhabitat Use by Arable Wood Mice." *J of Applied Ecology* 29 (1992): 352-59.

United States Dept. of Agriculture. *USDA Livestock Slaughter: 2013 Summary.* Apr 2014. Web. 1 July 2014.

"What Would Become of Domesticated Animals?" *veganforum*. 30 Dec 2010. Web. 1 July 2014.

Wishart, David J., ed. "Cattle Ranching." *Encyclopedia of the Great Plains*. U of Nebraska Press, 2011.

Wooley, J.B., et al. "Impacts of no-till row cropping on upland wildlife." *Trans North America Wildlife and Natural Resources Conference* 50 (1984): 157-68.

World Resources Institute. "Grain Fed to Livestock as a Percent of Total Grain Consumed." *Earthtrends: Database*. 2007. Web. 10 Aug 2013. Nearly 40% of world grain is fed to livestock; 50% in the USA.

Yogananda, Paramahansa. *Autobiography of a Yogi*. 1946. San Rafael, CA: Self Realization Fellowship, 2007. An account of Gandhi refusing eggs for his dying daughter-in-law appears on page 508.

37: The Killing Fields

Behmer, S.T., et al. "Post-ingestive feedbacks and associative learning regulate the intake of unsuitable sterols in a generalist grasshopper." *Journ of Exp Biology* 202.6 (1999): 739-48.

Chittka, Lars, et al. "What is comparable in comparative cognition?" *Philosophical Transactions of the Royal Society, Biological Sciences* 367.1603 (2012): 2677-85.

-----, and T.D. Doring "How human are insects and does it matter?" *Formos Entomologist* 31 (2011): 85-99.

-----. Interview. 4 Mar 2015.

Collett, M., et al. "Spatial memory in insect navigation." *Current Biology* 23.17 (2013): R789-800.

Godlovitch, Roslind, Stanley Godlovitch, and John Harris, eds. "*Animals, Men and Morals: An Inquiry into the Maltreatment of Non-humans*." London: V. Gollancz, 1971. Oxford intellectuals demand veganism.

Hance, Jeremy. "Uncovering the intelligence of insects, an interview with Lars Chittka." *mongabay*. 29 Jun 2010. Web. 15 Apr 2013.

Koch, C. "Exploring Consciousness: the Study of Bees." *Scientific American* 26 Nov 2008. Web. 9 Apr 2013.

McEwen, Melissa. Refer to Southan, Rhys (below): "Interview with an Ex-Vegan."

Southan, Rhys. "Forget Sentience: Here's the Real Reason We Grant Rights." *Let Them Eat Meat*. 31 Aug 2011. Web. 23 Mar 2012.

-----. "Interview with an Ex-Vegan: Melissa McEwen." *Let Them Eat Meat*. Web. 16 Apr 2010.

Tomasik, Brian. "Do Bugs Feel Pain?" *Utilitarian-essays*. 8 Jun 2014. Web. 12 Oct 2014.

Tulku, Ringu. *Confusion Arises as Wisdom: Gampopa's Heart Advice*. Boston: Shambhala, 2012, p. 123.

38: Death to Factory Farms

Belli, Brita. "Rice Paddies Have a Methane Problem." *E Magazine*. 22 Oct. 2012. Web. 28 Nov 2013.

Black, Robert, et al. "Maternal and child undernutrition: global and regional exposures and health consequences." *The Lancet* 371.9608 (2008): 243-60.

Carus, Felicity. "UN urges global move to meat and dairy-free diet." *The Guardian*. 2 Jun 2010. Web. 2 Nov 2013. Yet another example of a pro-vegan headline that does not match the article's content.

"Don't Blame Cows for Climate Change." *U of C Davis, News & Information*. 7 Dec 2009. Web. 5 Jan 2014.

Energy Conservation. State of Texas. "Biomass Energy: Manure for Fuel." 23 Apr 2009. Web. 3 Oct 2013.

"Fish oils reduce greenhouse gas emissions from flatulent cows." *Phys.org*. 30 Mar 2009. Web 7 Jan 2014.

Freetag, Amy. "Short Grass Prairie." *Southern Fried Science*. 23 Feb 2011. Web. 12 Dec 2013.

Friend, Catherine. *The Compassionate Carnivore*. Boston: Da Capo Press. 2008.

Gennarini, S. "UN Engages in Major Population Control Debate." *LifeNews* 31 Jan 2013. Web. 11 Dec 2013.

"Good Science with Less Animal Experimentation." *3R Research Foundation*. 2005. Web. 20 Nov 2013.

Goodin, J.R. and David K. Northington. *Plant Resources of Arid and Semiarid Lands: A Global Perspective*. Orlando, FL: Academic Press, 1985.

Groenigen, K. van, et al. "Increased greenhouse-gas intensity of rice production under future atmospheric conditions." *Nature Climate Change* 3 (2013): 288-91.

Hunt, Thomas, and Charles Burkett. *Farm Animals: Covering the General Field of Animal Industry*. New York: Orange Judd, 1923, p. 29.

Jamieson, Alastair. "UN admits flaw in report on meat and climate change." *The Telegraph*. 24 Mar 2010. Web. 15 Jan 2014. Falsely claimed that meat contributes more to global warming than transportation.

Johnson, J. "Mob Grazing Produces Healthy Soil and Livestock." USDA. Natural Resources Conservation Service, 2014. Source of farmer Bill Totemeier's testimony.

Johnson, K., and D. Johnson. "Methane emissions from cattle." *J of Animal Science* 73 (1995): 2483-92.

Kerston, Chris. Savory Institute. Interview. 18 Feb 2014.

Khan, A. "Holistic Grazing Has Huge Impact on Water." *Regenerating Grasslands.* 2014. Web. 27 Dec 2014.

Koba, K., and T. Yanagita. "Health benefits of conjugated linoleic acid (CLA)." *Obesity Res Clinical Practice* 8.6 (2014): 525-32.

Lala-Pritchard, T. "A Systems Approach for Reversing Land Degradation." *Research Program on Dryland Systems.* 29 Mar 2015. Web. 2 Apr 2015.

Manning, R. *Against the Grain: How Agriculture Has Hijacked Civilization.* New York: North Point, 2004.

Olsson, L., and J. Ardo. "Soil carbon sequestration in degraded semiarid agro-ecosystems: perils and potentials." *Ambio* 31.6 (2002) 471-77.

Painter, Kristen, L. "Rise of grass-fed meat forces industry to shift." *Star Tribune.* 18 Dec 2017. Web. 30 Dec 2017. Sales of grass-fed beef soared from $17 million in 2012 to $272 million in 2016, according to cited Nielsen data.

Robinson, Jo. *Why Grass-fed is Best.* Vashon, WA: Island Press, 2000.

Safriel, U., et al. "Dryland Systems." *Ecosystems and Human Well-being.* unep.org. n.d. Web. 2 Mar 2013.

Savory, Allan. "How to green the desert and reverse climate change." *TED.com.* Feb 2013.

Schwartz, Judith D. *Cows Save the Planet: And Other Improbable Ways of Restoring Soil to Heal the Earth.* White River Junction, VT: Chelsea Green, 2013.

United Nations. Environment Program. *Assessing the Environmental Impacts of Consumption and Production.* 2010. Web. 12 Feb 2013.

-----. Food and Agriculture Organization. *Tackling Climate Change Through Livestock: a global assessment of emissions and mitigation opportunities.* Rome, 2013. Web. 5 Jan 2014.

-----. Food and Agriculture Organization. *State of Food Security and Nutrition in the World.* Rome, 2017. Enough food is produced in the world every year to feed everyone, yet 815 million people go hungry.

Webber, Michael, and Amanda Cuellar. "Cow Power: The Energy and Emissions Benefits of Converting Manure to Biogas." *Enviro Research Letters.* 24 July 2008. Web. 10 Mar 2013.

"Why labels?" *The Veg Blog/archives.* 24 Oct 2007. Web. 5 Apr 2012.

Zhang, Y., et al. "Quantifying methane emissions from rice paddies in NE China by integrating remote sensing mapping with biogeochemical model." *Biogeosciences.* 19 Dec 2010.

39: Local Food: Growing a Revolution

Anderson, Kevin. "Climate Change: Going Beyond Dangerous: brutal numbers and tenuous hope." Tyndall Centre for Climate Change Research. July 2011. *Vimeo.* Web. 19 Oct 2013.

Andrews, Avital, and Reed McManus. "Raise a Fish, Save the World." *Sierra.* Apr 2015, p. 49.

Astyk, Sharon, and A. Newton. *A Nation of Farmers: Defeating the Food Crisis on American Soil.* Gabriola Island, BC: New Society Publishers, 2009.

Badgley, Catherine, et al. "Organic agriculture and the global food supply." *Renewable Agriculture & Food Systems* 22.2 (2007): 86-108.

Berry, Wendell. *The Unsettling of America: Culture & Agriculture.* San Francisco: Sierra Club Books, 1996.

Brown, Lester R. *Full Planet, Empty Plates: The New Geopolitics of Food Scarcity.* New York:: W.W. Norton, 2012.

———"Many Countries Reaching Diminishing Returns in Fertilizer Use." *Earth Policy Institute.* 8 Jan. 2014.

Brownlee, M. *Local Food Revolution: How Humanity Will Feed Itself in Uncertain Times.* Berkeley: N. Atlantic Books, 2016.

Crawford, John. "Graduation Address." University of Sydney. 15 Jun 2011. Web. 9 Mar 2013.

-------- "What if the Soil Runs Out?" *World Economic Forum.* 14 Dec 2012. Web. 3 Apr 2013.

Delate, Kathleen, et al. "The long-term agroecological research (LTAR) experiment supports organic yields, soil quality, and economic performance in Iowa." *Crop Management.* 29 Apr 2013. Web. 18 Jun 2013.

George, Amy. "Warrior Up." *Vancouver Media Co-op.* Video. 28 May 2014. Web. 12 Aug 2014.

Gorelick, Steven. "Facing the Farm Crisis." *The Ecologist.* 5 Jun 2000. Web. 20 Apr 2013.

Grogg, Patricia. "No-till Farming Holds the Key to Food Security." *Interpress Service News.* 20 Feb 2013. Web. 29 Aug 2013.

Gurian-Sherman, D. *Failure to Yield: Evaluating the Performance of Genetically Engineered Crops.* Union of Concerned Scientists. 2009. Web. 17 Aug 2013.

Herrero, M., et al. "Biomass use, production, feed efficiencies, and greenhouse gas emissions from global livestock systems." *Proc of the Natl Academy of Sciences* 110.52 (2013): n.p. Web. 2 Apr 2015.

Heyes, J.D. "Sedgwick, Maine is first town to declare food sovereignty, opposing state and federal laws." *NaturalNews.* 25 Mar 2013. Web. 8 Aug 2013.

Huff, Ethan A. "GMO multi-toxin crops continue to backfire as more insects become resistant to crop chemicals." *Natural News.* 29 Apr 2013. Web. 30 May 2013.

Kumar, R. "Urban Agriculture is Revitalizing Local Economies." *Huff Post.* 4 Jun 2013. Web. 23 Jun 2013.

Lotter, D., et al. "The performance of organic and conventional cropping systems in an extreme climate year." *American Journal of Alt Agriculture* 18.3 (2003): 146-54.

Martin, Ben. "Palm oil: the hidden ingredient causing an ecological disaster." *The Ecologist.* 14 Mar 2012. Web. 16 Jan 2014.

Montgomery, David R. *Dirt: The Erosion of Civilizations.* University of California Press. 2012.

O'Brien, Robyn. "Grocery Stores Say 'No' to Genetically Engineered Salmon, as Demand for Organic Food Grows." *Prevention.* 10 Mar 2014. Web. 2 May 2014.

O'Hara, J. *Market Forces: Creating Jobs through Public Investment in Local and Regional Food Systems.* Union of Concerned Scientists. Aug 2011. Web. 15 Jun 2013.

Ohlson, Kristin. *The Soil Will Save Us: How Scientists, Farmers, and Foodies Are Healing the Soil to Save the Planet.* New York: Rodale, 2014.

"Organic Farming Is Superior to Conventional Agriculture According to 30-Year Comparative Study." *Business Wire.* 16 Sept 2011. Web. 18 Jun 2013.

Pimentel, David. "Soil Erosion: A Food and Environmental Threat." *Enviro, Develop and Sustainability.* 8 (2006): 119-37.

Plumer, Brad. "After a steep and continuous decline, the number of U.S. farms is up for the first time since 1935." *Washington Post.* 2 Oct 2012. Web. 23 Jun 2013.

Pollan, Michael. *The Omnivore's Dilemma: A Natural History of Four Meals.* New York: Penguin, 2006.

Robinson, Jo. *Why Grass-fed is Best: The Surprising Benefits of Grass-fed Meat, Eggs, and Dairy Products.* Vashon, WA: Island Press, 2000.

Salatin, Joel. *Holy Cows and Hog Heaven: The Food Buyer's Guide to Farm Friendly Food.* Swoope, VA: Polyface, 2004, pp. 4, 8, 9, 11, 16.

Savitz, Eric. "Agroterrorism: Managing Risk in Food Supply Chain." *Forbes.* 19 Apr 2011. Web. 1 Nov 2013.

Sooby, J. "Five Years Later, Scientist Still Thinks Organic Can Feed the World." Organic Farming Research Foundation. 27 July 2013. Web. 28 Aug 2013.

Sullivan, C. "Can Livestock Grazing Stop Desertification?" *Scientific Americ.* 5 Mar 2013. Web. 9 Aug 2013.

United Nations. World Food Program. "Climate change is about the poorest, most vulnerable and food insecure people." 2014. Web. 23 Mar 2014.

United States. Dept. of Agriculture. "Growing Organic Demand Provides High-Value Opportunities." Economic Research Service. 6 Feb 2017. Web. Updated 25 Mar 2017.

-----. "Fertilizer Use and Price: 1960-2014." Economic Research Service. 2015. Web. 19 Aug 2015.

Weber, Keith, and Shannon Horst. "Desertification and Livestock Grazing: The Roles of Sedentarization, Mobility and Rest." *Pastoralism* 1:19 (2011): 1-11.

White, Courtney. "Pasture cropping: A regenerative solution." *Acres.* 21 Feb 2013. Web. 20 Mar 2013.

40: Ancestral Hunters/The Animal as Sacred

Bennett, J. and S. Rowley, eds. *Uqalarait: Oral History of Nunavut, Canada.* McGill-Queen's U Press, 2004.

Borre, Kristen. "Seal Blood, Inuit Blood, and Diet: A Biocultural model of physiology and cultural identity." *Medical Anthropology Quarterly* 5 (1991): 48-62.

Brower, R.H., Sr. "Cultural Uses of Alaska Marine Mammals." *Alaskool.org.* Dec 2001. Web. 14 Oct 2013.

Budiansky, S. *Covenant of the Wild: Why animals chose domestication*. New York: William Morrow, 1992.

Bunn, H.T. "Meat Made Us Human." *Evolution of the Human Diet*. Ed. P. Ungar, Oxford U Press, 2006.

Chan, Laurie, and Harriet Kuhnlein. "Traditional food and participatory research: a Canadian experience." *GRID Arendal*. n.d. Web. 8 Sept 2012.

Collura, Randall. "What is our Natural Diet and Should We Really Care?" *Food for Thought: The Debate Over Eating Meat*. Ed. Steve Sapontiz. Amherst, NY: Prometheus, 2004, pp. 36-45.

Cordain, Loren, et al. "Plant-animal subsistence ratios and macro energy estimations in worldwide hunter-gatherer diets." *Am Journal of Clinical Nutrition* 71.3 (2000): 682-92.

Courage, Katherine H. "Early Meat-Eating Human Ancestors Thrived While Vegetarian Hominin Died Out." *Scientific American*. 8 Aug 2012.

Dwyer, Helen, and Michael Burgan. *Inuit History and Culture*. New York: Gareth Stevens, 2012.

Forget, Dominique. "Largest study on Inuit health in Canada takes the pulse of a people afflicted with illnesses uncommon, until recently, in the North." *Can Geographic*. Jan/Feb 2010. Web. 17 Jan 2014.

Goodall, Jane. *The chimpanzees of Gombe: patterns of behaviour*. Harvard University Press, 1986.

Grinnell, George Bird. *Pawnee Hero Stories and Folk Tales*. U of Nebraska Press, 1961, pp. 245, 272.

Harris, Marvin. *Good to Eat: Riddles of Food and Culture*. Waveland Press, 1998, p. 29.

Harrod, Howard. *The Animals Came Dancing: Native Americans sacred ecology and animal kinship*. U of Arizona Press, 2000, pp. 46, 47.

Herculano-Houzel, S. "What Is So Special About the Human Brain?" *TED Talks*. Jun 2013. 12 Aug 2013.

Institution of Mechanical Engineers. *Global Food: Waste Not, Want Not*. Jan 2013. Web. 2 Apr 2015.

James, G.D. "Climate-related morphological variation and physiological adaptations in Homo sapiens." Ed. C.S. Larsen. *A Companion to Biological Anthropology*. Malden, MA: Wiley-Blackwell, 2010, pp. 153-166.

Kruuk, Hans. *Hunter and Hunted: Relationships Between Carnivores and People*. Cambridge U Press, 2002.

Lordkipanidze, David, et al. "A Complete Skull from Dmanisi, Georgia, and the Evolutionary Biology of Early *Homo*." *Science* 342 (2013): 326-31.

Mails, Thomas E. *Mystic Warriors of the Plains*. New York: Marlowe & Co., 1972, pp. 190-91.

Miles, Rosiland. *Who Cooked the Last Supper? The Women's History of the World*. New York: Three Rivers Press, 1988.

Milloy, John S. *The Plains Cree: Trade, Diplomacy and War, 1790-1870*. U of Manitoba Press, 1990, p. 103.

Nabokov, Peter. *Where the Lightning Strikes: American Indian Sacred Places*. New York: Viking, 2006.

"Nature's Laws: Sundance." Heritage Community Foundation, 2004. Web. 28 Oct. 2013.

Mitani, J., and D. Watts. "Why do chimpanzees hunt & share meat?" *Animal Behavior* 61.5 (2001): 915-24.

Palmater, P. "Idle No More: What do we want & where are we headed?" *Rabble*. 4 Jan 2013. 13 Dec 2013.

Palsson, G. "Legacy of Vilhialmur Stefansson." *The Arctic*. Stefansson Arctic Inst. 2000. Web. 2 Mar 2014.

Snyder, Gary. *The Practice of the Wild*. Berkeley: Counterpoint, 1990, pp. 21-22.

-----. *The Real Works: Interviews & Talks*. New York: New Directions, 1980, p. 89.

-----. *The Old Ways*. San Francisco: City Lights, 1977.

Spencer, Colin. *Vegetarianism: A History*. New York: Four Walls Eight Windows, 2000.

Spitzer, Aaron. "People for the Un-Ethical Treatment of Inuit." *Up Here: Life in Canada's Far North*. 20 Mar 2009. Web. 10 Dec 2013.

Stanford, Craig B. *Chimpanzee and Red Colobus: The Ecology of Predator and Prey*. Harvard U Press, 1998.

-----. *The Hunting Apes: Meat-eating and the Origins of Human Behavior*. Princeton U Press, 1999.

-----, et al. "Risk-prone hunting by chimpanzees increases during periods of high diet quality." *Behavioral Ecology and Sociobiology* 61 (2007): 1771-79.

Stefansson, Vilhjalmur. "Adventures in Diet: Eskimos Prove an All Meat Diet Provides Excellent Health." *Harper's*. Nov 1935. Web. 9 Mar 2014.

Stolzenburg, William. *Where the Wild Things Were: Life, Death, and Ecological Wreckage In a Land of Vanishing Predators*. New York: Bloomsbury, 2008, pp. 185, 190.

"Two Brave Men Who Ate Nothing but Meat for an Entire Year." *Inhuman Experiment*. 10 Sept 2009. Web. 8 Nov 2013.

Wanjek, Christopher. "Meat, Cooked Foods Needed for Early Human Brain." *LiveScience.* 19 Nov 2012.
Web. 18 Jan 2014.
Yardley, William, and Erik Olsen, "With Powerboat and Forklife, A Sacred Whale Hunt Endures." *New York Times.* 16 Oct 2011. Web. 3 Dec 2013.

41: Your Ancient Animal Self
Barthel, Margaret. "More Women are Hunting." *The Cultureist.* 11 Nov 2013. Web. 3 Jan 2014.
Bass, Rick. "Why I Hunt." *Sierra.* July/Aug 2001.
Kruuk, Hans. *Hunter and Hunted: Relationships Between Carnivores and People.* Cambridge U Press, 2002.
Pier, Carol. *Tainted Harvest: Ecuador's Banana Plantations.* Human Rights Watch. New York, 2002.
Pirog, Rich S., et al. *Food, Fuel, and Freeways.* Leopold Center. Iowa State University, 2001, p. 2.
Ripple, William, et al. "Status and Ecological Effects of World's Largest Carnivores." *Science* 343 (2014):
n.p. Web. 21 Dec 2014.
-----, et al. "Trophic cascades: wolves to grizzly bears in Yellowstone." *J of Animal Eco* 83 (2013): 223-33.
Schaller, George B. *Golden Shadows, Flying Hooves.* U of Chicago Press, 1983, p. 141.
Shore, Randy. "Ethical killing: Hipsters, hippies and women are taking up hunting." *Vancouver Sun.* 14
Apr 2013. This is the source of recovering-vegetarian-turned-hunter Kesia's quote.

42: The Food Chain, Including You, My Friend
"Another New World: Seeing Biology at the Atomic Level." *SciTech.* 7 Jun 2010. Web. 5 Apr 2014.
Blake, William. *Songs of innocence and experience: showing the two contrary states of the human soul.*
1789-1794. W. Blake. London: Oxford Press, 1977.
Bly, Robert. "The Slim Fir-Seeds." *Turkish Pears in August.* Eastern Washington University Press, 2007.
Eisenberg, B. "Engineering channels: Atomic biology." *Proc Nat Acad of Sciences.* 105.17 (2008): 6211-12.
Grand, Steve. "Where do those damn atoms go?" *Artificial Life in Real Life.* 12 Jan 2009. Web. 3 Apr 2014.
His Holiness the Dalai Lama. *Becoming Enlightened.* Trans. J. Hopkins. New York: Simon & Schuster, 2009.
Holy Bible, King James Version. Isaiah 40:6. The verse: "The voice said, Cry. And he said, What shall I cry?
All flesh is grass, and all the goodliness thereof is as the flower of the field."
Kelder, Peter. *The Eye of Revelation: The Ancient Tibetan Rites of Rejuvenation.* Ed. J.W. Watt, 1946.
Bradenton, FL: Booklocker, 2008.
Kinnell, Galway. "The Quick and the Dead." *Strong Is Your Hold.* New York: Houghton Mifflin, 2006.
Sambhava, Padma. *Tibetan Book of the Dead: The Great Book of Natural Liberation Through Understand-
ing in the Between.* Trans. R. Thurman. New York: Viking Penguin, 2006.
Schulz, M., et al. "Three-dimensional imaging of atomic four-body processes." *Nature* 422 (2003): 48-50.
Schwarzbein, D., MD, and N. Deville. *The Schwarzbein Principle.* Health Communications, 1999, p. 33.
Shah, Bipin. "Sky Burial Tradition of The Ancients From Anatolia (Turkey), Persia, India, Tibet, Thailand, Sri-
Lanka and China." *Academia.edu.* 2014. Web. 25 Mar 2014.
Snyder, Gary. *The Practice of the Wild.* Berkeley: Counterpoint, 2003, p. 20.
Trungpa, Chogyam. *Cutting Through Spiritual Materialism.* Boston: Shambhala, 1973.
Zajonc, Arthur. *The New Physics and Cosmology: Dialogues with the Dalai Lama.* Oxford U Press, 2004.

43: Autobiography of a Veg'n
Crandall, Russ, PhD. *The Ancestral Table.* Las Vegas: Victory Belt Publishing, 2013.
Keston, Deborah. *The Healing Secrets of Foods: A Practical Guide for Nourishing Body, Mind, and Soul.*
Novato, CA: New World Library, 2001.
Linebaugh, K. "A Lesson From Dalai Lama on Meat Eating." *Samvid Beauty* 12 Feb 2013. Web. 3 Mar 2014.
NhaMinerva, Erin. "Food in Ancient Ireland." 1996. *Black-Rose.* Web. 5 Mar 2014.
Yogananda, Paramahansa. *Autobiography of a Yogi.* San Rafael, CA: Self Realization Fellowship, 2007.
-----. "Meat Eating Versus Vegetarianism." *Inner Culture.* Apr/May, 1935. Reprinted in *MyBountifulHealth.*
2012. Web. 5 Mar 2014.

ACKNOWLEDGMENTS

To all former vegans and vegetarians whose struggles and stories inspired me to write this book, I say *un grand merci,* thank you. May you continue to honor the wisdom of your own beautiful, highly individual body. An abundance of gratitude as well to the many fine teachers, scientists, naturalists, poets, farmers and caretakers of the earth who helped shape my beliefs and values. These include among many others: Dr. Charles Jonkel, Dr. Ron Erickson, Dr. Patricia Baulbach, Dr. William Ripple, Dr. Lars Chittka, Dr. Craig Stanford, Dr. Jane Goodall, Aldo Leopold, Gary Snyder and Terry Tempest Williams.

Many respected dietary experts helped guide my argument for moderation and time-honored traditions: Diane Schwarzbein, MD, Ron Rosedale, MD, Jody Shevins, ND, John Douillard, DC, Mary Enig, PhD, Sally F. Morrell and Amelia Greacen. As well, I am indebted to Colin Spencer, Rod Preece, and Marcel Detienne for their impeccable research and scholarly writings on the history of vegetarianism and Pythagoras. A sincere thanks to my editor Barbra Brady for her gracious and sensible advice. And to all the amazing and colorful characters who graced my youthful, adventurous life—Ramona, Maité, Linda, Moon, Nolan, Mary, John, Barb, Carol, rompin' stompin' Buck, Lee, Joe, Jim, Ilene, Karen, wise Carlos, crazy Larry, elegant David and many more—happy trails to you.

For putting up with my all-day research excursions, thank you Laura, Yohan, Emma and Lucas. Daughter: for your brave journey in recovering your health and studying nutritional science in order to help others find their individual path to well-being, I dedicate this book to you. And to all the animals I have loved, whose lives I have saved and whose flesh has saved me: *ka utua te name.* "The debt will be repaid." Our good earth will see to that.

ABOUT THE AUTHOR

Mara Kahn, MS, is an ecologist, college teacher, and professional journalist who specializes in health issues, the environment, and human-animal ethics. She lives in the snowy northern Rockies with her family and a wandering tribe of elk, cougars, and black bears.

CPSIA information can be obtained
at www.ICGtesting.com
Printed in the USA
BVHW071102311018
531765BV00004B/534/P